Manures, Fertilizers and Pesticides

Theory and Applications

Manures, Fertilizers and Pesticides

Theory and Applications

Amitava Rakshit PhD
Priyankar Raha PhD
Nirmal De PhD

Faculty
Department of Soil Science and Agricultural Chemistry
Institute of Agricultural Sciences
Banaras Hindu University
Varanasi, UP

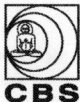

CBS

CBS Publishers & Distributors Pvt Ltd

New Delhi • Bengaluru • Chennai • Kochi • Kolkata • Mumbai
Bhopal • Bhubaneswar • Hyderabad • Jharkhand • Nagpur • Patna
• Pune • Uttarakhand • Dhaka (Bangladesh) • Kathmandu (Nepal)

Manures, Fertilizers and Pesticides
Theory and Applications

ISBN: 978-81-239-2540-0

Copyright © Authors and Publisher

First Edition: 2015

Reprint: 2020

Published by Satish Kumar Jain and produced by Varun Jain for

CBS Publishers & Distributors Pvt Ltd

4819/XI Prahlad Street, 24 Ansari Road, Daryaganj, New Delhi 110 002, India.
Ph: 23289259, 23266861, 23266867   Website: www.cbspd.com
Fax: 011-23243014   e-mail: delhi@cbspd.com; cbspubs@airtelmail.in.
Corporate Office: 204 FIE, Industrial Area, Patparganj, Delhi 110 092

Ph: 011-4934 4934   Fax: 011-4934 4935   e-mail: publishing@cbspd.com; publicity@cbspd.com

Branches

- **Bengaluru:** Seema House 2975, 17th Cross, K.R. Road, Banasankari 2nd Stage,
  Bengaluru 560 070, Karnataka
  Ph: +91-80-26771678/79   Fax: +91-80-26771680   e-mail: bangalore@cbspd.com
- **Chennai:** 7, Subbaraya Street, Shenoy Nagar, Chennai 600 030, Tamil Nadu
  Ph: +91-44-26260666, 26208620   Fax: +91-44-42032115   e-mail: chennai@cbspd.com
- **Kochi:** 68/1534, 35, 36, Power House Road, Opp. KSEB, Kochi 682018, Kerala
  Ph: +91-484-4059061-65   Fax: +91-484-4059065   e-mail: kochi@cbspd.com
- **Kolkata:** No. 6/B, Ground Floor, Rameswar Shaw Road, Kolkata 700014 (West Bengal), India
  Ph: +91-33-2289-1126, 2289-1127, 2289-1128   e-mail: kolkata@cbspd.com
- **Mumbai:** 83-C, Dr E Moses Road, Worli, Mumbai 400018, Maharashtra
  Ph: +91-22-24902340/41   Fax: +91-22-24902342   e-mail: mumbai@cbspd.com

Representatives

• Bhopal	0-8319310552	• Bhubaneswar	0-9911037372	• Hyderabad	0-9885175004
• Jharkhand	0-9811541605	• Nagpur	0-9421945513	• Patna	0-9334159340
• Pune	0-9623451994	• Uttarakhand	0-9716462459	• Dhaka	01912-003485
• Kathmandu	977-9818742655			(Bangladesh)	
(Nepal)					

Printed at India Binding House, Noida, UP, India

to

our wives

Foreword

The phenomenal growth in agricultural production since independence has been triggered by higher input use, particularly purchased inputs as well as technology-induced productivity enhancement. The key inputs which changed the complexion of agriculture include a high yielding variety of seeds, chemical fertilizers, irrigation, pesticides, farm machinery and equipment, credit and labor. In order to step up agricultural production to meet the demands of the ever-increasing population, chemical fertilizers should be used along with organic manures and pesticides in a right proportion for a particular agroecological unit. In the light of present-day knowledge and practices, agriculture differs much in our own from that of earlier times, invention of new inputs and tools and improvement of the old, better methods of application, and superior educational facilities raising the general plane of intelligence are among the more potent forces that have affected the change. The book, Manures, Fertilizers and Pesticides—Theory and Applications aims at documentation of huge comprehensive almost all aspects of inputs used in agriculture, from traditional farming to the latest developments. Further, a monumental coverage of inorganic and organic chemicals quite encyclopedic in nature facilitating communication among the agricultural stakeholders.

As an aid of improving scientific communication for everyone from students to public decision-makers, the book could prove to be a comprehensive guide on inputs in agriculture. The book bridges the gap among diverse branches of the agricultural sciences and will facilitate as a ready reference in the broad spectrum of agriculture. Significant and relevant issues pertaining to all spheres in agriculture and natural resource have also been discussed in the book. The authors of the book have made an attempt to arrange different areas of input management in a concise but comprehensive manner and deserve commendation for their painful efforts. It is hoped that this book will be a valuable source of information for students and teachers engaged in various applications of agriculture. The authors deserve appreciation for bringing out highly useful and relevant publication of immense use.

Dr S Ayyappan
Secretary and Director General
Government of India
Department of Agricultural Research and Education and
Indian Council of Agricultural Research
Ministry of Agriculture, Krishi Bhawan, New Delhi

Preface

Agricultural production has increased dramatically in India and elsewhere in the past five decades as agricultural practices have evolved. But this success has been costly: water pollution, soil depletion, and a host of human (and nonhuman) health and safety problems have emerged as important side effects associated with modern agricultural practices. Because of increased concern with these costs, an alternative view of agricultural production has arisen that has come to be known as sustainable agriculture. In other words, current agricultural research centers not only on increasing production but also on finding ways for improving the environmental sustainability of agriculture. The idea for a comprehensive book associated with the rapidly expanding fields related to agriculture. The book aims to provide a balanced scientific review of the environmental and sustainability issues relating to different agrochemicals, i.e. manure, fertilizer and pesticide use and how their environmental impact can be minimized. The text is designed to fulfill the needs of the students studying soil, crop and environmental science, and general readers. No other book in this field covers such a wide range of topics and can be applied to as many geographic areas as agriculture, manures, fertilizers, pesticide and the environment. The book is divided into five chapters. Chapter 1 deals with different fertilizers and their role in sustainability in agriculture and the challenges to produce enough food while caring for the environment. Chapters 2 and 3 discuss the benefits and prospects of manure and beneficial microorganisms used in agriculture and Chapter 4 covers the benefits and problems of pesticides, their possibilities and challenges for increased food production in future. A thorough overview has been included the important agricultural applications of natural products and synthetic compounds derived from natural products. Detailed information on the isolation, structural studies, biological activity and toxicology of these compounds is provided. Chapter 5 covers organic farming in detail, providing a balanced scientific review of the issues relating to inorganic and organic inputs use and how their impact can be minimized.

Anyone interested in the environment will find this book helpful as well as those studying soil, crop and environmental science. The suggestions and comments from students, teachers and researchers for further improvement of this book are always welcome.

Amitava Rakshit
Priyankar Raha
Nirmal De

Preface

Acknowledgments

A t the outset we would like to thank God. In the process of putting this book together, we realized how true this gift of writing is for us. He has given us the power to believe in our passion and pursue our dreams. We could have never done this without the faith we have in the Almighty.

We would like to express our gratitude to many people who knew us through this book; to all those who provided support, talked over things, read, wrote, offered comments, allowed us to quote their works, and assisted us in the editing, proofreading and design. This book was not only inspired by our learned colleagues but also directly improved by their active involvement in its development.

We would like to thank Mr Sunil for enabling us to publish this book. Finally, the editorial and production team of CBS Publishers & Distributors, New Delhi, deserves our special appreciation for guiding us through the process of publishing this new work. Above all, we want to thank our family members who supported and encouraged us in spite of all the time it took us away from them. It was a long and difficult journey for them.

Amitava Rakshit
Priyankar Raha
Nirmal De

Contents

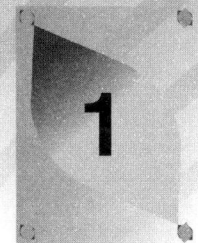

Inorganic Fertilizers

1.1 CONCEPT

Everywhere in the world and over many thousands of years, farming has been a hit-and-miss affair. Land was cleared and farmed. If it failed, the land reverted back to scrub and forest or was lost altogether, leaving the bones of the land, the naked rock, behind. In developing countries, rapid improvements in agricultural productivity, especially after the 1950s, were required to achieve food security for an increasing population. There was little information on the existing fertility of many soils. Following the trends, that were evolving at that time in developed countries, there was a considerable increase in N fertilizer use that was not matched by an appropriate increase in the application of P and K fertilizers. This has led to soil nutrient mining, especially of K, in many parts of the developing world. The present situation is exacerbated by the fact that many small farmers in developing countries lack adequate resources to purchase manufactured fertilizers, especially P and K fertilizers. In consequence, they have sought to use locally available rock phosphates to supply P.

Agricultural systems using inputs of added nutrients have developed slowly since the mid-1800s. Such systems now rely on inputs of plant nutrients from fertilizers to supplement the supply from the soil and nutrients returned in organic materials. A series of events can be identified in the use of fertilizers in European agriculture. The history have been chronologically presented in Table 1.1. First, widespread P deficiency in soils (Europe) had to be corrected and this was made possible by the industrial scale production of superphosphate in the mid-1800s. At that time, limited amounts of N were available as ammonium sulphate and sodium nitrate from the natural deposits in Chile. By the mid-1850s, wood ash was the main source of K, the large deposits of K-bearing salts in Germany were not discovered until the 1860s. Emigrants from Europe to North America took European methods of agriculture with them. These included crop rotations, which optimized the use of indigenous plant nutrients in soil. It was not until the early years of the 20th century that the industrial fixation of atmospheric N was achieved (ammonia synthesis by Haber–Bosch; urea synthesis by Wöhler). Even then, however, large amounts of N were not used in agriculture because the available crop cultivars did not have the yield potential to respond to large applications. It was not until after

Table 1.1: History of fertilizer

Year	Scientist involved	Location	Material
1730	Viscount Charles Townshed	Flanders	Fertilizing value of crop rotation
1745	Johann Friedrich Mayer	Germany	Gypsum
1840	Jnstos von Liebig	Germany	Posphate of lime + $H_2SO_4 \rightarrow$ Fertilizer
1838	Jean Baptiste Boussingault	France	N-ous fertilizer
1903	Kristian Birkeland	Norway	HNO_3
1927	Erling Johnson	Norway	Nitrophosphate
1850	Fison, Packard, Hadfield	UK	SSP
1761	Wallerius	Sweden	Fertilizing value of humans
17th century	Gauber, Francis Bacon	The Netherlands	KNO_3

the 1950s, that N fertilizer use increased greatly, a time that also saw a large increase in the use of P and K fertilizers. Today, agricultural productivity in many developed countries relies heavily on the input of nutrients from fertilizers. The financial returns allow these and other inputs to be purchased by farmers. Increasing agricultural production in India by area increasing process is no longer possible as cultivable land left over is only marginal. Further a considerable cultivable land is being diverted year after year for industrial purpose and housing, etc. Hence, self sufficiency in food lies in increasing the yield per unit area per unit time through adoption of modern agricultural technology.

It is universally accepted that the use of chemical fertilizers is an integral part of the package of practices for raising the agricultural production to a higher place. Studies conducted by the food and agricultural organization of the United Nations (FAO) have established beyond doubt that there is a close relationship between the average crop yields and fertilizer consumption level. Moreover the nutritional requirement of different crops could not be fully met with the use of organic manures like FYM and other bulky organic manures like neem cake, castor cake, groundnut cake, etc. for want of their availability in adequate quantities.

Use of fertilizers is needed for all types of long-term crop production in order to achieve yield levels which make the effort of cropping worthwhile. Modern fertilizer practices, first introduced more than a century ago and based on the chemical concept of plant nutrition, have contributed very widely to the immense increase in agricultural production and have resulted in better quality food and fodder. As a beneficial side-effect, the fertility of soils has been improved resulting in more stable yield levels, as well as in a better resistance to some biotic and abiotic stress. Furthermore, the farmer's economic returns have increased due to more effective production. The purpose of fertilizer use, especially for higher yields, is identical in temperate and tropical climates, i.e. to supplement the natural soil nutrient supply in order to satisfy the demand of crops with a high yield potential, to compensate for the nutrients lost by the removal of plant products or by leaching, etc. and to improve unfavourable or to maintain good soil conditions for cropping.

There are five principal reasons for applying fertilizer:

- **Balancing the soil:** To bring the composition of nutrients in a soil up to the ratio required by crops, or to add nutrients that are in short supply. By analyzing the base rocks from which the soil is weathered, and knowing the requirements of the standing crop or mix of crops over a few seasons, the nutrients in shortest supply can be determined and these can be added in the form of artificial fertilizer. In traditional soil testing, a sample of the A horizon is analysed, rather than the C or B horizons. This is done because the composition of the A horizon, the plough and root zone, is of immediate interest for the season's production. By analysing the C or B horizons as well, the original nutrients in shortest supply can be detected and added to improve the future soil composition.
- **Replacing:** To replace the nutrients that have been harvested. In small-scale primitive societies, human and animal wastes were returned to the cropland where they originated from, but in commercial agriculture where the produce is sold and consumed very far away, this can no longer be achieved. Artificial fertilizer is then necessary to maintain the soil's natural fertility.
- **Rapid response:** Quick release fertilizer is applied to meet the sudden need of a fast growing monoculture.
- **Optimising:** Artificial fertilizer is added to optimise some economic parameter, usually the amount of profit from the operation.
- **Feeding soil organisms:** The most important aspect often overlooked is the use of fertilizer to feed soil organisms.

Further, fertilizers have the advantages of smaller bulk, easy transport, relatively quick in availability of plant-food constituents and the facility of their application in proportion suited to the actual requirements of crops and soils. Hence, there is need for an efficient use of fertilizers as a major plant nutrient resource in enhancing the farm productivity.

1.2 WHAT IS A FERTILIZER?

Any natural (mined) or manufactured material, which contains at least 5% of one or more of the three primary nutrients (N, P_2O_5, K_2O) can be called fertilizer. Fertilizer is generally defined as "any material, organic or inorganic, natural or synthetic, which supplies one or more of the essential chemical elements required for the plant growth". Industrially manufactured fertilizers are called *mineral fertilizers*.

1.3 NUTRIENTS REQUIRED BY PLANTS

Plants contain practically large number of natural elements but need only sixteen for good growth. Sixteen elements are identified as essential elements for plant growth, of which nine are required in macro and seven in micro quantities. Thirteen of these are essential mineral nutrient elements, commonly abbreviated, though with less precision, to "nutrients". They must be provided either by the soil or by manure or mineral fertilizer. Some other mineral nutrient elements, e.g. Na, Si, Co, have a beneficial effect on some plants but are not essential. Essential mineral nutrients are required for normal growth metabolism and development. The essential elements exist as structural components of a cell, maintain cellular organizations, function in energy transformations and in enzyme reactions. Carbon, Hydrogen and Oxygen are three naturally occurring nutrients and form about 94 per cent of the dry weight of plants. These are the major components of carbohydrates, proteins and fats. Besides their structural role, they provide energy required for growth and development of plants by oxidative breakdown of carbohydrates, proteins and fats during cellular respiration. Nitrogen, phosphorus and potassium are three major or primary nutrients which are to be made available in larger quantities. Calcium, magnesium and sulphur are secondary nutrients which are required in relatively smaller but in appreciable quantities. Iron, zinc, manganese, copper, boron, molybdenum and chlorine are required by plants in small quantities for their growth and development. Hence, they are known as micronutrients or trace elements. It is an established fact that the micronutrient elements are required by plants in very low concentration suggests that they all function as catalysts or at least closely linked with some catalytic processes in plants.

Macronutrients of which the critical contents in plants dry matter are 2–30 g/kg of dry matter:

Major nutrients applied in fertilizers for almost all crops on most soils:
- N = nitrogen (taken up as NO_3^- or NH_4^+)
- P = phosphorus (taken up as $H_2PO_4^-$ or HPO_4^{2-} or PO_4^{3-})
- K = potassium (taken up as K^+)

Secondary nutrients applied in fertilizers mainly for certain crops on some soils:
- S = sulphur (taken up as SO_4^{2-})
- Ca = calcium (taken up as Ca^{2+})
- Mg = magnesium (taken up as Mg^{2+})

Micronutrients of which the critical contents in plants are 0.3–50 mg/kg of dry matter:

Heavy metals:
- Fe = iron
- Mn = manganese
- Zn = zinc
- Cu = copper
  Fe, Mn, Zn, & Cu are taken up as divalent cation or chelate
- Mo = molybdenum taken up as molybdate MoO_4^{2-}

Non-metals:

- Cl = chlorine, taken up as Cl^-
- B = boron, taken up as $H_2BO_3^-$, etc.

Some **beneficial nutrients** useful for some plants:

- Na = sodium
  (taken up as Na^+; can partly replace K for some crops)
- Si = silicon
  (taken up as silicate, etc., e.g. for strengthening cereal stems to resist lodging)
- Co = cobalt
  (mainly for N-fixation of legumes)
- Cl = chlorine
  (useful for some crops in greater than essential amounts, for osmotic regulation and improved resistance to some fungi)
- Al = aluminium (perhaps beneficial for some plantation crops, e.g. tea)

Fertilizer use must also take into account the nutritional requirements of animals and human beings consuming the crops. It is necessary to supply, for the larger benefit of grazing animals, increased amounts of elements which are not essential to the plants, e.g. Na, Co or Se. Since hardly any soil can supply all the nutrients needed in sufficient amounts to meet the demands of high-yielding superior crops, the deficit must be made good by adding fertilizers and/or manures.

As a general rule, nutrient uptake should always be ahead of the production of plant dry matter during the vegetative period. The total amount needed at a given stage can be estimated from the internal plant requirement. In fact the nutrient contents of crops are usually somewhat higher than the critical levels (Fig. 1.1). On the contrary, a large surplus or luxury supply is unwanted, not only because of the

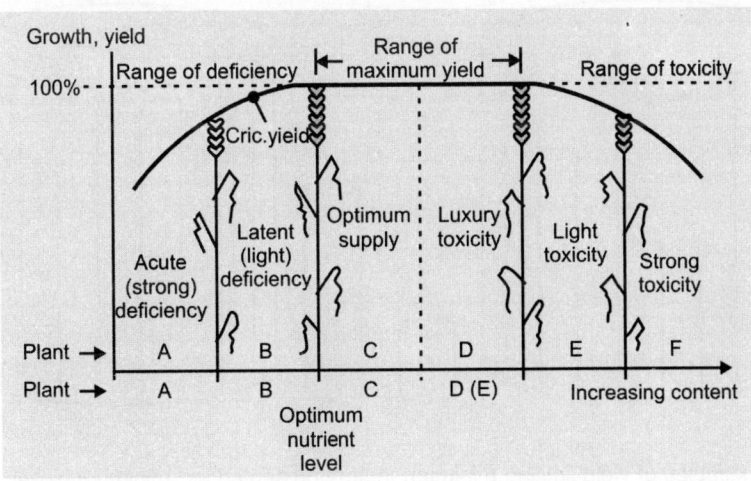

Fig. 1.1: Growth dependency of plants on nutrient supply (Courtesy: IFA, Paris)

considerations but also because it may upset the nutrient balance, economic and environmenal tuning.

Plants, in general, contain maximum amounts of nutrients in the reproductive stages of growth shortly before maturity, but nutrient balance calculations for the most part based on the somewhat smaller amounts that are, or could be, removed from the field at the time of harvest. Pertinant nutrient removal data should be established for all crops and farming systems under different agroecology.

The amounts of nutrients which need to be added in fertilizers and manures depend on:

- The nutrient requirement of a crop for the desired yield level,
- The fertility status of soil which can be estimated by diagnostic methods.

No fertilizer or manure is needed if the uptake of a nutrient from the soil does not lead to any significant depletion of the soil reserves. This is often the case with micronutrients. Fertilizer use should concentrate especially on the so-called minimum factor which, according to the Law of the Minimum, critically limits plant growth (Fig. 1.2).

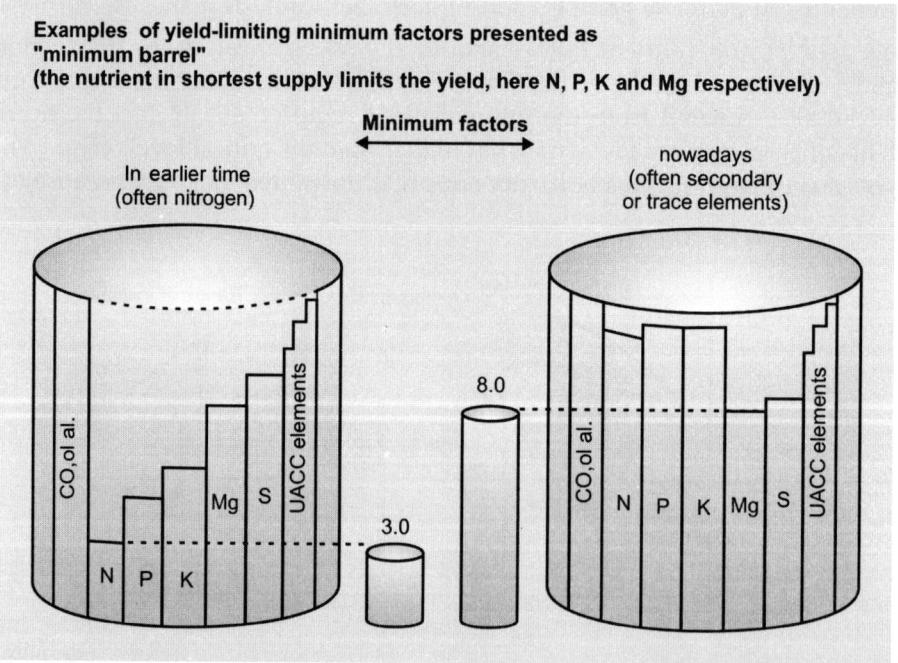

Fig. 1.2: Examples of yield-limiting minimum factors presented as "minimum barrel" (Courtesy: IFA, Paris)

1.4 CLASSIFICATIONS

Fertilizers are classified on the basis of following parameters:

i. **Method of production**
- **Natural** (as found in nature or only slightly processed): Naturally occurring inorganic fertilizers include chilean sodium nitrate, mined rock phosphate, and limestone.
- **Synthetic** (manufactured by industrial processes): Urea, SSP, MOP, DAP, NPK.

ii. **Chemical nature**
- **Organic** (composed of organic matter): Urea, calcium cynamide
- **Inorganic** (made of simple, inorganic chemicals or minerals): Urea, SSP, MOP, DAP, NPK.

iii. **Number of nutrients**
- **Single-nutrient** or straight fertilizers/incomplete (whether for major, secondary or micro nutrients): Urea, MOP, Borax.
- **Multinutrient** (multiple nutrient) or compound fertilizers/complete, with 2, 3 or more nutrients: SSP, DAP, NPK, Boronated NPK.

iv. **Concentrations in plant dry matter**
- **Macronutrients fertilizer** containing nitrogen, phosphorus, potassium, calcium, magnesium and sulphur.
- **Micronutrients fertilizer** containing iron, manganese, boron, copper, molybdenum, nickel, chlorine, and zinc.

v. **Type of combination**
- **Mixed** fertilizers, i.e. either a physical mixture of two or more single-nutrient or multinutrient fertilizers (for granular products this may comprise a mixture of separate granules of the individual ingredients, or granules each containing these ingredients): Urea mixed with MOP; Urea, SSP, MOP mixed –2:1:1
- **Complex** fertilizers, in which two or more of the nutrients are chemically combined (e.g. nitrophosphates, ammonium phosphates): DAP, NPK (10:26:26); boronated NPK

vi. **Physical condition**
- **Solid** (crystalline, powdered, prilled or granular) of various size ranges: Urea, SSP, MOP, DAP, NPK
- **Liquid** (solutions and suspensions): Urea, UAN
- **Gaseous** (liquid under pressure): Ammonia

vii. **Mode of action**
- **Quick-acting** (water-soluble and immediately available): Urea, SSP, MOP, DAP, NPK
- **Slow-acting** (transformation into soluble form required): Rock phosphate, pyrite

viii. **Nutrient content**
- **High analysis** (>25%): Urea, MOP, NPK
- **Low analysis** (<25%): SSP, RP

ix. **Residual effect on soil**
- **Acid forming** (leaving acidic residue in soil): NH_3 (148); AC (128); AS (110); ASN (93); AP (86); Urea (80); AN (60)
- **Basic forming** (leaving basic residue in soil): $CaCN_2$ (63); $NaNO_3$ (29); DCP (25); $Ca(NO_3)_2$ (20)
- **Neutral** (leaving no residue in soil): CAN Kisan khaad (O)

Inorganic Fertilizers

Inorganic fertilizers are chemicals, which provide plant-food in ample quantities. Fertilizers also have the advantage of smaller bulk, the resultant easy transport. Inorganic fertilizers are grouped into nitrogenous fertilizers, phosphatic fertilizers, potassic fertilizers and so on.

Nitrogen Fertilizers

They are valued according to their total N-content, the different N-forms (which determine the rate of action) and side-effects if any. According to the manner in which their nitrogen is combined with other elements, the nitrogenous fertilizers are divided into four groups; nitrate, ammonia, and ammonium salts, chemical compounds containing nitrogen in the amide form, and plant and animal by-products.

I. Inorganic Nitrogenous Fertilizers

Inorganic substances containing large amount of nitrogen come under this category. It is further divided into following groups according to the form of nitrogen they contain:

- **Nitrate fertilizers (NO_3^-):** Nitrogen present in these fertilizers are in nitrate form, NO_3^- which are rapidly dissociated to release NO_3^- ions and readily absorbed by the plants. Nitrate ions are highly reactive and mobile and are susceptible to losses due to leaching and under water-logged conditions by dentrification. All are quick-acting and increase soil pH. They are alkaline in their residual effect in soil. Following are the nitrate fertilizers:

Fertilizer	%NO_3^- N
Sodium nitrate ($NaNO_3$)	16% N
Calcium nitrate $Ca(NO_3)_2$	15.5% N
Chilean nitrate ($NaNO_3$)	16% N
Potassium nitrate (KNO_3)	13% N

- **Ammonium fertilizers (NH_4^+):** Ammonium fertilizers are soluble in water and, as such, absorbed on the soil colloids and thus protected from being washed away by runoff or by leaching. All ammonium fertilizers are moderately quick-acting. Uptake by plants can be retarded by addition of nitrification inhibitors, e.g. N-serve, dicyandiamide (DCD). Some crops like rice, sugarcane, tuber crop, seedlings directly utilize ammonium form of these fertilizers. The absorbed ammonium ions on soil collections are transformed to nitrate slowly and taken up by most of the crops. They are acidic in their residual effect in soil. Following are the ammonium fertilizers:

Fertilizer	$\%NH_4-N$
Ammonium bicarbonate – NH_4HCO_3	18%
Ammonium sulphate – $(NH_4)_2SO_4$	20.6%
Ammonium chloride – NH_4Cl	25%
Ammonium phosphate – $NH_4 (H_2PO_4)$	20%
Anhydrous ammonia – NH_3	82%
Ammonia solution – NH_3 in water	20-25%

- **Nitrate and Ammonium fertilizers (Nitrate, NO_3^- and ammonium, NH_4^+):** These fertilizers contain nitrogen in both nitrate (NO_3^-) and ammonium forms (NH_4^+). The nitrate nitrogen is readily available to plants for immediate need, whereas ammonium nitrogen becomes available to plants at a later stage, when it is transformed by microbiological process to nitrate. They are soluble in water and suitable for most of the crops and soils. They are acidic in its residual effect.

Fertilizer	%N
Ammonium nitrate – NH_4NO_3	33 to 34% N
Calcium ammonium nitrate (CAN)$Ca(NO_3)_2NH_4NO_3$	25% N with calcium carbonate
Ammonium sulphate nitrate (ASN)$(NH_4)_2SO_4NH_4NO_3$	26% N

- **Solutions containing more than one form of N:** Urea ammonium nitrate solution (28–32%N).
- **Multinutrient fertilizers containing N, NPK:** Nitrophosphate, NP (20-23% N, 20–23% P_2O_5); monoammonium phosphate, MAP (11% N, 50% P_2O_5); diammonium phosphate, DAP (18% N, 46% P_2O_5); liquid ammonium polyphosphates (e.g. 12% N, 40% P_2O_5); NK and NPK.

Fertilizer	Total nitrogen (N)	Neutral ammonium citrate soluble phosphate (P_2O_5)	Water soluble phosphate (P_2O_5)	Water soluble potash (K_2O)
Ammonium phosphate				
11-52-0	11.0	52.0	44.2	
18-46-0	18.0	46.0	41.0	

Contd.

(Contd.)

Fertilizer	Total nitrogen (N)	Neutral ammonium citrate soluble phosphate (P$_2$O$_5$)	Water soluble phosphate (P$_2$O$_5$)	Water soluble potash (K$_2$O)
Ammonium phosphate sulphate				
16-20-0	16.0	20.0	19.5	
20-20-0	20.0	20.0	17.0	
18-9-0	18.0	9.0	8.5	
Ammonium phosphate sulphate nitrate				
20-20-0	20.0	20.0	17.0	
Nitrophosphate				
20-20-0	20.0	23.0	12.0	
23-23-0	23.0	23.0	18.5	
Ammonium nitrate phosphate				
23-23-0	23.0	23.0	20.5	
Urea ammonium phosphate				
28-28-0	28.0	28.0	25.2	
24-24-0	24.0	24.0	20.4	
20-20-0	20.0	20.0	17.0	
Potassium nitrate (cystalline/prilled)				
13-0-45	13.0			45.0
Monopotassium phosphate				
0-52-34			52.0	34.0
NPK fertilizers				
15-15-15	15.0	15.0	4.0	15.0
10-26-26	10.0	26.0	22.1	26.0
12-32-16	12.0	32.0	27.2	16.0
22-22-11	22.0	22.0	18.7	11.0
14-35-14		35.0	29.0	14.0
17-17-17	17.0	17.0	14.5	17.0
14-28-14	14.0	28.0	23.8	14.0
19-19-19	19.0	19.0	16.2	19.0
17-17-17	17.0	17.0	13.6	17.0
20–10–10	20.0	10.0	8.5	10.0

II. Organic Nitrogenous Fertilizers

These fertilizers contain nitrogen in organic form. These include plant and animal by-products. These fertilizers are relatively slow-acting but they supply nitrogen for a longer period.

- **Amide Fertilizers (Amine, NH_2 or amide, CN_2):** These fertilizers contain nitrogen in organic compounds as amide-NH_2 or -CN_2 not directly available to plants, as such, but quickly converted by soil microbes to ammoniacal and nitrate form and then utilized. Amide fertilizers are:

Fertilizer	% N
Urea $CO(NH_2)_2$	46% N
Calcium cyanamide $CaCN_2$	21% N

- **Slow release nitrogenous fertilizers:** Either derivatives of urea with N in large molecules, or granular water-soluble N fertilizers encased in thin plastic film, but slow or very slow-acting according to type of coating; partly including a quick-acting component or other means of slow release, e.g. sulphur coated urea (SCU). These are newly developed fertilizers which release nitrogen in soil very slowly so that it may be available to the plants for longer period of time. Use of these materials result in better utilization of applied nitrogen by the growing crop plants and reduce losses.

Fertilizer		% N
Urea-form (Urea+formaldehyde)		38% N
Oxamide H_2NCO—$CONH_2$		31.8% N
Isobutylidene diurea (IBDU) (Urea+Isobutylaldehyde) $(CH_3)_2$—$CH=CH$—$(NH$—CO—$NH_2)_2$		32.2% N
Crotonilidine diurea (CDU) (Urea+acetaldehyde)		32% N
Guanyl urea (GU)		37% N
N-lignin (Ammonified lignin)		18% N
Sulphur coated urea (SCU)		36 to 40% N
Metal-ammonium phosphate $Me.NH_4PO_4 \times H_2O$		
If Me is	Mg	8.3% N
"	Fe	7.5% N
"	Cu	7.2% N
"	Zn	7.8% N
"	Mn	7.5% N
"	Co	6.1% N
Nutricate, osmocate		Mixed fertilizers coated with various resin containing release controlling agents, additives

Phosphate Fertilizers

These are classified as natural phosphates, treated or processed phosphates, and by-product phosphates and chemical phosphates. P_2O_5 content in phosphatic fertilizer refers to available portion, except for rock phosphate where it means total content.

Types of P Fertilizers

Water-soluble types (quick-acting):

- single superphosphate (18–20% P_2O_5);
- triple superphosphate (45% P_2O_5).

Partly water-soluble types (quick and slow-acting):

- partly acidulated phosphate (23–26% P_2O_5, at least one-third water-soluble).

Slow-acting types:

- dicalcium phosphate (34% P_2O_5 citrate-soluble);
- basic slag (3–8% P_2O_5 citric acid-soluble).
- bone meal (20% P_2O_5)

Very slow-acting types:

- rock phosphate (finely-powdered soft type, e.g. 30% P_2O_5), with reactivity indicated by formic acid-solubility; permitted minimum is about one-half of total P_2O_5 content).
- imported (30–40% P_2O_5) Egypt, Zordan, Australia
- indigenous (18–35% P_2O_5) Udaipur, Mussorie, Jhabua, Purulia

Multinutrient fertilizers containing P:

- NP;
- PK (mixtures very commonly used).

NPK (may contain about one-third or more water-soluble P for quick supply and two-thirds slow-acting P for continuous supply).

Straight phosphatic fertilizers are as follows:

Fertilizer	Water soluble phosphate P_2O_5 (per cent by weight)	Neutral ammonium citrate soluble phosphates (per cent by weight)	2% citric soluble phosphate (per cent by weight)
Single superphosphate (16%)	16.0	16.5	–
Single superphosphate (14%)	14.0	14.5	–
Triple superphosphate	42.5	44.0	–
Dicalcium phosphate	46.0	–	–

Contd.

(Contd.)

Fertilizer	Water soluble phosphate P_2O_5 (per cent by weight)	Neutral ammonium citrate soluble phosphates (per cent by weight)	2% citric soluble phosphate (per cent by weight)
Bonemeal (raw) (Total P_2O_5 = 20%) (Total N = 3%)	–	–	8.0
Bonemeal steamed (Total P_2O_5 = 22%)	–	16.0	–
Rock phosphate (Total P_2O_5 = 40%)	–	26.0	–
Fused calcium magnesium phosphate	–	–	16.5
Pelophos (Total P_2O_5 = 17.0%)	–	16.0	–

Potash Fertilizers

These are mainly derived from geological saline deposits. Although low-grade, unrefined materials can be used directly, most fertilizer use is now in the form of higher-concentration products, all of which are water-soluble and quick-acting:

- potassium chloride, or muriate of potash (40–60% K_2O), the lower grades providing Na in addition to K_2O, with or without Mg;
- potassium sulphate (50% K_2O), for Cl-sensitive crops (e.g. potatoes, tobacco);
- potassium magnesium sulphate, also known as sulphate of potash magnesia (e.g. 40% K_2O, 6% Mg).
- potassium nitrate (45% K_2O)

Recently, several industrial residues containing K, e.g. filter dust, have been developed for use as slower-acting forms, especially where it is desired to avoid loss by leaching. Seaweed, particularly bladderwrack, kelp or laminaria contains all soil nutrients especially potassium in higher content (1.0% K). Potash fertilizers should generally be applied at sowing time. The K^+ ions are adsorbed in the soil and thus remain available, yet largely protected against leaching. However, split application is advisable (e.g. part autumn, part spring) in sandy soils where higher leaching losses may be expected. Some immobilization into clay lattice layers reduces availability but strong fixation into completely unavailable forms is fortunately restricted to a few special soil types. The utilization rate of K in fertilizers is about 50–60% during the first year.

Straight potassic fertilizers are as follows:

Fertilizer	Potash content (per cent by weight)	Total chloride (per cent by weight)	Sodium chloride content (per cent by weight)
Potassium chloride (muriate of potash) (KCl)	60.0	–	3.5
Potassium sulphate (K_2SO_4)	48.0	2.5	2.0
Potassium schoenite ($K_2SO_4.MgSO_4.6H_2O$)	23.0	2.5	1.5
Potassium magnesium sulphate ($K_2SO_4. 2MgSO_4$)	22.0	–	–

Micronutrients Fertilizer

Micronutrient fertilizers are required by plants in very low concentration. Micronutrients, required in concentrations ranging from 5 to 100 parts per million (ppm) by mass. The average concentration of these nutrient in soil are Mn 1000 ppm, Cl 480 ppm, Zn 80 ppm, Cu 70 ppm, B 10 ppm, Mo 2 to 3 ppm, iron 140 ppm. Plant micronutrients include Fe, Mn, B, Cu, Mo, Ni, Cl, and Zn.

The micronutrient deficiency occurs under conditions of:

1. Soils with a very high organic matter content (peat and muck soils)
2. Soils with very high or very low pH.
3. High doses of commercial fertilizers.
4. Highly leached acid and sandy soil.
5. Soils with impeded drainage or high water table.
6. Over liming of the soil.
7. Intensive cultivation.

The deficiencies may be overcome by addition of more than one micronutrients. If more than one micronutrients are applied it is called multinutrients. Specific sources include:

Name of the micronutrient	Source (formula)	Nutrient
Copper	Copper sulphate ($CuSO_4.5H_2O$)	25–35% Cu
Zinc	Zinc sulphate ($ZnSO_4.7H_2O$) Chelated Zn	22–35% Zn 12% Zn
Boron	Borax or sod. borate ($Na_2B_4O_7.10\ H_2O$) Disodium octaborate tetrahydrate	10.6% B 20% B
Manganese	Manganese sulphate ($MnSO_4.4H_2O$)	23% Mn
Molybdenum	Ammonium molybdate [$(NH_4)_6Mo_7O_{24}.4H_2O$]	54% Mo
Iron	Ferrous sulphate ($FeSO_4.7H_2O$)	20% Fe

1.4.1 Manufacturing Processes

Fertilizers are a basic component of efficient and sustainable crop production. In agricultural and horticultural crops, fertilizers can be the largest variable cost production component. During the past year, fertilizer prices have risen dramatically. Prices have increased due to increased energy costs for production, especially natural gas, precursor (sulphur, sulphuric acid, phosphoric acid) increased transportation costs, and increased demand.

The history of the Indian fertilizer industry dates back to 1906, when the first fertilizer factory opened at Ranipet (Tamil Nadu). Since then, there have been major developments in terms of both the quantity and types of fertilizers produced, the technologies used and the feedstocks employed (Table 1.2). The fertilizer industry in India is in the core sector and second to steel in terms of investment. Prior to 1960/61, India produced only straight nitrogenous fertilizers [ammonium sulphate, urea, calcium ammonium nitrate, ammonium chloride and single superphosphate]. The production of NP complex fertilizers commenced in 1960/61. Currently, India produces a large number of grades of NP/NPK complex fertilizer. In addition, India produces various grades of simple and granulated mixtures.

Table 1.2:   History of fertilizer production in India

Year of manufacture	Fertilizer product	Total number of units
1906	SSP	65
1933	AS	10
1959	Ammonium sulphate nitrate	No longer manufactured
1959	Urea	29
1959	Ammonium chloride	1
1960	Ammonium phosphate	3
1961	CAN	3
1965	Nitrophosphate	3
1967	DAP	11
1968	TSP	No longer manufactured
1968	Urea ammonium phosphate	2
1968	NPK complex fertilizers	6

Common Products

There are many solid, soluble, and liquid products used as fertilizers in India. The products may have organic or mineral origin. The majority of the major nutrients nitrogen (N), phosphorus (P), and potassium (K) are applied as solid mineral fertilizers. Little quantities of nitrogen are also applied as anhydrous ammonia in commercial orchards. Anhydrous ammonia is a gas that is sold in liquefied form under pressure in the same way that LPG is stored and transported.

1.4.1.1 Nitrogen Fertilizer Production

Nitrogen helps make plants green and plays a major role in boosting crop yields. Nitrogen plays a critical role in protein formation and is a key component of chlorophyll. Plants with adequate nitrogen show healthy vigorous growth, strong root development, dark green foliage, increased seed and fruit formation and higher yields. Nitrogen comes from the air and is the primary building block for all life. The air we breathe is of about 78 per cent nitrogen, but there are very few plants that can make direct use of nitrogen in the air. To make this nitrogen available to support life, nitrogen from the atmosphere is converted into a form plants can easily use.

All major nitrogen (N) fertilizer sources begin with the fixation of non-plant available atmospheric N_2 molecules into anhydrous ammonia molecules (NH_3). Nitrogen fertilizer manufacturing captures naturally occurring nitrogen from the atmosphere, and combines it with hydrogen from natural gas under heat (400–500 °C) and pressure (150–250 atm) to form anhydrous ammonia. Ammonia is used in two ways: it is applied directly to crops as a nitrogen fertilizer and it is used as a building block to make other nitrogen fertilizer products, including urea, ammonium nitrate, ammonium sulfate and water-based liquid nitrogen fertilizers.

The top five nitrogen producing countries in the world are China, India, the United States, Russia and Canada and top nitrogen consuming countries are China, USA, France, Germany and Brazil (Table 1.3).

Table 1.3: Countrywise total N consumption in the world

Country	Total N consumption (Mt/pa)
China	18.7
India	12.5
USA	9.1
France	2.5
Germany	2.0
Brazil	1.7
Canada	1.6
Turkey	1.5
UK	1.3
Mexico	1.3
Spain	1.2
Argentina	0.4

Ammonia : Ammonia is the basis for all of the major, manufactured nitrogen fertilizers. The hydrocarbon source provides a source of energy for the production of heat and compression in the manufacturing process as well as hydrogen. Natural gas is the most commonly used hydrocarbon feedstock for new plants; other feedstocks that have been used include naphtha, oil, and gasified coal. Natural gas is favored over the other feedstocks from an environmental perspective. Water contributes hydrogen, and air is the source of nitrogen. Ammonia contains 82% nitrogen. Ammonia (NH_3) is produced from atmospheric nitrogen and hydrogen from a hydrocarbon source (Fig. 1.3). Ammonia production from natural gas includes the following processes: desulfurization of the feedstock; primary and secondary reforming; carbon monoxide shift conversion and removal of carbon dioxide, which can be used for urea manufacture; methanation; and ammonia synthesis. Catalysts used in the process may include cobalt, molybdenum, nickel, iron oxide/chromium oxide, copper oxide/zinc oxide, and iron.

Air (N_2) + Natural gas (CH_4) = Anhydrous ammonia (NH_3)

The final stage, which is the actual Haber process is the synthesis of ammonia using magnetite, iron oxide, as catalyst:

$N_2(g) + 3H_2(g) = 2NH_3(g)$, $\Delta H = -92.4$ kJ/mol (Pt catalyst; 400–500 °C)

This is done at 150–250 atmospheres (atm) and between 300 and 550 °C, passing the gases over four beds of catalyst, with cooling between each pass to maintain a reasonable equilibrium constant. On each pass only about 15% conversion occurs, but any unreacted gases are recycled, so that eventually an overall conversion of 98% can be achieved.

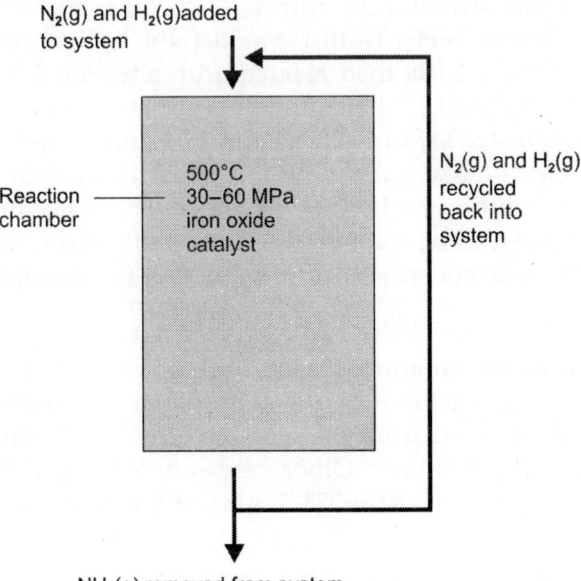

Fig. 1.3: Diagram of an iron oxide catalyst used in industries to produce ammonia economically

Urea: Urea (46% N, dry granular) is manufactured by reacting carbon dioxide and anhydrous ammonia at 200 atmospheres (atm) and 180 °C. Two principal reactions take place in the formation of urea from ammonia and carbon dioxide. The first reaction is exothermic:

$2 NH_3 + CO_2 \leftrightarrow H_2N\text{-}COONH_4$ (ammonium carbamate)

whereas the second reaction is endothermic:

$H_2N\text{-}COONH_4 \leftrightarrow (NH_2)_2CO + H_2O$

Carbon dioxide (CO_2) + Anhydrous ammonia $(2NH_3)$ = Urea $[CO(NH_2)_2]$ + Water

Both reactions combined are exothermic. The process, developed in 1922, is also called the Bosch-Meiser urea process after its discoverers.

Urea fertilizers production process steps include solution synthesis, where ammonia and carbon dioxide react to form ammonium carbamate, which is dehydrated to form urea; solution concentration by vacuum, crystallization, or evaporation to produce a melt; formation by-product from the petrochemical industry.

Urea manufacture is associated with anhydrous ammonia production in modern plants because carbon dioxide is a by-product of ammonia production and is thus readily available to react with ammonia. The urea can either be dried and granulated into 46% N urea fertilizer, or dissolved in water with ammonium nitrate to make urea ammonium nitrate (UAN) solution.

Ammonium nitrate: Ammonium nitrate (34% N) is manufactured by first transforming ammonia (NH_3) to nitric acid (HNO_3) with oxygen from the atmosphere. The nitric acid is then reacted with additional ammonia to form ammonium nitrate (NH_4NO_3). The ammonium nitrate produced in this process can be dried and granulated to form 34% N ammonium nitrate fertilizer, or dissolved in water with urea to make UAN solution. Heat is used to concentrate the ammonium nitrate solution by boiling-off water. The concentrated solution is sprayed into the top of a rising column of air in the prill tower, where the droplets cool and freeze into solid spheres called prills as they fall through the air.

$$HNO_3 + NH_3 = NH_4NO_3$$

Urea-ammonium nitrate solution (UAN): Urea-ammonium nitrate solutions (28, 30 and 32% N) are manufactured by dissolving urea and ammonium nitrate in water, and thus are derived from the manufacture of anhydrous ammonia to produce liquid nitrogen fertilizer. Other grades of UAN solution, for example 24-0-0-3 S, are made by diluting 30 or 32% UAN solution with water and dissolving a sulfur source.

Ammonium sulfate: Ammonium sulfate (21-0-0-24S) can be manufactured by synthetically reacting anhydrous ammonia with sulfuric acid and as a coke by-product. Sulphuric acid is produced by burning molten sulphur is burned to produce sulphur dioxide, which passes over vanadium oxide catalyst to oxidize into sulphur trioxide. The gas is absorbed in water to form 93% sulphuric acid. $(S + 2O_2 + H_2O = H_2SO_4)$.

$$H_2SO_4 + 2NH_4 = (NH_4)_2 SO_4$$

Sulphuric acid is reacted with ammonia in a pipe reactor located inside the granulator. The reaction between ammonia and sulfuric acid produces an ammonium sulfate solution that is continuously circulated through an evaporator to thicken the solution and to produce ammonium sulfate crystals. The crystals are separated from the liquor in a centrifuge, and the liquor is returned to the evaporator. The crystals are fed either to a fluidized bed or to a rotary drum dryer and are screened before bagging or bulk loading. The resulting slurry is sprayed onto a seed bed of small granular particles to form product size granules. Since ammonium sulfate is used mainly for its sulfur content, changes in price are associated with demand for sulfur and/or price increases for other N fertilizer sources.

1.4.1.2 Phosphate Fertilizer Production

Phosphorus is present in all living cells and is essential to all forms of life. Phosphorus is the second most abundant of all the mineral nutrients contained in our bodies. It can be found in every cell, but nearly 80 per cent of phosphorus found in people is concentrated in teeth and bones.

The source of phosphorus in fertilizer is fossilized remains of ancient marine life found in rock deposits in North America and North Africa, and volcanic activity in China. The phosphate manufacturing process combines phosphate rock from these natural geological deposits with sulfuric acid to produce a concentrated phosphorus solution. The countries with abundant phosphorus resources are the United States, China, India, Russia and Brazil.

The major phosphate (P) fertilizer sources that we currently use are diammonium phosphate (DAP), ammonium polyphosphate (APP), monoammonium phosphate (MAP), and triple superphosphate.

The process involved in the production of various phosphatic fertilizers are schematically shown in Fig. 1.4.

Rock phosphate $[Ca_{10} (PO_4)_6 (F, Cl, OH)_2/CO_3]$ is the raw material used in the manufacture of most commercial phosphate fertilizers on the market. In the past, ground rock phosphate (0.15 mm IS sieve) itself has been used as a source of P for acid soils. However, due to low availability of P in this native material, high transportation costs, and small crop responses, very little rock phosphate is currently used in agriculture. This agricultural grade phosphoric acid is then utilized to make the phosphorus fertilizers that are used in agricultural applications.

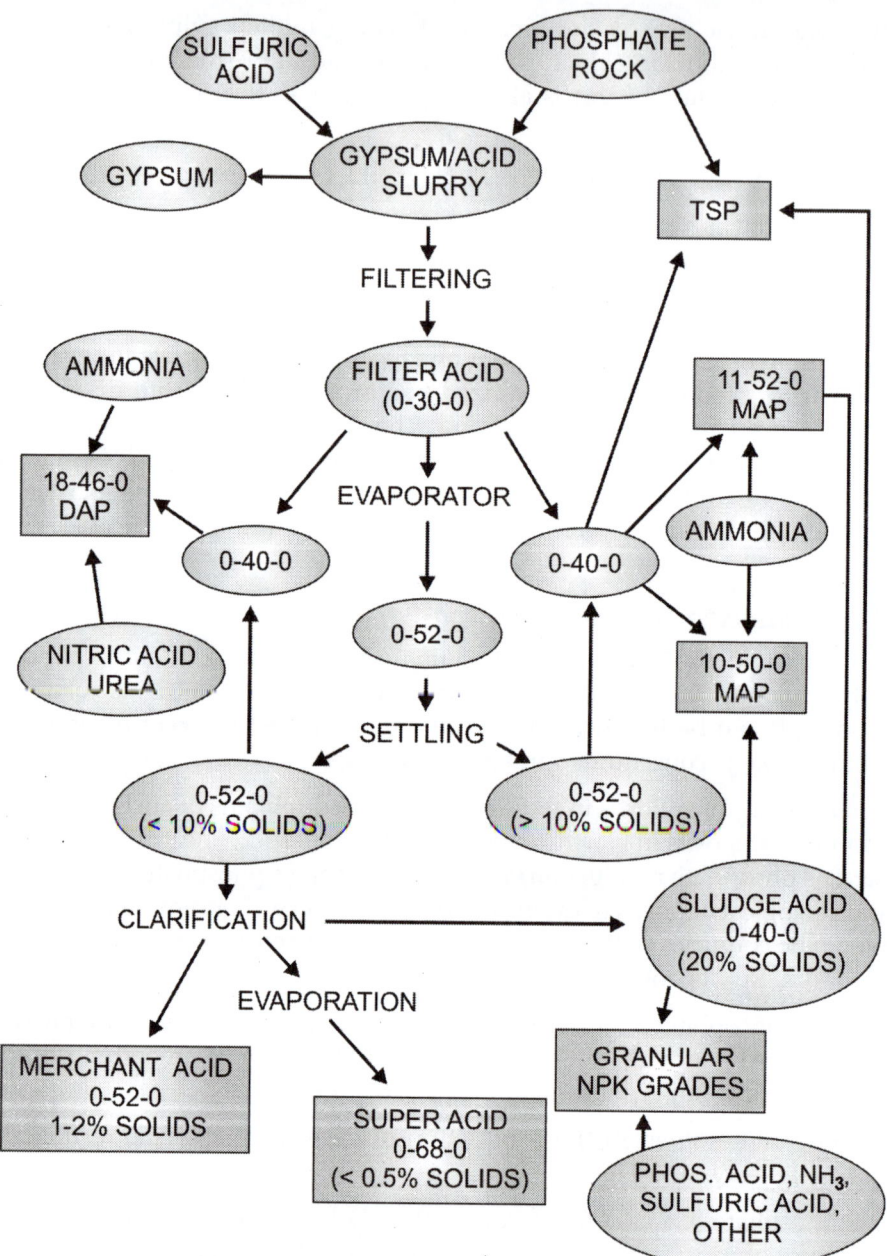

Fig. 1.4: The process used in the manufacture of various phosphate fertilizers

The cost of converting rock phosphate to the individual phosphate fertilizers varies with the process used (Figs. 1.4 and 1.4(a)). More importantly, the processes used have no effect on the availability of P to plants. The manufacture of most commercial phosphate fertilizers begins with the production of phosphoric acid. A generalized diagram showing the various steps used in the manufacture of various phosphate fertilizers is provided in Figs. 1.4 and 1.4(a). Phosphoric acid is produced by either a dry or wet process. In the dry process, rock phosphate is treated in an electric furnace. This treatment produces a very pure and more expensive phosphoric acid (frequently called white or furnace acid) used primarily in the food and chemical industry. Fertilizers that use white phosphoric acid as the P source are generally more expensive because of the costly treatment process.

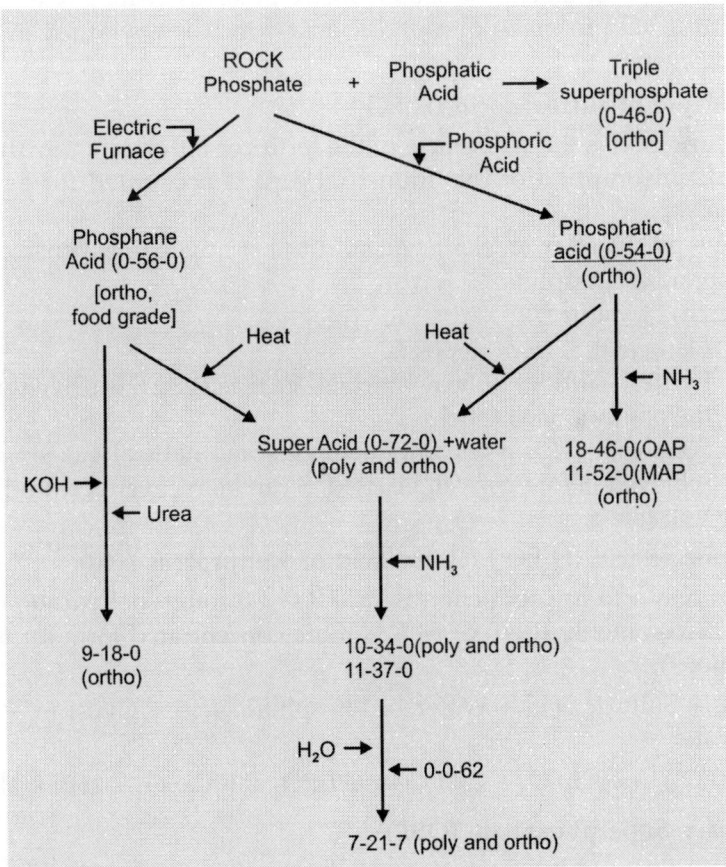

Fig. 1.4(a): The process used in the manufacture of various phosphate fertilizers (Courtesy: IFA, Paris)

The wet process involves treatment of the rock phosphate with acid producing phosphoric acid (also called green or black acid) and gypsum which is removed as a by-product. The impurities which give the acid its color have not been a problem in the production of dry fertilizers. Either treatment process (wet or dry) produces orthophosphoric acid—the phosphate form that is taken up by plants.

The phosphoric acid produced by either the wet or dry process is frequently heated, driving-off water and producing a superphosphoric acid. The phosphate concentration in superphosphoric acid usually varies from 72 to 76%. The P in this acid is present as both orthophosphate and polyphosphate. Polyphosphates consist of a series of orthophosphates that have been chemically joined together. Upon contact with soils, polyphosphates revert back to orthophosphates.

The phosphate fertilizer production process involves treating with rock phosphate with sulfuric acid to make phosphoric acid which is envisaged in the following systematic steps:

a. Production of sulfuric acid (H_2SO_4)

   i. Sulfuric acid is the workhorse of the fertilizer industry; more than 60% of the total consumption of this industrial acid is accounted for by the fertilizer industry.

  ii. Easily produced from elemental sulfur (a relatively inexpensive raw material in abundant supply).

 iii. Sources of sulfur:

    1. Elemental S, from deposits.

    2. Pyrites - sulfides of heavy metals, such as FeS_2; S is driven-off by burning the ore (not used much).

    3. Sour gas - H_2S is a component of some natural gas sources; must be removed before gas can be used; S can be recovered from H_2S.

    4. Volcanic S.

b. Phosphoric acid (H_3PO_4) (Green acid or wet process acid)

Wet process acid at production is 28% P_2O_5; through dehydration it is brought up to 54% (commonly used) or 64% (a more concentrated form for use in making NP solutions)

Apatite + Sulfuric acid + Water → Phosphoric acid + Gypsum + Hydrofluoric acid + Water

$$Ca_{10}F_2(PO_4)_6 + 10H_2SO_4 + 20H_2O \rightarrow 6H_3PO_4 + 10CaSO_4 + 2HF + 2H_2O$$

c. Ordinary Superphosphate (OSP)

It is manufactured by reacting ground phosphate rock with 65 to 75 per cent sulfuric acid.

Apatite + Sulfuric Acid + Water → Monocalcium phosphate + Gypsum + Hydrofluoric acid

$$Ca_{10}F_2(PO_4)_6 + 7H_2SO_4 + 3H_2O \rightarrow 3Ca(H_2PO_4)_2 + 7CaSO_4 + 2HF$$

This process was patented in 1842. Previous to that time, phosphate was obtained from ground-up bones or animal manure.

i. superphosphate is referred to as SP, normal super, single super, or superphosphate.

ii. SP contains 20% P_2O_5.

iii. Gypsum ($CaSO_4$) is an integral part of monocalcium phosphate; it cannot be separated out, thus if OSP is applied as fertilizer, gypsum is applied along with it; gypsum is a source of sulfur in the soil; OSP is 12% S and 20% Ca.

iv. The hydrofluoric acid (HF) produced can be trapped and sold.

v. Will get uranium cake (about 6.6 kg/ton) from OSP production.

vi. Problems with forming monocalcium phosphate: impurities such as Al, Fe, and Mg (most deleterious); these are picked up especially in lower grade ores; their presence will precipitate out P and will not let manufacturing reaction proceed.

vii. Monocalcium phosphate as SP is 80% water- and citric-acid soluble.

d. Concentrated superphosphate (CSP)

These fertilizers are made by reacting anhydrous ammonia (NH_3) with phosphoric acid.

$$H_3 PO_4 + NH_3 \rightarrow NH_4H_2 PO_4$$

These are 100% water soluble, and have the following analysis and properties:

DAP (18-46-0) — Dry granular

MAP (11-52-0) — Dry granular

APP (10-34-0) — Clear liquid

These are the most widely used P fertilizers, with DAP being the single most widely used P source.

This fertilizer is made by reacting rock phosphate with phosphoric acid to produce a P fertilizer with an analysis of 0-46-0. This is a dry granular fertilizer utilized in bulk blending for making zero N grade complete fertilizers. This fertilizer also serves as the P source for ammoniation plants where granular N-P-K fertilizers that contain all nutrients in each granule are manufactured. These fertilizers are generally marketed in vegetables and other high value crops.

Apatite + Phosphoric acid + Water → Monocalcium phosphate + Hydrofluoric acid

$$Ca_{10}F_2(PO_4)_6 + 14H_3PO_4 + 10H_2O \rightarrow 10Ca(H_2PO_4)_2 + 2HF$$

i. This reaction produces no gypsum because no S is added as sulfuric acid.

ii. This material is referred to as triple superphosphate (TSP), or triple super.

iii. TSP contains 46% P_2O_5.

iv. TSP is 90 to 95% water- and citric-acid soluble.

e. Manufacture of superphosphoric acid (polyphosphate)

i. Removes two H_2O molecules from 3 molecules of wet process acid to form polyphosphoric acid (106 to 115% H_3PO_4, or 76 to 85% P_2O_5); reaction requires high temperature and centrifugation.

ii. Principally used in production of liquid polyphosphate fertilizers.

f. Monoammonium phosphate (MAP) $NH_4(H_2PO_4)$ 11-48-0

Ammonia (NH_3) + Phosphoric acid (H_3PO_4) → $NH_4(H_2PO_4)$ (MAP)

g. Diammonium phosphate (DAP) $(NH_4)_2HPO_4$ 18-46-0

Ammonia (NH_3) + Phosphoric acid (H_3PO_4) → $(NH_4)_2HPO_4$ (DAP)

i. DAP is the single most popular fertilizer in the world.

ii. Both MAP and DAP are 100% water- and citric-acid soluble.

Phosphate Fertilizer Terminology

Because of the prevalence of number of products on the market, the selection of a phosphate fertilizer can be confusing. An explanation of some terminology may help to avoid some of the confusion. Some important terms are:

- **Water-soluble:** Fertilizer samples analyzed by a control laboratory are first placed in water and the percentage of the total phosphate that dissolves is measured. This percentage is referred to as water-soluble phosphate.
- **Citrate-soluble:** The fertilizer material that is not dissolved in water is then placed in an ammonium citrate solution (2%). The amount of P dissolved in this solution is measured and expressed as a percentage of the total in the fertilizer material. Phosphate measured with this analytical procedure is referred to as citrate-soluble.
- **Available:** The sum of the water-soluble and citrate-soluble phosphates is considered to be the percentage that is available to plants and is the amount guaranteed on the fertilizer label. Usually, the citrate-soluble component is less than the water-soluble component (Table 1.4).

Table 1.4: Percentage of water-soluble and available phosphate in several common fertilizer sources

P_2O_5 source	N	P_2O_5 Total	P_2O_5 Available	P_2O_5 Water soluble
Superphosphate (OSP)	0	21	20	85
Concentrated superphosphate (CSP)	0	45	45	85
Monoammonium phosphate (MAP)	11	49	48	82
Diammonium phosphate (DAP)	18	47	46	90
Ammonium polyphosphate (APP)	10	34	34	100
Rock phosphate	0	34	3-8	0

1.4.1.3   Potassium Fertilizer Production

Potassium is the seventh most abundant element in the earth's crust and is found in every cell of plants and animals. Potassium helps plants grow strong stalks, in the same way that calcium gives people strong bones. More than 85 per cent of the body's potassium is found in the muscles, skin, blood, digestive tract and liver.

Fertilizer produces mine potassium, or potash, from naturally occurring ore deposits that were formed when seas and oceans evaporated, many of which are covered with several thousands of feet of earth. Potassium (K) salts [Sylvite (KCl); Sylvinite (KCl, NaCl); Kainite (KMg(SO$_4$)Cl . 3H$_2$O; Carnalite (KMgCl$_3$. 6H$_2$O); Schoenite (K$_2$SO$_4$ MgSO$_4$. 6H$_2$O)] used in manufacturing K fertilizers are mined from deposits (5000 ft deep) that occur beneath the earth's surface, like coal, or from brines. Once the ore is brought to the surface, unwanted minerals are removed in the manufacturing process and the product is then granulated for application. These deposits are mined and then refined by crystallization (based on solubility) or flotation (based on difference in specific gravity).

Most of the world's potash deposits are found in Canada, Russia, Belarus, Germany and the United States. Recently geological survey of India (GSI) found deposit in India (Leh, Jammu, Bikaneer, Rajasthan) too. The major K fertilizers manufactured are potassium chloride, potassium sulfate, and potassium magnesium sulfate. Commercial-scale production of K fertilizers began in Germany around 1861; salt deposits from old inland seas were mined for the production of common table salt, but mined material also contains KCl; the KCl needed to be upgraded (beneficiated) before it could be used as fertilizer. Beneficiation processes were developed by German chemists.

Potassium Chloride: Potassium chloride (KCl), or potash, is most widely sold as a dry, granular fertilizer that is red, pink, or white in color. A powdered grade of KCl is utilized in manufacturing liquid fertilizers. These fertilizers are water-soluble and are the most widely utilized K sources in the world. The major restriction for KCl use is that some crops such as potatoes, tobacco, and citrus are sensitive to high levels of chloride.

Potassium sulfate: This fertilizer is manufactured by reacting potassium chloride with sulfuric acid or other S sources. Produced by the reaction of KCl with sulfuric acid: 2KCl + H$_2$SO$_4$ → K$_2$SO$_4$ + 2HCl or it can also be produced from langbeinite: K$_2$SO$_4$· 2MgSO$_4$ + 4KCl → 3K$_2$SO$_4$ + 2MgCl$_2$. It is widely used in tobacco and potato production, is a dry granular product that is water-soluble, and is an excellent sulfur source as well as K source.

Potassium magnesium sulfate: This is a naturally occurring mineral that is mined from nature. It is a dry granular fertilizer that is water soluble and is a source of K, Mg and S for crops. However, it is more expensive than potassium chloride and is used in situations where magnesium and/or sulfur are needed in addition to potassium.

Potassium nitrate: This fertilizer is manufactured by the reaction of KCl and nitric acid:

$KCl + HNO_3 \rightarrow KNO_3 + HCl$. It contains 44% K_2O and 13% N.

Other products: Waste products from tobacco processing (stems and ribs of leaves) are ground and sold for use as fertilizers; these contain 4 to 8% potassium and 2 to 4% nitrogen. Again sea water contains vast amounts of K (one cubic milimeter contains the equivalent of 1.6 million tons of K); extraction of K from this source is not yet economically feasible. Seaweeds, particularly bladderwrack, kelp or laminaria, can be used as a source for K as it contains all soil nutrients (0.3% N, 0.1% P, 1.0% K, plus a full range of trace elements).

1.4.1.4 Fertilizer Industry

Agriculture the backbone of Indian economy still holds its relative importance for more than a billion people. The Government of India from time to time has taken considerable steps for the upliftment of agriculture sector. The fertilizer industry in India started its first manufacturing unit of single superphosphate (SSP) in Ranipet near Chennai with a capacity of 6000 MT a year. The sector experienced a faster growth rate and presently India is the third largest fertilizer producer in the world.

Basically the fertilizer industry in India consists of three major players; The Government owned public sector Undertakings, Co-operative societies like IFFCO, KRIBHCO and units from private sector. There are about 33 major producers producing N and NP/NPK fertilizers in the country at present. The fertilizer industry of India had made constructive use of the fertilizer subsidy provided by the Government of India to ensure that the country achieved reasonable self-sufficiency in foodgrain production. The fertilizer industry has organized itself through fertilizer association of India (FAI) in co-ordination with the Government of India to achieve the macro-economic objectives related to agricultural sector and to provide other services.

Public sector fertilizer companies

- National Fertilizers Limited (NFL)
- Paradeep Phosphates Limited (PPL)
- Fertilizers & Chemicals Travancore Limited (FACT)
- Pyrites Phosphates & Chemicals Limited (PPCL)
- Rastriya Chemical Fertilizers Limited (RCF)
- Steel Authority of India Limited (SAIL)
- Hindustan Fertilizer Corporation Limited (HFC)
- Hindustan Copper Limited (HCL)
- Fertilizer Cooperation of India Limited (FCIL)
- Neyvelli Lignite Co-operation Limited (NLC)

- Brahmaputra Valley Fertilizer Corporation Limited (BVFC)
- FCI Aravali Gypsum and Minerals India Limited

Co-operative sector

- Indian Farmers Fertilizer Co-operative Limited (IFFCO)
- Krishak Bharati Co-operative Limited (KRIBHCO)

Private sector fertilizer companies

- Basant Agro Tech India Limited
- Gujarat State Fertilizer and Chemical Limited
- Coromandel Fertilizers Limited
- Godavari Fertilizer & Chemicals Limited
- Bharat Fertilizer Industries Limited
- Chambal Fertilizers and Chemicals Limited
- Chemfert Traders
- Deepak Fertilizer and Petrochemicals Corporation Limited
- Duncans Industries Limited
- Gujarat State Fertilizers and Chemicals Limited
- Indo-Gulf Fertilizers and Chemicals Corporation Limited
- The Maharashtra Agro Industries Development Corporation Ltd. (MAIDC)
- Mangalore Chemicals and Fertilizers Limited
- Meerut Agro Chemical Private Limited
- Dharamsi Morarji Chemical Co. Limited
- Multiplex Fertilizer Private Limited
- Nagarjuna Fertilizers and Chemicals Limited
- Gujarat Narmada Valley Fertilizer Co. Limited
- Shriram Fertilizers and Chemicals
- Southern Petrochemical Industries Corporation Ltd.
- Tuticorin Alkali Chemi and Fertilizer Limited
- United Phosphorous Limited
- Zuari Industries Fertilizer Limited

1.4.2 Properties of Major Nitrogenous, Phosphatic, Potassic Complex and Mixed Fertilizers

Many different physical and chemical forms of commercial fertilizer are available. Fertilizer materials can be solids, liquids, or gases. Each physical form has its own uses and limitations, which provide the basis for selecting the best material for the job.

Granulated fertilizer: These materials are solid, homogenous mixtures of fertilizer materials generally produced in ammoniation granulation plants by combining raw materials such as anhydrous ammonia, phosphoric acid, and potassium chloride. Granulated materials are N-P or N-P-K grades of fertilizer. Each uniform size fertilizer particle contains all of the nutrients in the grade. For example, each particle in a 10-26-26 granulated fertilizer theoretically contains 10 per cent nitrogen, 26 per cent phosphate, and 26 per cent potash. The principle advantage of granulated materials is the uniform distribution of nutrients. There is no segregation of the nutrients in handling or spreading, and plant roots absorb a complete set of the applied nutrients. Granulated fertilizers generally have good handling properties, with little tendency to cake or dust.

Blended fertilizers: These are simple physical mixtures of dry fertilizer materials. The ingredients of a blended fertilizer can be straight materials, such as urea or potassium chloride; can be granulated compound fertilizer materials mixed together; or can be a combination of the two. In blended fertilizers, the individual particles remain separate in the mixture, and there is a potential for segregation of the nutrients. This problem can be reduced by using materials that are of the same size. Properly made blends are generally equal in effectiveness to other compound fertilizers. Blends have the advantage of allowing a very wide range of fertilizer grades that makes it possible to match a fertilizer exactly to a soil test recommendation. Blends have been used effectively as starter fertilizers; however for this purpose, urea and diammonium phosphate should be avoided because both materials produce free ammonia, which can hinder seed germination and seedling growth.

Fluid fertilizers: These are commonly used. Fluids can be either straight materials, such as nitrogen solutions, or compound fertilizers of various grades. Fluid fertilizers are categorized into two groups: (1) clear solutions, and (2) suspensions.

1. In clear solutions, the nutrients are completely dissolved in water. The major advantage is ease of handling. In addition, the phosphorus in these materials is highly water soluble. The disadvantages are that only relatively low analyses are possible, especially when the material contains potassium, and the cost per unit of nutrients is generally higher. Clear solutions are equal in agronomic effectiveness to other types of fertilizers, when equal amounts of plant food are compared.

2. Suspension fertilizers are fluids in which solubility of the components has been exceeded and clay has been added to keep the very fine, undissolved, fertilizer particles from settling out. The major advantage is that they can be handled as a fluid. Another advantage of suspensions is that they can be formulated at much higher analyses than clear solutions. Analyses as high as those of dry materials are possible. The major disadvantages are that suspensions require constant agitation, even in storage, and suspension fertilizer cannot be used as a carrier for certain chemicals, for example Paraquat. As in the case of clear solutions, the agronomic effectiveness of suspensions is

equal to other types of fertilizer materials when equal amounts of plant food are compared.

Gaseous fertilizer: This fertilizer requires some special considerations in handling and use. Anhydrous ammonia is a high nitrogen content gaseous material used both in the manufacture of all other common nitrogen-containing fertilizers and in direct applications to the soil. Once applied, anhydrous ammonia behaves similarly to any other ammonium nitrogen source. However, special handling methods and safety precautions are required because anhydrous ammonia is stored as a compressed liquid. When expansion occurs during application to the soil, it immediately becomes a gas. Thus, it must be injected into the soil to prevent the gas from escaping.

Some hazards are involved in handling anhydrous ammonia. Since the material can cause serious chemical burns and asphyxiation, proper safety percautions are necessary. Anhydrous ammonia is an excellent nitrogen fertilizer, but it must be handled properly.

Organic Materials

That are commonly used as fertilizers have many varied properties. Therefore, the physical properties of these materials should be evaluated on an individual basis. Since the specific chemical properties of fertilizers also are very complex and varied, a detailed discussion of several important chemical properties should be considered in selecting a fertilizer material. These properties are solubility, particle size, soil pH, chemical form, and soluable salts.

Solubility: It indicates how readily nutrients are dissolved in the soil water and taken up by plants. Since the nitrogen and potassium in fertilizers are essentially completely soluble in water (Table 1.5), their solubility is not a major consideration for the common fertilizer sources. Only phosphorus that is soluble in neutral ammonium citrate (this includes the water-soluble phosphorus) is counted as available phosphorus on the fertilizer label.

Phosphorus must be dissolved in water to be taken up by plants. However, the water solubility of the available phosphorus can vary from 0 to 100 per cent. Generally, the higher the water solubility the more effective the phosphorus source is for short-season fast-growing crops, for crops with restricted root-systems, for starter fertilizers, and for situations where less than optimal rates of phosphorus are applied to low fertility soils. Water solubility of the available phosphorus is less important in other applications. Fortunately, most common phosphorus sources (triple superphosphate and the ammonium phosphates) contain highly water-soluble forms of phosphorus. There is no apparent difference in agronomic effectiveness when a highly water soluble phosphorus source is applied as a fluid fertilizer or as a dry fertilizer. Materials such as raw rock phosphate have a very low water solubility.

Table 1.5: Solubility of some fertilizer materials

Material	Solubility (g/litre)
Ammonium nitrate	1,617
Urea	902
Ammonium sulfate	623
Diammonium phosphate	574
Monoammonium phosphate	312
Muriate of potash	283
Potassium nitrate	263
Sulfate of potash	92

Particle size: Particle size of a fertilizer material can be important for both agronomic and handling reasons. Agronomically, particle size is most important for the sparingly soluble materials such as rock phosphate. These materials must be very finely ground to ensure sufficient solubility. For most soluble fertilizers, particle size is not critical for agronomic purposes but is very important in determining ease of handling of the materials. Very fine materials, which often become dusty and can cake, are difficult to handle; granular materials are sized to avoid these problems and to promote handling convenience. While there is no standard for particle size, most fertilizers are sized to pass through a 2.8 mm IS sieve but be retained on a 1 mm IS sieve. Particle size is most critical for materials that are used in blended products. Materials of different sizes tend to segregate as the fertilizer is handled and spread. Particle size has been identified as the most important factor in producing a stable, high quality, blended fertilizer.

Soil pH: It can be changed by the reaction of fertilizer materials. The most important reaction is the microbial oxidation of ammonium nitrogen to nitrate nitrogen. This occurs regardless of the source of ammonium nitrogen (fertilizer, manure, or organic residues). The acidity of a fertilizer is usually given by convention as the amount of pure limestone that would be required to offset the acidity produced by the reaction of the fertilizer.

Material	Equivalent acidity (kg. $CaCO_3$ per kg. of N)
Anhydrous ammonia	1.8
Urea	1.8
Ammonium nitrate	1.8
Manure	1.8
Diammonium phosphate (DAP)	3.5
Ammonium sulphate	5.3
Monoammonium phosphate (MAP)	5.3

Equivalent acidities can be used to compare materials, but the actual amount of limestone required to neutralize the acidity from the fertilizer is probably greater than shown here. Remember the residual effect of the materials. Many of these materials greatly, but temporarily, increase the soil pH. Another example of this temporary pH change is the reaction of the superphosphate materials. The initial reaction is a drastic lowering of the pH around the fertilizer particle, but the residual effect of the superphosphates changes the soil pH very little. The common potassium materials are neutral salts that have no effect on the soil pH.

Chemical forms: Chemical forms of the nutrient itself are critical for agronomic crops only in special situations. There is generally little practical difference for example between an ammonium and a nitrate nitrogen source (if leaching or denitrification are serious potential problems, then the ammonium form is preferred) or between orthophosphates and polyphosphates (unless insoluble micronutrients are added to a liquid fertilizer, in which case the polyphosphates are preferred) or between potassium chloride and potassium sulfate (some crops such as potato and tobacco are sensitive to chloride, in which case the sulfate is preferred).

Soluble salts: Soluble salts at high concentrations in soil solution, can cause injury or death to plants or prevent germination of seeds. Under normal conditions, fertilizers uniformly distributed at recommended rates do not cause soluble salt levels that are high enough to damage plants. However, a concentrated application of fertilizer or manure placed in contact with the seed or in a band near the germinating seed or growing plant can cause damage. An estimate of potential salt injury from different fertilizers is given as the salt index for that material. The salt index is a relative scale useful for comparing materials for special placement (such as for drilling with the seed, banding at high rates, and for pop-up treatments) when a low salt index is preferred. The salt index for several common fertilizer materials is given here:

Table 1.6: Salt index of some fertilizer materials

Material	Salt index*
Nitrogen (N)	
Ammonium sulfate	54
Ammonium nitrate	49
Urea	27
Anhydrous ammonia	10
Phosphate (P$_2$O$_5$)	
Triple superphosphate	4
Monoammonium phosphate (MAP)	7
Diammonium phosphate (DAP)	8
Superphosphate (9% P)	6.4

Contd.

Table 1.6: Salt index of some fertilizer materials *(Contd.)*

Material	Salt index*
Phosphate (P_2O_5)	
Superphosphate (21% P)	3.5
Potash (K_2O)	
Potassium chloride	32
Potassium sulfate	14

*The salt index assumes equal weights of the primary nutrient are being compared.

1.5 RAW MATERIALS AND ENERGY REQUIREMENTS FOR FERTILIZER PRODUCTION

Raw Materials

Domestic raw materials are available only for nitrogenous fertilizers. For the production of urea and other ammonia-based fertilizers, methane presents the major input which is gained from natural gas/associated gas, naphtha, fuel oil, low sulfur heavy stock (LSHS) and coal. In the more recent past, production has more and more switched over to the use of natural gas, associated gas and naphtha as feedstock. Out of these gas is most hydrogen rich and easiest to process due to its light weight and fair abundance within the country. However, demand for gas is quite competitive since it serves as a major input to electricity generation and provides the preferred fuel input to many other industrial processes. For production of phosphatic fertilizer most raw materials have to be imported. India has no source of elemental sulfur, phosphoric acid and rock phosphate. Yet, some low-grade rock phosphate is domestically mined (Udaipur, Mussorie, Purulia, Jhabua) and made available to rather small-scale single superphosphate fertilizer producers. Sulfur is produced as a by-product by some of the petroleum and steel industries.

Energy Use

Agriculture produces biomass in the form of vegetables, cereals and feed, which are the energy sources for humans and animals. Biomass and the processed food (e.g. bread made from wheat grain) have a defined energy content, which is measured in joules or calories. Today, questions are often asked about the energy efficiency of modern agriculture. This is mainly because of the high consumption of energy in the production of farm inputs, in particular mineral nitrogen fertilizers, and the high degree of mechanization on the farms.

Fertilizer production is one of the most energy intensive processes in the Indian industry. In this high energy intensive energy category we have iron and steel, alumunium, paper, cement and glass.

Energy is consumed in the form of natural gas, associated gas, naphtha, fuel oil, low sulfur heavy stock and coal. The choice of the feedstock is dependent on the availability of feedstock and the plant location. It is generally assigned to the plants by the government. Production of ammonia has greatest impact on energy use in fertilizer production. It accounts for 80% of the energy consumption for nitrogenous fertilizer. The feedstock mix used for ammonia production has changed over the past. Since new capacity in the form of gas-based fertilizer plants was added in the 1980s, the share of gas has increased substantially. The shift towards the increased use of natural/associated gas and naphtha is beneficial in that these feedstocks are more efficient and less polluting than heavy fuels like fuel oil and coal. Furthermore, capacity utilization in gas-based plants is generally higher than in other plants. Therefore, gas and naphtha present the preferred feedstocks for nitrogenous fertilizer production. Energy intensity in India's fertilizer plants has decreased over time. This decrease is due to advances in process technology and catalysts, better stream sizes of urea plants and increased capacity utilization. Capacity utilization is important as losses and waste heat are of about the same magnitude no matter how much is actually produced in a plant at a specific point of time. Actual energy consumption in a plant depends on the age of the technology and the scale of the plant. For example, a typical ammonia plant established in 1970s would consume more than a plant established in early 1990s. The production of phosphatic fertilizer requires much less energy than nitrogenous fertilizer. And similarly potassic fertilizer requires less lenegy than phosphatic fertilizer (Table 1.6).

It is evident form the above discussion that inorganic fertilizers are major consumers of energy in the agricultural sector. Inorganic fertilization accounts considerable amount to the total energy input to crop production. In contrast to tractors, irrigation pumps, and other types of equipment, fertilizers are indirect energy consumers. That is, the bulk of energy use associated with fertilizers is not consumed directly at the agricultural site, but indirectly during its production, packaging, and transportation to the site. Additional energy is then used onsite during fertilizer application. Most fertilizer energy use is attributable to the production of nitrogen fertilizers with natural gas. Natural gas is the principal energy resource for creating anhydrous ammonia, a key nitrogen fertilizer. The natural gas provides a source of hydrogen in the synthesis of ammonia by the Haber process. Over 90% of nitrogenous fertilizers contain ammonia and/or other fertilizer elements derived from ammonia (e.g. ammonium nitrate, sodium nitrate, calcium nitrate, ammonium sulfate, ammonium phosphates, and urea). Producing ammonia is a very energy intensive process; it requires about 1090 to 1250 m^3 of natural gas to produce 1 metric ton of anhydrous ammonia. Natural gas is also used in other ways in the fertilizer industry. For example, natural gas as a fuel provides the process heat for producing other types of fertilizers. It is estimated the natural gas supplies between 70 and 80% of all energy for fertilizer production. Each of the three primary nutrients in inorganic fertilizers has a different set of energy requirements during its lifecycle. However, these requirements can be separated into four main stages: production, packaging, transportation, and application. Table 1.7 summarizes the world average energy requirements by nutrient type and lifecycle stage for inorganic fertilizers and clearly shows the relatively high energy intensity of nitrogen production. Nitrogen production requires roughly 70,000 kJ per pound of nutrient (30,000 Btu per kg). This corresponds to almost 90% of nitrogen's total energy requirement. In contrast, the production of phosphate and potash account for only about 45% of the total energy requirement for these nutrients. Moreover, the energy requirement for nitrogen fertilizer is 4.5 times that of phosphate fertilizer, and 5.7 times that of potash fertilizer.

Table 1.7: Energy requirements to produce, package, transport, and apply inorganic fertilizers

Energy requirement (world average) (MJ/kg)			
	Nitrogen	**Phosphate**	**Potash**
Produce	69.5	7.70	6.40
Package	2.6	2.60	1.80
Transport	4.5	5.70	4.60
Apply	0.69	1.50	1.00
Total	78.2	17.5	13.8

Source: Data compiled from Helsel ZR (1992). Energy and alternatives for fertilizer and pesticide use. *Energy in Farm Production*, Volume 6 (ed. RC Fluck), p. 177–201 New York: Elsevier.

1.6 COMPOSITION

The major mineral fertilizers have been discussed before and are also listed in the table below with composition. Many of the solid products can be mixed to create blends that meet specific nutrient needs of crops and pastures.

Fertilizer	Approximate percentage of principal elements				
	N	**P**	**K**	**S**	**Ca**
Anhydrous ammonia	82	–	–	–	–
Aqua ammonia	20.5	–	–	–	–
Urea	46	–	–	–	–
Ammonium nitrate	34	–	–	–	–
Calcium ammonium nitrate	21–27	–	–	–	8–14
Calcium nitrate	15.5	–	–	–	19
Ammonium sulfate	20–21	–	–	24	–
Ammonium phosphate sulfate	14–18	7–12	–	12–17	–
Mono-ammonium phosphate (MAP)	10–12	22	–	1–2	–
Sulfur coated MAP	9	19	–	12	1.7

Contd.

(Contd.)

Fertilizer	Approximate percentage of principal elements				
	N	P	K	S	Ca
Di-ammonium phosphate (DAP)	18	20	–	1–3	–
Sulfur coated DAP	16	18	–	12	0.6
Sodium nitrate	16	–	–	–	–
Ground phosphate rock/reactive phosphate rock	–	11–16	–	–	30–37
Single superphosphate	–	8–9	–	11	18–20
Sulfur fortified single superphosphate	–	5–8	–	25–45	12–17
Double/triple superphosphate	–	17–20	–	1–4	15–16
Sulfur coated triple superphosphate	–	16	–	20	11.8
Powdered sulfur	–	–	–	100	–
Potassium chloride (muriate of potash)	–	–	48–51	–	–
Potassium nitrate	13	–	37–38	–	–
Potassium sulfate (sulfate of potash)	–	–	40–42	16	–

1.7 FERTILIZER USAGE

India is the fourth largest producer as well as consumer of fertilizer in the world. With population growing at a fast rate, food production was given highest priority in India since the 1960. Although India's soil is varied and rich, it is naturally deficient in major plant nutrients (nitrogen, phosphate and potassium). Growth in chemical fertilizer production and consumption therefore reveals the single largest contributor to agricultural progress, its technological transformation and commercialization. Fertilizer production in India has been growing at an accelerating rate, from very low levels after independence and still low levels in the early 1970s to a total production of 21 million tonnes in 2020. Currently, India produces various kinds of both nitrogenous and phosphatic fertilizers domestically. These include straight nitrogenous fertilizers (urea and ammonium), straight phosphatic fertilizers (single superphosphate) and complex fertilizers (like DAP). Potassic fertilizers are not manufactured domestically due to lack of indigenous reserves of potash (Leh in J&K; Bikaneer in Rajasthan by GSI, India), the main input. The capacity of nitrogenous fertilizer has almost doubled with the commissioning of large-sized gas-based fertilizer plants in the 1980s. While most of the nitrogenous fertilizer production capacity can be found in the public sector, phosphatic fertilizer capacity is mainly installed in the private sector.

For nitrogenous fertilizer capacity the share of the public sector has been declining over time. With the introduction of co-operative units (IFFCO, KRIBHCO) and policy changes towards greater investment in the private sector the share of the public sector started to decline and that of the private and co-operative sector to improve. Regarding phosphatic fertilizer production, throughout the year, the private sector has always enjoyed the highest share of up to more than 70%. Today, the co-operative sector assumes a major role within the fertilizer industry not only in fertilizer distribution but also in the provision of other general services to farmers such as credit programs, capital management, technical assistance, etc.

Although the Indian fertilizer sector progressed considerably over the past, there are various problems associated with the sector. These problems mainly relate to investment into capacity upgradation and expansion, to profitability of operation, and to availability, storage and transportation of raw materials and finished products.

Fertilizer consumption in India has increased significantly in the last three decades. Total NPK (N, P_2O_5 and K_2O) consumption increased nine-fold (from 2 million to 30.5 million tonnes) between 1969/1970 and 2011/12. Per-hectare NPK consumption increased from 11 to 143.13 kg in the same period. After reaching a record level in 1999/2000, fertilizer consumption in India has been irregular up to 2003/04. From 2005/06 onwards the consumption increased at a steady rate (Table 1.8).

Table 1.8:   Growth in fertilizer consumption in India

Year	Fertilizer (NPK) consumption	
	(million tonnes)	(kg/ha)
1969/70	1.98	11.04
1979/80	5.26	30.99
1989/90	11.57	63.47
1999/2000	18.07	94.90
2000/01	16.70	89.30
2001/02	17.36	92.80
2002/03	16.09	86.01
2003/04	16.80	89.80
2004/05	18.39	104.5
2005/06	20.34	112.76
2006/07	20.67	113.4
2007/08	22.57	121.6
2008/09	23.78	127.2
2009/10	26.48	135.27
2010/11	28.3	141.3
2011/12	30.5	143.13

Source: Fertilizer Association of India

Fertilizer Use by Agro-ecological Zone (AEZ)

Fertilizer consumption varies widely between the AEZ owing to the substantial differences in soil type, fertility status, crop, weather, rainfall, irrigation facilities, etc. AEZ 4 (Semi-Arid) was the most important region in terms of fertilizer use and consumption. In six AEZs namely 2 (Arid), 4, 6, 7 (Semi-Arid), 9 and 13 (Sub-Humid) the annual fertilizer consumption has exceeded one million tonnes and together they accounted for about 65 per cent of total fertilizer consumption.

Fertilizer Use by Crop

Before the 1950s, fertilizer use was very low and was confined to plantation crops. The introduction of fertilizer-responsive HYVs and expansion in the irrigated area led to a sharp increase in fertilizer application on field crops. Per-hectare fertilizer consumption is higher in the case of crops with a larger proportion of irrigated area. About 40 per cent of the agricultural area in India is irrigated, accounting for 68.5 per cent of total fertilizer consumption. Six crops (rice, wheat, cotton, sugarcane, rapeseed and mustard) are estimated to account for more than two-thirds of the total fertilizer consumption in the country.

Past and Future Demand

Fertilizer consumption depends on various factors. These include agricultural related factors such as geographical aspects, calamities, rainfall and irrigation patterns, soil quality, farming methods, availability of technology and information, varieties and qualities of seeds as well as access to capital and other inputs. Additionally, fertilizer consumption depends on more macro-oriented factors such as market forces and policies regarding demand and supply. The introduction of high-yielding varieties of seeds and the greater awareness of the benefits of fertilizers – spread out through government initiated extension networks that started in the 1960s – significantly spurred the production and consumption of fertilizers. As shown in Table 1.8 fertilizer consumption more than doubled between 1980 and 1990. Imports during the same time period did not increase. Rising consumption could entirely be met by increasing production. The increase in consumption and production in the 1980s was made possible to a large extent by tremendous subsidies provided by the government. However, the consumption of phosphatic fertilizers which cannot be produced domestically remained rather stagnant. The optimal mix of fertilizer components depends on the variety of seeds to be grown and the soil quality specific to the region. To assure more efficient use of fertilizer the government has promoted the setting up of soil testing laboratories throughout the country at district level KVK. However, more recently in the progress of liberalization, industry policy and subsidy schemes moved towards supporting nitrogenous fertilizers relatively more than phosphatic and potassic fertilizers. This has led to a shift in the consumption of nutrients away from a generalized ideal fertilizer balance of 4:2:1 NPK to a ratio of 5.9:2.4:1 NPK in nineties and further to 8.5:2.5:1 NPK in the present era reducing the economic and ecological productivity of fertilizer substantially. Due to continued increase in population and food requirements, demand for fertilizer is expected to further grow at an optimistically stable mix of nutrients (6.8:2.1:1 NPK). This will help to substantiate agricultural growth.

1.8 FATE AND REACTIONS IN THE SOIL

Reactions of Nitrogenous Fertilizer

Urea and ammonium sulphate are widely used in the tropics and are best applied in bands or placed or given as split applications. Urea is also applied as a foliar spray. However, urea applied as a foliar spray provides the quickest possible N supply, but for this purpose the biuret content must be below 0.3%. Calcium nitrate is not widely used commercially because it is deliquescent. However, it has been used in experiments to supply nitrate (NO_3) for comparison with ammonium (NH_4) fertilizers. Amide N, e.g. as urea, must first be transformed to ammonium as a result of microbial action which is dependent upon temperature.

Decomposition of urea ($CO(NH_2)_2$) to NH_4 through the ubiquitously present enzyme urease is temperature-dependent and takes about a week. Transformation from NH_4 to nitrite (NO_2) by *Nitrosomonas* bacteria, depends on soil pH and temperature, whereas further oxidation of NO_2 to NO_3 by the bacteria *Nitrobacter* and *Nitrosolobus* is rapid.

$$CO(NH_2)_2 + H_2O \xrightarrow{\text{Urease}} 2NH_3 + CO_2$$

$$2NH_4^+ + 3O_2 \xrightarrow{\text{Nitrosomonas}} 2NO_2^- + 2H_2O + 4H+$$

$$2 NO_2^- + O_2 \xrightarrow{\text{Nitrobacter}} 2NO_3^-$$

Nitrate N in the soil solution is immediately available and thus acts quickly but is most liable to leaching. Plants take up N mainly in nitrate form. Ammonium N, although fully available, has a somewhat slower effect, because it is first adsorbed and then only gradually released and nitrified. When urea and urea-ammonium-nitrate (UAN) solutions are applied to bare soil, there is a risk of large losses of ammonia (NH_3) by volatilization. To minimize such losses, such fertilizers should be immediately incorporated into at least the top few centimetres of soil. The efficiency with which urea is used in the tropics can be improved by addition of a urease inhibitor, such as heavy metals (Cd, Cr, Pb, As) N-(n-butyl) thiophosphoric triamide (NBTPT) or phenylphosphodiamidate (PPD), which inhibits the activity of urease for about two weeks. In an experiment with ^{15}N-labelled urea, the loss of NH_3 from the soil was less with urea plus PPD than from calcium ammonium nitrate (CAN), but the largest loss was from urea alone. Such inhibitors have gained practical and commercial importance.

Nitrification can be delayed for several weeks by adding special nitrification inhibitors to the fertilizer. This can be useful for preventing an undesirable accumulation of nitrate in vegetable crops or reducing loss by leaching. The efficiency of urea and NH_4-containing N fertilizers such as AS and ASN can also be improved through the addition of a nitrification inhibitor such as dicyandiamide (DCD), DCD/1,2,4-Triazol (a mixed stabilizer) or 3,4- dimethylpyrazole-phosphate (DMPP). When such inhibitors are incorporated in NH_4-containing fertilizers such as AS and ASN or urea, the efficiency of N use is improved. The rates (1% relative to the content of NH_4N/Amide-N) used vary according to the specific activity of the inhibitor. In addition, the pH rise (>8) during urea hydrolysis may promote NH_3 volatilization losses.

The NO_3 and NH_4 supplied through mineral N fertilizers have quite different effects in the soil-plant continuum in arid region as compared to humid region. When taken up by crops, NO_3 causes an increased efflux of bicarbonate ions (HCO_3) and an increase in soil pH, while that of NH_4 leads to an enhanced proton release and a decrease in soil pH (Fig. 1.5). This acidifying effect of NH_4 can be increased when a nitrification inhibitor is applied and this increased acidity can improve Zn uptake.

Most N fertilizers tend to act rather too quickly. This means that high rates given wholly at sowing time often provide too much for the young plant but not enough during the later stages. This can be compensated by dividing the total N application between a basal application at sowing and one or more topdressings. The N supply from slow release fertilizers is theoretically better adapted to the curve of N uptake but depends on temperature. Being more expensive, they are mostly confined to high value crops.

N dynamics in soils are very complex (Fig. 1.6). The important process of nitrification (microbial mediated transformation of ammonium to nitrate) proceeds rather quickly when temperatures are warm. At temperatures of 20–25 °C an application supplying 50–100 kg/ha N would nitrify in about one to two weeks. The utilization rate of N in fertilizers is mostly about 50–70% during the first year.

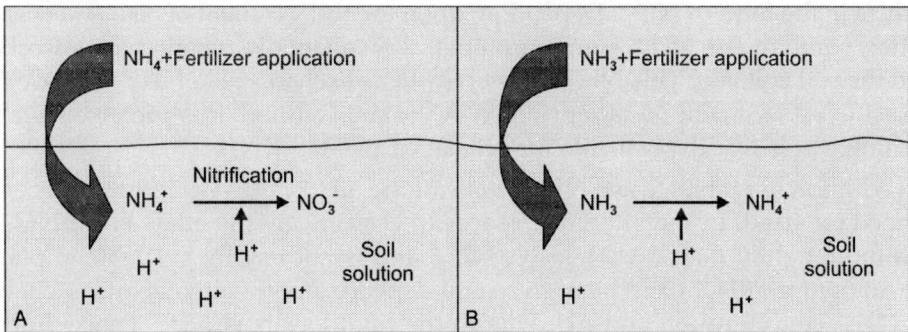

Fig. 1.5: Effects of NH_4^+(A) and NH_3 (B) fertilizer applications on pH. Through nitrification, H^+ ions are released to the soil, there by decreasing pH(A). In contrast conversion of NH_3 to NH_4^+ takes up H^+ from soil solution, thereby temporarily increasing soil pH (B)

In terms of energy the production of 1 kg N in fertilizer requires the equivalent of about 1 litre of oil. On the contrary, the energy output of the principal crops is about two to three times the energy input. More effective fertilizer use, particularly of N fertilizers, therefore means a saving in energy.

Factors Affecting the Efficient Use of Nitrogen Fertilizers

The supply of N limits the growth and productivity of non-leguminous crops more often than the supply of any other mineral nutrient.

When fertilizer N is applied to soil, the N changes from one form to another, or is transformed. Most of the transformations are brought about by microorganisms in the soil. The nature and extent of the transformations ultimately determine the fate of the fertilizer N, its availability to the crop, and its pollution potential. Among the possible transformations that can occur are:

1. Fixation of ammonium (NH_4^+) by clay (2:1 expanding type).
2. Volatilization of NH_4^+, with gaseous loss of ammonia (NH_3) at high pH and temperature.
3. Nitrification – the conversion of NH_4^+ to nitrite (NO_2^-) and then nitrate (NO_3^-).
4. Immobilization – the uptake of NH_4^+ or NO_3^- by soil microorganisms.
5. Mineralization – the release of NH_4^+ from organic forms by microorganisms.
6. Denitrification – the conversion of NO_3^- or NO_2^- to gaseous forms of N, either dinitrogen (N_2) or nitrous oxide (N_2O).

The N transformations that occur after application of N fertilizer to soil depend upon many factors, including weather conditions (i.e. temperature and precipitation), soil properties (e.g. organic matter and clay content), and the type of fertilizer applied.

Ammonium Fixation: The number of possible N transformations is greater for NH_4^+ or NH_4^+-producing (e.g., urea) fertilizers, than for fertilizer in which all of the N is in the form of NO_3^-: Depending upon the soil's content of clay and organic matter, some of the NH_4^+ from ammoniacal fertilizers is retained, or adsorbed, onto the soil colloids. This NH_4^+ is referred to as exchangeable NH_4^+ because it is subject to replacement by other cations in the soil solution. It is protected against leaching, yet is readily available for uptake by plants.

In addition to exchangeable NH_4^+, some of the NH_4^+ added as fertilizer becomes trapped, or fixed, in the interlayer spaces of certain clay minerals. Fixed NH_4^+ is held more tightly than exchangeable NH_4^+ and is not readily available to plants. The amount of NH_4^+ fixed by a given soil depends upon many factors, including the NH_4^+ concentration and pH. Due to the high localized NH_4^+ concentration, fixation is likely to be greatest when an ammoniacal fertilizer is applied in a band, as in the case of anhydrous NH_3, or in the microsite surrounding a fertilizer granule. Fixation has been found to decrease markedly under acidic conditions, which suggests that very little fixation may occur when N is applied in the form of mono- or diammonium phosphate (MAP or DAP). However, experimental support for this view is lacking, as is evidence from a direct comparison that NH_4^+ fixation is greatest with anhydrous NH_3 or in the immediate vicinity of a dissolving fertilizer granule.

Ammonia Volatilization: Ammonia volatilization refers to the process by which gaseous NH_3 escapes from the soil into the atmosphere. It can occur whenever free NH_3 is present near the soil surface. The NH_3 is derived from NH_4^+ in the soil solution via the equilibrium,

$$NH_4^+ \leftrightarrow NH_3(\text{solution}) + H^+$$

Volatile loss of NH_3 results from the reaction,

$$NH_3(\text{solution}) \leftrightarrow NH_3(\text{air})$$

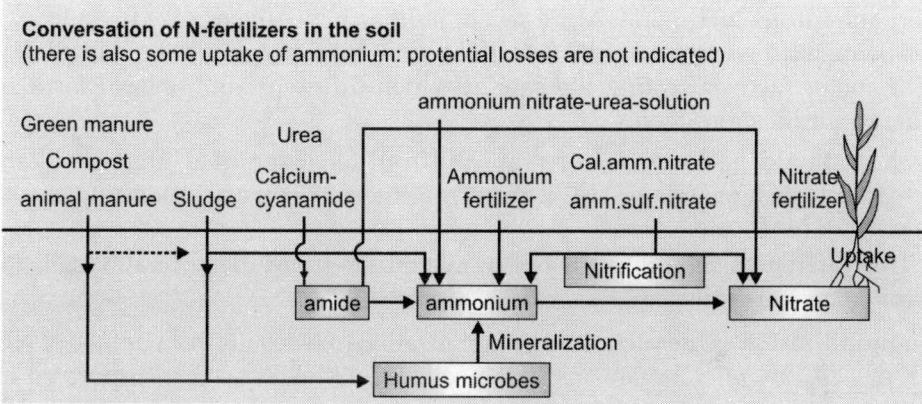

Fig. 1.6: Conversion of N-fertilizers in the soil (Courtesy: IFA, Paris)

Volatilization of NH_3, however, is governed by the chemical equilibrium between NH_4^+ and NH_3 and the equilibrium between aqueous and gaseous NH_3.

$$CO(NH_2)_2 + H_2O \xrightarrow{\text{urease}} (NH_4)_2 CO_3$$

$$(NH_4)_2 CO_3 \xrightarrow{H_2O} 2NH_3 + CO_2$$

$$NH_4^+ + OH \longrightarrow NH_3 + H_2O$$

$$NH_3(\text{aq}) \longrightarrow NH_3(\text{g})$$

Hydrolysis of urea increases the pH, resulting in higher concentrations of OH in the solution. This forces the equilibrium of NH_4^+ - NH_3 to the right, thus stimulating NH_3 production. The rate of volatilization of NH_3 is linearly related to the vapour pressure of NH_3 in the solution, which is linearly related to the concentration of NH_3 in the solution, and is furthermore temperature-dependent. The rate of volatilization also depends on wind speed.

The magnitude of loss depends upon the NH_4^+ concentration, pH, soil type, temperature, and mosisture content. Extensive loss of NH_3 can occur when anhydrous NH_3 is applied under conditions where the applicator slit does not seal properly, but losses can also be serious with other NH_4^+ or NH_4^+-producing fertilizers, particularly if they are applied to a neutral or calcareous soil or to a soil having a low cation-exchange capacity. In such cases, losses will be greater with urea than with an acidic material such as ammonium sulfate [$(NH_4)_2SO_4$] or DAP.

Nitrification: In most agricultural soils, NH_4^+ from fertilizer is readily converted to NO_3^- by the process of nitrification. The change occurs in two steps: NH_4^+ is first converted to NO_2^-, and the NO_2^- is then converted to NO_3^-. Nitrification is carried out largely by rather a select group of soil microorganisms and, for that reason, the process is quite sensitive to environmental conditions. Nitrification is favored by a high pH (the optimum is around 8.5), although it does not occur under the extreme conditions of high pH and high NH_4^+/NH_3 concentrations that exist at the center of an anhydrous NH_3 band. More recent studies have given mixed results, with urea being nitrified more rapidly than $(NH_4)_2SO_4$ in most cases, but not in all. If pH is the major factor affecting the rate at which different ammoniacal fertilizers undergo nitrification, then:

- NO_3^- should be formed more rapidly from fertilizers that give an alkaline reaction, such as urea or UAN, than from those that are acid-forming, such as MAP or DAP; and
- The differences should be greater in magnitude for acidic or neutral soils than for calcareous soils.

Immobilization-mineralization: Immobilization of N results from uptake of NH_4^+ and/or NO_3^- by microorganisms in the soil. The N taken up is incorporated into proteins, nucleic acids, and other organic N constituents of microbial cells and cell walls; as such, it becomes part of the biomass. As the microbes die and decay, some of the biomass N is released as NH_4^+ through the process of mineralization; the remainder undergoes conversion to more stable organic N compounds, ultimately becoming a part of soil organic matter. The stabilized organic compounds are not readily available to plants; therefore, the net result of immobilization-mineralization is a decrease in the availability of the N added to soil as fertilizer, and also the partial conversion of this N to a form that is not subject to loss from the soil, except by erosion. The microorganisms responsible for immobilization utilize NH_4^+ in preference to NO_3^- which accounts for reports that immobilization-mineralization is more extensive with ammoniacal fertilizers than with NO_3^- fertilizers. But it is also important to recognize that, like other biological N transformations, immobilization-mineralization is affected by environmental conditions, and this can lead to differences among ammoniacal fertilizers in the rate and extent of incorporation of NH_4^+-N into organic forms due to their effects on soil pH.

Denitrification: When soils are saturated with water, gaseous loss of N can occur as a result of bacterial denitrification. This process involves the conversion of NO_3^-

and NO_2^- to the gases, N_2 and N_2O, which escape from the soil. Ammonium-N is not subject to denitrification (it must first be converted to NO_2^- or NO_3^-), but there is evidence that N_2O can be produced during the conversion of NH_4^+ to NO_3^- by nitrifying microorganisms present in soils. Field studies indicate that emission of N_2O is greater for ammoniacal fertilizers than for NO_3^- fertilizers and that emission is much greater with anhydrous NH_3 than with other N fertilizers.

Reactions of Phosphate Fertilizer

Soil Phosphorus Reactions

a. *General considerations:* Phosphorus reactions and availability in soil: Phosphorus is generally very insoluble in soil; there is only a small concentration of soluble P in the soil solution; there is a whole array of possible soil reactions that take fertilizer P out of solution, making it less available to plants.

b. *Quantity and intensity factors*

   i. Quantity factor can be small or large, and can include all forms of P in the soil (including apatite, which is very insoluble).

   ii. Monocalcium phosphate (that form of P in SSP and TSP) is the only calcium phosphate compound that is water-soluble. Plants absorb either $H_2PO_4^-$ or $H(PO_4)_2$.

   iii. The first reaction of monocalcium phosphate (MCP) in the soil is to form dicalcium phosphate, $CaHPO_4$, which is somewhat soluble; weak acids do dissolve this material, so it may or may not be available depending on soil conditions.

   iv. The quantity factor is directly related to soil solution P; soil solution P may range from 0.03 to 0.5 ppm; 0.5 ppm is very high; 0.2 ppm is considered adequate or sufficient.

   Example: if the soil solution P concentration was 0.25 ppm and citrus needs to take up 160 kg P_2O_5 per acre, how many times would the quantity factor equilibrium need to turn over to make that amount of P available?

   (0.25 ppm P) × 2.29 = 0.6 ppm P_2O_5 or 1.2 kg P_2O_5/acre

   160 kg P_2O_5 required/acre ÷ 1.2 kg P_2O_5/acre in solution = 134

   Thus, the soil solution has to be renewed 134 times by the quantity factor.

   v. Soil solution P moves by diffusion to the root; the distance over which this occurs is 1/8 to 1/4 inch; the P must be this close or it will become tied up before it gets to root; roots must "grow" towards the soil P.

   vi. The temperature influences the release of soil P into solution P because it affects the solubility of the various forms of soil P; thus, P is more available during the warmer seasons.

c. *Forms of phosphorus in soil*
   i. *Acid soils* (pH less than 5):
      1. If soluble phosphorus is added, it ends up as aluminum or iron phosphate ($AlPO_4$ or $FePO_4$):
         a. $AlPO_4.2H_2O$ Variscite (insoluble)
         b. $FePO_4.2H_2O$ Strengite (insoluble)
      2. Can have many different combinations of Al, NH_4, K, Ca, Fe with phosphate.
   ii. *Calcareous soils* (pH greater than 7)
      1. Get transformations of phosphate over time; each transformation results in a compound that is less water soluble than the one before:
         a. $Ca(H_2PO_4)$ Monocalcium phosphate (sol. 15 g/L)
         b. $CaHPO_4$ Dicalcium phosphate (sol. 0.25 g/L)
         c. $Ca_3(PO_4)_2$ Tricalcium phosphate (sol. 0.02 g/L)
         d. $[Ca_3(PO_4)_2]_3 . Ca(OH)_2$ Hydroxy apatite
         e. $[Ca_3(PO_4)_2]_3 . CaF$ Apatite
      2. Time affects P availability to plants; calcium phosphate is converted to less and less available forms of P; if excess Ca is available in the soil, it will react with P.
   iii. Best pH for soil phosphorus availability is 6.6 to 7.3 (same as the best pH range for agronomic crops).

d. *Factors influencing phosphorus retention in soils*
   i. Nature and amount of soil components
      1. Iron and aluminum compounds (in acid soils) and calcium (in alkaline soils) will precipitate P (phosphorus fixation).
      2. Phosphorus retention increases as soil clay concentration increases.
      3. The activity of phosphorus will be lower in soils with a large concentration of highly-reactive calcium carbonate.
   ii. *Cation effects*: Soils containing large amounts of Ca_2^+ can retain greater amounts of phosphorus than if other ions like K^+ or Na^+ are present.
   iii. *Organic matter*: Phosphorus bound to organic matter or in organic compounds can move to greater depths in the soil than can dissolved inorganic phosphorus.
   iv. Coated vs. uncoated sands
      1. Some sands are coated with iron and aluminum oxides, so they are able to trap and fix phosphorus through formation of Fe/Al phosphates.
      2. Uncoated sandy layers (usually white in color) have no mechanism to fix phosphorus, so P is able to leach until encountering a soil layer that can trap it (a clay or spodic layer).

For phosphatic fertilizer, availability is measured by solubility in specified extractants as an indication of the rate of transformation under various soil conditions. Water-soluble P (e.g. mono-calcium phosphate) is easily available to plants and remains available, though to a somewhat lesser extent after immobilization into other forms, this transformation being retarded by granulation and placement of the fertilizer. Citrate/citric acid-soluble P is moderately available to plants and is suitable for many purposes over a wide range of acidic to neutral soil conditions except where quick action is required. Formic acid-soluble P in soft powdery rock phosphate is only very slowly available to plants; its reactivity (release of soluble P) is somewhat better where soils are warmer, moister and more acidic, but still above the acidity damage range.

A fascinating, complex series of chemical events takes place when a soluble P fertilizer contacts the soil. Almost immediately the P is converted to the most stable form possible in the soil. These stable forms are less available to plants, because they do not dissolve easily in the soil water. Instead they react with other soil components and become part of the soil solids. In essence, the fertilizer P becomes soil P. The conversion from "fertilizer" P to "soil" P is called fixation. In some soils the fixation process is very rapid, and the final forms of soil P are quite unavailable to plants. In most soils the conversion occurs more slowly, and the final forms are more available. Phosphorus from fertilizer is most available immediately after application. However, residual benefits occur in most soils for many years. Phosphorus from livestock manure reacts similarly. However, most of the P from the source is in organic forms and must be broken down by microbes (PSB, mycorrhiza) to be available to plants. Once this breakdown occurs, the P from manure is subject to the same chemical reactions in the soil as is fertilizer P. Also, at this point, there is no difference in the P derived from soil organic matter and manure and that supplied in commercial fertilizer. The tendency of P to react quickly with the soil greatly limits its mobility in the soil. It does not move appreciably from the point of application and is not subject to being leached from the root zone. It is lost only through crop removal and soil erosion.

On acid soils containing a large amount of clay, however, the soluble P can be rapidly converted into more stable P compounds and this reduces the opportunity for immediate uptake by the plant. By comparison, in a weekly buffered soil, a good response can even be obtained when 35 kg/ha P_2O_5 is applied to crops. Root crops, have a larger demand for P. Placement (banding) (Fig. 1.7) of phosphate close to the seeds or roots enhances response, while coating seeds with phosphate can help satisfy the plant's large demand for P during early growth.

Under conditions of intensive farming on well, or quite well supplied soils, for most purposes, the common phosphate fertilizers give about an equal yield response per unit of 'available' P_2O_5. Water-soluble P, however, is superior for crops with a short growing season and limited root system in deficient soils. The dynamics of phosphate fertilizers in soil is illustrated in Fig. 1.8.

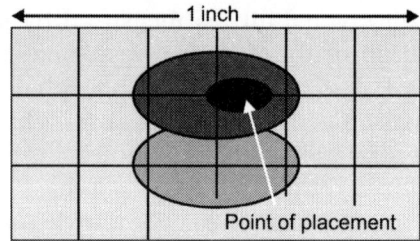

Fig. 1.7: Phosphorus fertilizer moves very little in the soil, so it must be placed where the plant roots can intercept it

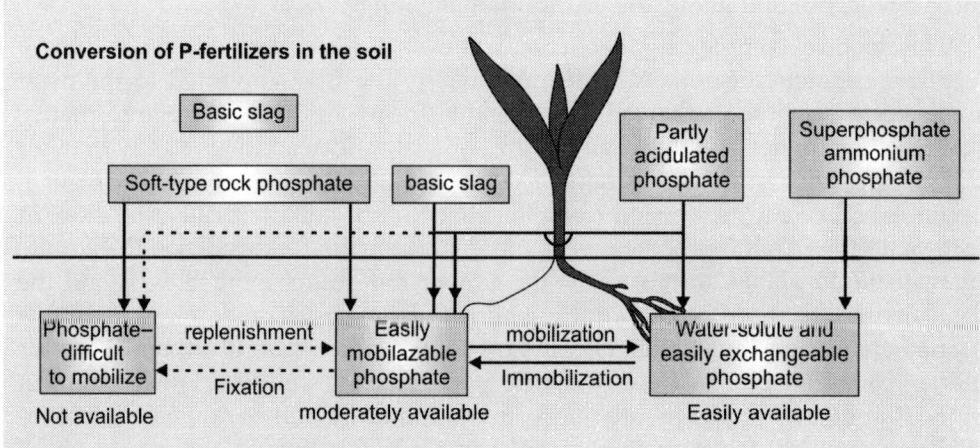

Fig. 1.8: Conversion of P-fertilizers in the soil (Courtesy: IFA, Paris)

NP fertilizers are generally superior in placement application; gaseous losses may occur from surface-applied diammonium phosphate on neutral soils. The utilization rate of P in fertilizers is usually about 15% in the first year but only 1–2% per year thereafter, with the result that only about two-thirds is taken up by the end of thirty years.

Most polyphosphate fertilizers will have 40 to 60% of the phosphorus remaining in the orthophosphate form. In the soil, polyphosphate ions readily convert to orthophosphate ions in the presence of soil water. This conversion is rapid and, with normal soil temperatures, can be complete in days or less. This conversion process is enhanced by an enzyme called pyrophosphatase, which is abundant in most soils.

In Africa, South America and many parts of India there are many indigenous PR deposits of sedimentary and igneous origin with a total P content of about 25% P_2O_5. Although not all are suitable for upgrading to soluble P fertilizers, some are quite reactive, as measured by their solubility in 2% citric or formic acid. Such PRs can be used to supply both P and Ca provided that they contain only small amounts of impurities, like cadmium. The effectiveness of a PR depends not only on its reactivity but also on the degree of fineness of the particles. Finely ground PRs of high reactivity are suitable for direct application on acid soils giving a long-lasting effect of P and Ca provided that sufficient PR is applied.

Significant increase in the availability of P in PRs can be achieved by partial acidulation, i.e. by treating the PR with less sulphuric acid than the amount required to make SSP. There are other ways also. These include mixing the PR with elemental S or compacting the PR with AS to which a nitrification inhibitor has been added. They can also be added to compost of organic wastes, like straw, molasses and manure, from plant or animal production. During microbial decomposition of the organic material, organic acids and chelates are produced. Organic acids like oxalic and tartaric acid will solubilize PRs directly and chelates will combine with Ca ions from apatites. Both processes increase P availability. Although PRs are only sparingly soluble in neutral to alkaline soils, in the presence of active plant roots, the pH in the rhizosphere can drop by 2 pH units and, in the acid conditions, the solubility of the PR, and hence plant availability of the P, will increase. To achieve such an effect, the PR must be placed near to the roots to minimize the interaction of the P that has been released with soil components.

Reactions of Pottasic Fertilizer

Potassium chloride (muriate of potash, MOP) as fine crystals can be readily incorporated into granular compound fertilizers. As compacted particles it can be used in blends of different fertilizers to give required ratios of N:P:K. Potassium sulphate (sulphate of potash, SOP) is more expensive per tonne K_2O than MOP but it contains two nutrients, K and S. It tends to be used for high value crops and those where it can be shown to improve crop quality, e.g. starch levels in potatoes and the smoking quality of tobacco. It can also be used to advantage on saline soils in arid and semi-arid areas. Potassium nitrate (NOP) also contains two nutrients, K and N as NO_3, which is readily available for uptake by plant roots. Both SOP and NOP are idealy suited for use in fustigation systems because they can be obtained as very pure salts and they are readily soluble in water.

Adding potassium fertilizer causes a rapid increase in the concentration of solution potassium. As a result, potassium ions can enter clay particles through openings in the layers (2.8 A°) a process known as potassium fixation. Although some potassium can enter deep into the interlayer space (especially if it is held open by larger ions), most of the potassium ends up deposited towards the outer margin of the layer. This potassium can be slowly released over time. How much potassium can be fixed by any one soil depends on the type of clays within that soil, and on how much potassium they already contain. Hydrous micas and 2:1 illite clays have a high capacity for fixing potassium.

Some potassium added to soil will bind to negative sites on the surface of soil particles. The amount of this exchangeable potassium in a soil depends on the cation exchange capacity (CEC) of the soil, and on the levels of other cations (positively charged ions) in the soil. The CEC is simply a measurement of a soil's potential to bind cations. It reflects the amount of negative charge in the soil. This in turn is dependent upon the blend of organic matter and types of clay minerals in the soil, as well as the pH. Exchangeable potassium can easily be released into soil solution.

Soil solution potassium is available for uptake by plants or micro-organisms. However, it is also vulnerable to loss by leaching. This is particularly an issue in soils that do not have a large capacity to fix potassium (i.e. are low in hydrous micas and illite clays), and in soils that have a low CEC (because there is little space available for potassium to bind). Leaching of potassium is common in sandy and silty soils, with the greatest losses occurring when soils at field capacity are further wetted by irrigation or rainfall. When this happens, drainage occurs, and potassium ions are leached out in this drainage water.

There is no shortage of K fertilizers worldwide and K has no adverse environmental impact. However, K fertilizers are not used as widely as they should be in many countries in the tropics and subtropics. Where increase in crop yield has not been observed in many field experiments. This would imply that sufficient K has been available from soil reserves to meet the requirements of the crops grown. However, this process of soil mining cannot go on forever without seriously jeopardizing soil fertility and food security. Efforts are required through knowledge transfer with reference to moblization of fixed K^+ through microbial mediation.

1.9   SECONDARY MICRONUTRIENT FERTILIZERS

Secondary Nutrient Fertilizers

Magnesium: Magnesium fertilizers are either quick-acting soluble salts (mainly sulphates) or in slow-acting form (their nutrient content may be expressed in terms of either Mg or MgO).

Quick-acting types:
- Magnesium sulphate, in the forms of Epsom salts (10% Mg) or Kieserite (16% Mg);
- Potassium magnesium sulphate.

Slow-acting:
- Magnesium carbonate (dolomitic lime).

The utilization rate and potential leaching loss of water-soluble Mg are similar to K. For soils needing liming, the cheapest source of Mg is a lime containing Mg, of which a high rate of application can ensure a good supply of Mg for several years without detrimental effect.

Common Magnesium Sources

Material	Per cent Mg
Dolomitic limestone (Mg Carbonate)	3–12
Magnesia (Mg oxide)	55-60
Basic slag	3
Magnesium sulphate	9–20
Potassium-magnesium sulphate	11
Magnesium chloride	7.5

Sulphur: The increasing incidence of sulphur deficiency, especially in crops with high requirements such as oilseed rape and legumes, has considerably increased the use of sulphur fertilizers. Water-soluble sulphates, e.g. potassium sulphate or magnesium sulphate (18% S), are most effective for the treatment of growing crops, as also is ammonium sulphate (24% S) where its acidifying effect can provide an added benefit. Slower-acting types such as pure gypsum (18% S) or the by-product calcium sulphate of superphosphate (14% S) should be used if leaching poses a problem. Elemental (yellow) sulphur (100% S) may be applied either in powdered form or as the coating in sulphur-coated urea (10–20% S). Both the water-soluble and slower-acting forms are suitable for application at sowing time.

Common Sulphur Sources

Material	Chemical formula	Per cent S
Ammonium sulphate	$(NH_4)_2 SO_4$	24
Ammonium thiosulphate	$(NH_4)S_2O_3 \, 5H_2$	26
Ammonium polysulphide	$(NH_4)_2S_x$	40-50
Potassium sulphate	K_2SO_4	18
Potassium-magnesium sulphate	$K_2SO_4 . 2MgSO_4$	22
Elemental sulphur	S	>85
Gypsum	$CaSO_4 . 2H_2O$	12–18
Magnesium sulphate	$MgSO_4 . 7H_2O$	14

Calcium: Calcium is only applied other than for liming in cases of definite deficiency. Sources which do not raise the pH are:

Quick-acting:

- Calcium chloride, solid or in solution;
- Ca components of foliar sprays.

Slow-acting: gypsum.

Soil application, though simple, is often disappointing because of restricted translocation within the plant; in such cases a foliar spray is preferable.

Common Calcium Sources

Material	Per cent Ca	Relative neutralizing value*
Calcitic limestone	32	95–108; 85–100
Dolomitic limestone	29	50–70
Basic slag	22	None
Gypsum	22	15–85
Mari	24	120–135
Hydrated lime	46	150–175
Burned lime	60	150–175

*Based on pure calcium carbonate at 100%

Sixteen elements are essential for plant growth out of these Fe, Zn, Mn, Cu, B, Mo, Cl are required in small quantities. They are called tertiary or micronutrient. The average concentration of these nutrient in soil are Mn 1000 ppm, Cl 480 ppm, Zn 80 ppm, Cu 70 ppm, B 10 ppm, Mo 2 to 3 ppm, iron 140 ppm. Apart from the widespread recognized areas of natural deficiencies of micronutrients, attention should be given to the possibility that they may become critical "minimum factors" as other critical factors are amended and yield levels rise. They may be applied either as single-nutrient fertilizers or as supplements in macronutrient fertilizers. The quickest and commonest method of correcting deficiencies is by foliar application.

Development of micronutrient deficiency: The micronutrient deficiency occurs under conditions of:

1. Soils with a very high organic matter content (peat and muck soils)
2. Soils with very high or very low pH.
3. High doses of commercial inorganic fertilizers.
4. Highly leached acid and sandy soil.
5. Soils with impeded drainage or high water table.
6. Overliming of the soil.
7. Intensive cultivation.

The deficiencies may be overcome by addition of more than one micronutrients. If more than one micronutrients are applied it is called multinutrients. The information on sources of micronutrients, their formulae, solubility and nutrient content is given in Table 1.9.

Copper: Copper deficiency may most easily be corrected for a longer period by soil application of 5 kg/ha Cu as Cu sulphate or oxides, etc. Chelates or neutralized Cu sulphate (25% Cu) are suitable for foliar spraying of deficient crops.

Zinc: Zinc is usually applied to deficient crops as a foliar spray of Zn sulphate (e.g. 23% Zn) or Zn chelate (e.g. Zn-EDTA) @ 0.5 g/L water, for soil application a rate of 5–10 kg/ha Zn is recommended.

Boron: Boron needs vary widely. As a prophylactic treatment for crops with high demands, soil application of borax (11% or 22% B) is advisable, the rate depending on the crop (0.5–2.0 kg/ha B), or foliar (solubor - 1 g/L 20% B) but no more should be given than needed for that crop in order to avoid the risk of a damaging surplus affecting a succeeding crop with a low requirement. A better distribution can be obtained by incorporating the boron in e.g. phosphate or multinutrient fertilizers. Polyborates seem to be superior to borax for foliar application (at about 1 kg/ha).

Manganese: Manganese deficiency occurs mainly in slightly acidic to neutral soils. Both Mn sulphate (24–32% Mn) and Mn-EDTA (13% Mn) are water-soluble and quick-acting, and are suitable for foliar or soil application; Mn oxides may be used as a means of increasing the soil's reserves. Indirect improvement of the soil supply may be achieved by using acidifying N fertilizers.

Molybdenum: Molybdenum is required in only very small amounts: 0.5–1.0 kg/ha Mo for soil application of water-soluble Na molybdate or ammonium molybdate (40–50% Mo); less than 100 g/ha Mo for foliar application.

Iron: Iron is usually applied as a foliar spray in the form of chelates such as Fe-EDTA (9% Fe) or Fe-EDDHA (6% Fe). For soil application the latter has the advantage that it is more stable in neutral soils.

Table 1.9: Micronutrient fertilizer sources, and water solubility

Source	Per cent B	Water soluble	Source	Per cent Cu	Water soluble
Borax	11.3	Yes	Copper sulphate	22.5–24	Yes
Sodium pentaborate	18.0	Yes	Copper ammonium Phosphate	30.0	Slight/ sparingly
Fertilizer Borate 46	14.0	Yes	Copper chelates	Variable	Yes
Fertilizer Borate 65	20.0	Yes	Other organic	Variable	Yes
Boric acid	17.0	Yes	**Source**	**Per cent Mn**	
Colemanite	10.0	Low	Manganese sulphate	26–30.5	
Solubor	20.0	Yes	Manganese oxide	41–68	
Boronated Single Superphosphate	0.18	Yes	Manganese chelate	12	

Contd.

Contd.

Source	Per cent Fe				
Iron sulphate	19–23		Manganese carbonate	31	
Iron oxide	69–73		Manganese chloride	17	
			Source	**Per cent Mo**	**Water soluble**
Iron ammonium sulphate	14		Ammonium molybdate	54	Yes
Iron ammonium polyphosphate	22		Sodium molybdate	39–41	Yes
Iron chelates	5–14		Molybdic acid	47.5	Slight/ sparingly
Other organics	5–10		**Source**	**Per cent Zn**	
			Zinc sulphate (hydrated)	23–36	
			Zinc Oxide	78	
			Basic Zinc sulphate	55	
			Zinc-ammonia complexes	10	
			Zinc chelates	9–14	
			Other organics	5–10	

Source	% Nutrient
Copper sulphate ($CuSO_4.5H_2O$)	25–35% Cu
Zinc sulphate ($ZnSO_4.7H_2O$)	22–35% Zn
Borax or Sod. Borate ($Na_2B_4O_7.10H_2O$)	10.6% B
Manganese Sulphate ($MnSO_4.4H_2O$)	23% Mn
Ammonium Molybdate ($(NH_4)_6Mo_7O_{24}.4H_2O$)	54% Mo
Ferrous sulphate ($FeSO_4.7H_2O$)	20% Fe

Multinutrient Fertilizers

Since crops often require an additional supply of several nutrients, special combinations with different nutrient ratios offer a considerable simplification and facilitation of fertilizer application. Most combinations are of the complex NPK-type, which contains N in part as ammonium and part as nitrate, one-third of the phosphate in water-soluble form and K mostly as chloride. Most multi-nutrient fertilizers produced are either complex fertilizers, each granule of which contains a uniform ratio of nutrients, or blends. Typically, complex NPK fertilizers are manufactured by producing slurries of ammonium phosphates, to which potassium salts are added prior to granulation or prilling. PK fertilizers, on the other hand, are generally produced as compounds by the steam granulation of superphosphates (SSP or TSP) with potassium salts.

In this category another approach is some compound has been deliberately added with any fertilizer with an aim for enhancing its nutrient value. Several common fertilizers can be fortified with compounds of nutrients such as Zn, S, B, Mo. Additional advantage of fortification is that small amounts of micronutrients needed can be uniformly applied over a field with ease. Example: single superphosphate fortified with boron (boronated SSP), urea fortified with zinc (zincated urea) and NP/NPK complexes fortified with boron or zinc.

1.10 FERTILIZER APPLICATION

Fertilizers may be applied on or into the soil or directly to the plants uniformly and effectively. The method will depend on the type of material (Fig. 1.9). The amount and timing of nutrient uptake depends on various factors, such as crop variety, planting date, crop rotation, soil and weather conditions. Timing and the quantity must be planned in such a way that as much as possible of the nutrients is used by the plants. For optimum crop use efficiency and minimum potential for environmental pollution, one must apply the nutrients as near to the time the crop needs them as is practical. This is of particular importance for mobile nutrients such as nitrogen, which can easily be leached out of the soil profile, if they are not taken up by the plant roots. In the cases of urea and DAP application, losses may occur through emission of ammonia to the air. Both these fertilizers must be incorporated into the soil immediately after application, if there is no immediate rainfall or irrigation to wash it into the soil. This is of particular importance on alkaline (calcareous) soils. All primary and secondary nutrients should be incorporated immediately after application in regions where intense rainfall is expected, to avoid losses due to run-off and erosion. When fertilizer is applied by hand, extreme care should be taken to distribute nutrients uniformly and at the exact rates. Where fertilizer application equipment is used, it should be adjusted to ensure uniform spreading and correct rates.

Mineral fertilizer application method depends according to the type of material used

- Solid water-soluble fertilizers are evenly distributed onto the soil surface or are placed directly into the root zone, e.g. beneath the seed at sowing time.
- Solid water-insoluble fertilizers are distributed on to the soil surface and mechanically mixed into the arable layer.
- Liquid fertilizers are either sprayed onto the soil surface in their original concentration and left to penetrate or mixed into the soil immediately after application or injected directly into the soil; or sprayed in diluted form directly onto the plants.
- Gaseous fertilizers are injected into the top layer of the soil at a depth of at least 10 cm.

Amendments should be evenly distributed on the soil surface to the extent possible and mixed into the arable layer, e.g. by harrow, disc harrow or plough, but some amendments need to be applied directly into the subsoil.

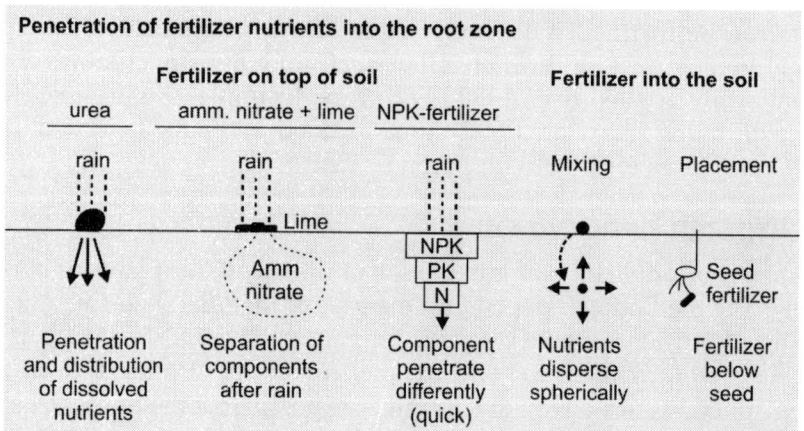

Fig. 1.9: Penetration of fertilizer nutrients into the root zone (Courtesy: IFA, Paris)

Theoretically, finely powdered material mixed thoroughly into the arable layer would give the most uniform distribution within the root zone but this is often not necessary and too costly. The use of granular fertilizer represents a compromise between uniformity of distribution and ease of application. The granule size of water-soluble fertilizers is standardized, for example 90% of the granules are at 2–5 mm. Since water-insoluble fertilizer in similar granules of this size would generally act too slowly, they are usually granulated in such a way that powdery material is only loosely connected and the granules therefore disintegrate rapidly.

The cost of distribution depends on the accuracy desired. Since medium accuracy suffices for most purposes, broadcasting by simple types of spinning disc distributors (with a spread of around 10–20 m) is very common. The amount of fertilizer to be distributed ranges from about 100 kg to more than 1500 kg per hectare.

For more precise distribution, and especially for the application of fertilizers with varying physical characteristics, pneumatic or similar types of distributors are preferred, which either blow or throw the fertilizer through a number of distribution tubes onto the soil. Such machines can cover a width ranging from 5 m up to 24 m.

Broadcasting

The broadcasting of fertilizer (i.e. applying it to the surface of a field) is used mostly on dense crops not planted in rows or in dense rows (small grains) and on grassland. It is also used when fertilizers should be incorporated into the soil after application to be effective (phosphate fertilizers), or to avoid evaporation losses of nitrogen (urea, DAP). Incorporation through tilling or ploughing-in is also recommended to increase the fertility level of the entire plough layer. Whether the fertilizer is broadcast by hand or with fertilizer spreading equipment, the spreading should be as uniform as possible.

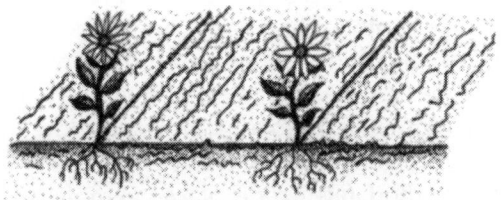

Fertilizer broadcasted between rows

Row or Band Placement

Inserting or drilling or placing the fertilizer below the soil surface by means of any tool or implement at desired depth to supply plant nutrients to crop before sowing or in the standing crop is called placement. With placement methods, fertilizers are placed in the soil irrespective of the position of seed, seedling or growing plants before sowing or after sowing the crops.

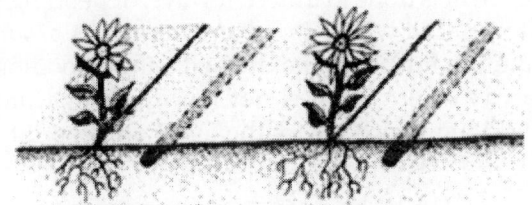

Fertilizer placed in bands beside rows

When localized fertilizer placement (putting the fertilizer only in selected places in the field) is used, the fertilizer is concentrated in specified parts of the soil during planting, which may be either in bands or strips under the surface of the soil or to the side of, and below, the seed. This can be done either by hand or by special planting and/or fertilizer drilling equipment (seed-cum-fertilizer drill). It is preferably used for row crops, which have relatively large spaces between rows (maize, cotton, and sugarcane); or on soils with a tendency to phosphate and potassium fixation; or where relatively small amounts of fertilizer are used on soils with a low fertility level.

Where crops are cultivated by hand and planted in hills, the recommended number of grams of fertilizer are placed in the row or planting hole under, or beside the seed, and covered with soil. Great care has to be taken that no fertilizer is placed either too close to the seed or to the germinating plant to avoid toxicity, i.e. salt damage to the seedling (burning of the roots). The following methods are most common in this category:

Plough-sole Placement

In this method, the fertilizer is placed in a continuous band on the bottom of the furrow during the process of ploughing. Each band is covered as the next furrow is turned. No attempt is usually made to sow the crop in any particular location with regard to the plough-sole bands. This method has been recommended in areas where the soil becomes quite dry up to a few inches below the soil surface during the growing season, and especially with soils having a heavy clay pan a little below the plough-sole. By this method, fertilizer is placed in moist soil where it can become more available to growing plants during dry seasons.

Deep Placement of Nitrogenous Fertilizers

This method of application of nitrogenous and phosphatic fertilizers is adopted in paddy fields. In this method, ammonical nitrogenous fertilizer like ammonium sulphate or ammonium forming nitrogenous fertilizer like urea, is placed in the reduction zone, where it remains in ammonia form and is available to the crop during the active vegetative period. Deep or sub-surface placement of the fertilizer also ensures better distribution in the root zone and prevents any loss by surface drain-off. Deep placement is done in different ways, depending upon the prevailing moisture. In irrigated tracts, where the water supply is assured, the fertilizer is applied under the plough furrow in the dry soil before flooding the land ready for transplanting. In areas where there is not too much of water in the field, it is broadcast before puddling which places the fertilizer deep into the root zone.

Sub-soil Placement

This refers to the placement of fertilizers in the sub-soil with the help of heavy power machinery in humid and sub-humid regions where many sub-soils are strongly acidic. Due to acidic conditions the level of available plant nutrients is extremely low. Under these conditions, fertilizers, especially phosphatic and potassic are placed in the sub-soil for better root development.

Localised Placement

This method refers to the application of fertilizers into the soil close to the seed or plant. Localised placement is usually employed when relatively small quantities of fertilizers are to be applied. Localised placement reduces fixation of phosphorus and potassium. Placement directly into the root zone ensures early accessibility of nutrients (e.g. N, P, micronutrients) to the roots of young plants and avoidance of close, overall contact between fertilizer and soil becomes feasible.

The benefit of placement is greatest, in the case of P, on P-deficient soils, in dry weather conditions, with crops in widely spaced rows (maize) and receiving relatively small amounts of fertilizer in comparison to narrower row-spacing crops (wheat) in humid areas. For micronutrients, placement can take the form of actual attachment to the seed.

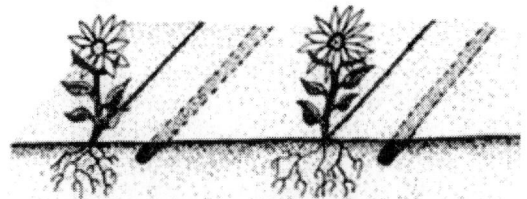

Fertilizer placed in bands beside rows

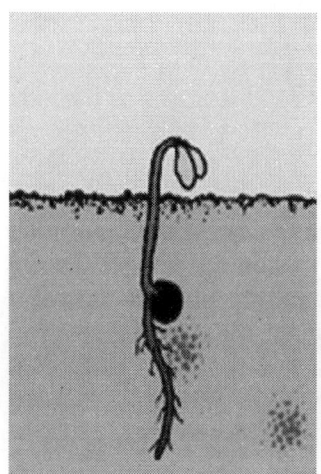 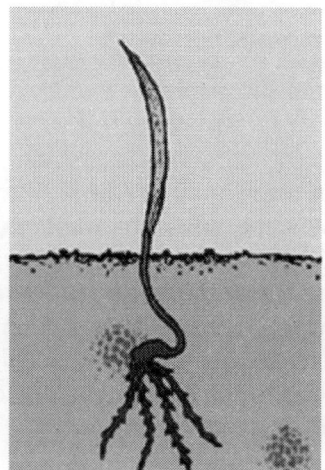 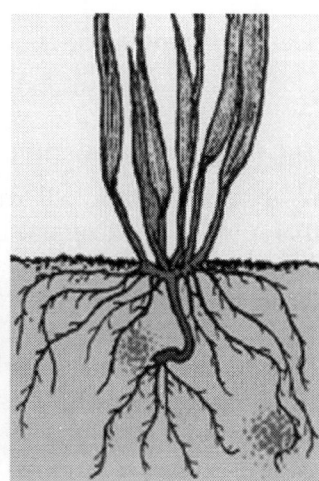

Top Dressing

Top-dressing (broadcasting the fertilizer on a standing crop) is mainly used for small and large grain crops and for forage crops. Top-dressing is a normal practice where there is a need for additional nitrogen on soils and with crops where a single application of the total nitrogen amount needed at sowing might lead to losses through leaching, or where the crops show a special need for nitrogen at certain stages of growth. The mobile nitrate moves downwards in the soil and can be taken up there by the plant roots. Top-dressing of potassium, which does not move in the soil to the same extent as nitrogen, might be recommended on light soils, i.e. applying the total amount divided into a basal dressing and top-dressing. Phosphate hardly moves in the soil at all. Hence, it is usually applied before or at sowing or planting time (basal application), preferably in combination with potassium and part of the nitrogen. The remaining nitrogen should then be applied as a top-dressing in one or more split applications.

Side Dressing

Applying fertilizer as side-dressing is the practice of putting it to the side of widely spaced plants grown in rows such as maize, cotton and sugarcane. Trees or other perennial crops also are normally side-dressed.

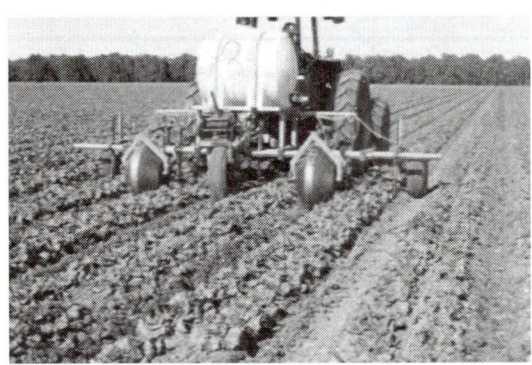

Seed cum Fertilizer Drill

Seed cum fertilizer drill is an implement useful to sow the seed in rows as well as to apply the fertilizers at the same time. The implement is designed to place the fertilizer 5 cm (2") below the seed and 5 cm (2") away from the seed avoiding fertilizer injury to the seed. Separate hoppers are provided for the seed and fertilizer. There is also arrangement to regulate the seed and fertilizer rates as per the crop requirement. This is efficient way of applying fertilizer and sowing the seed. Additionally, the drill ensures uniform stand and growth of plants. Using seed cum fertilizer drill almost all crops can be sown.

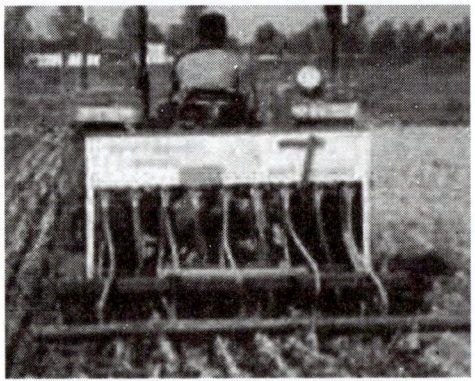

Foliar Application

Foliar application refers to the spraying on leaves of growing plants with suitable fertilizer solutions. These solutions may be prepared in a low concentration to supply any one plant nutrient or a combination of nutrients. It has been well established that all plant nutrients are absorbed through the leaves of plants and this absorption is remarkable rapid for some nutrients. Foliar application is the most efficient method of supplying micronutrients (but under a stress situation for the crop also N or NPK) which are needed only in small quantities and may become unavailable if applied to the soil. To minimize the risk of leaf scorch, the recommended concentration has to be respected and spraying should preferably be done on cloudy days and in the early morning or late afternoon.

Present research claims an efficiency ratio of between 7 or 10:1, foliar fertilizers over solid soil applied fertilizer. Plant leaves are where the all-essential photosynthesis, which turns the sun's energy, and carbon dioxide, water, nutrients and trace elements into sugars, occurs. At various stages during plant growth these sugars are converted to other complex foods required during the growth process. Foliar feeding bypasses the root-vein-leaf system and delivers vital ingredients directly to the energy conversion part of the plant an produces a quicker response to the nutrient feed. Compressed, cold or water-logged soil can kill small roots and small fragile root hairs and a foliar feed in times of plant stress can be a life-saver. The journey from the soil through the root and veins to the leaf is long and right through this process there is wastage either because of leaching from the soil, or fixation in the soil, or by the stress placed on the plant whilst achieving this process.

Foliar application does not result in a great saving of fertilizer but it may be preferred under the following conditions:

- When visual symptoms of nutrient deficiencies observed during early stages of deficiency.
- When unfavourable soil physical and chemical conditions, which reduce fertilizer use efficiency (FUE).
- During drought period where in the soil application could not be done for want of soil moisture.

There are certain difficulties associated with the foliar application of nutrients as detailed below:

- Marginal leaf burn or scorching may occur if strong solutions are used.
- As solutions of low concentrations (usually three to six per cent) are to be used, only small quantities of nutrients can be applied in single spray.
- Several applications are needed for moderate to high fertilizer rates, and hence foliar spraying of fertilizers is costly compared to soil application, unless combined with other spraying operations taken up for insect or disease control.

Spraying is most effective, and the risk of scorch is minimized, if the spray droplets do not dry too rapidly, i.e. on cloudy days and in the early morning or late afternoon. The amount of water used is often around 400 L/ha but progress is being made with lower volumes.

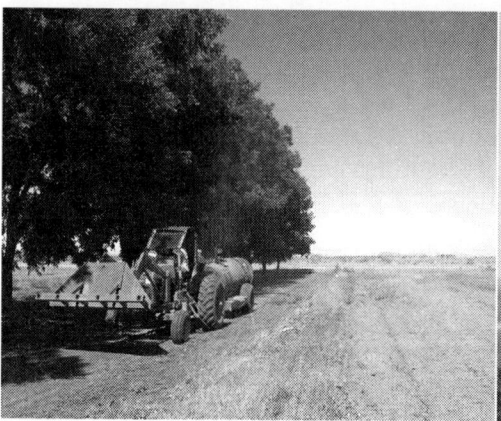 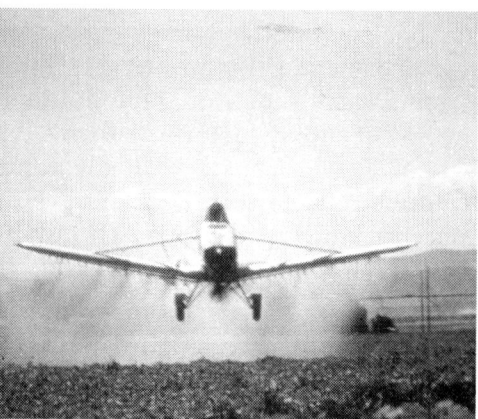

Liquid Fertilization

Liquid fertilizers are commonly described as "high energy fertilizers" provided in a form which can be readily mixed with water for application to the soil or direct to the plant. They feed the plant and the soil environment, are non-toxic and when used as directed are not harmful to beneficial insects, birds, livestock and soil micro-organisms. They can also be added to routine spray program so that two jobs can be completed with the one spraying. The use of liquid fertilizers as a means of fertilization has assumed considerable importance in foreign countries. Solutions of fertilizers, generally consisting of N, P_2O_5, K_2O in the ratio of 1:2:1 and 1:1:2 are applied to young vegetable plants at the time of transplanting. These solutions are known as 'Starter solutions'. They are used in place of the watering that is usually given to help the plants to establish. Only a small amount of fertilizer is applied as a starter solution. The starter solution has two advantages:

- The nutrients reach the plant roots immediately,
- The solution is sufficiently diluted so that it does not inhibit growth.

As such a starter solution helps rapid establishment and quick early growth. There are two disadvantages of starter solution, if watering is not a part of the regular operation–extra labour is necessary and the fixation of phosphate may be greater. Direct application of liquid fertilizers to the soil need special equipment. Special spraying machinery is needed, especially for suspensions.

Advantages of liquid fertilizations are:

- Easy transfer from one container to another by pumping,
- The accuracy of distribution,
- The speed of application (covering 5–10 ha/hr),
- The possibility of incorporating fungicides, etc. and,
- In irrigated agriculture, the ease of inclusion of fertilizer in irrigation water.

Process for Producing Liquid Fertilizers

The process for producing liquid fertilizers in high-concentration solution is characterised by reacting, under temperature and pH control, thermic polyphosphoric acid with potassium hydroxide solution to obtain a potassium polyphosphate solution which reacts with ammonium polyphosphate to give a ternary solution of ammonia nitrogen, phosphoric anhydride in ortho and polyphosphatic form, and potassium hydroxide, water being added in the quantity required by the fertilizer composition to be obtained.

Soil Application of Liquid Fertilizers

The fact that liquid fertilizers are dissolved in water and spread over the land means much more soil comes in contact with the fertilizer molecules than can happen with solid fertilizer. This is particularly relevant when spreading comparatively minute quantities of some trace elements over a large area. These molecules are attracted to the soil colloids (humus and clay) and held in a highly energetic readily available form.

1.11 COMPATIBILITY OF FERTILIZER MATERIALS

Mixtures of fertilizer shall only be used if there is no risk of chemical or physical reaction between fertilizers in the blend or mixture that may reduce application accuracy. The blend or mixture should be such that there is little or no physical separation or settling of the blended or mixed components in transport and handling operations. Expert advice should be sought before creating a blend as some fertilizers are not compatible.

Before mixing two or more different fertilizers varying in physical and chemical composition it has to be ensured that it does not yield any adverse effects. For this formulation certain additional materials called 'Fillers' and 'Conditioners' are used to improve the physical condition of the mixed fertilizer. This mixed fertilizer should be applied as top dressing. Instead of distributing single-nutrient fertilizers separately or making use of multinutrient fertilizers the farmer may wish either to mix the fertilizers himself or to avail himself of the services of retailers with mixing facilities. This provides the opportunity to prepare special blends with nutrient ratios to suit the particular farmer's needs appropriate to his own soils and crops. However, fertilizers which are to be mixed must be compatible both chemically and physically (Fig. 1.10):

- Chemically, so that no gaseous loss will occur nor any decrease in nutrient availability or caking due to chemical reactions.
- Physically, i.e. of similar granule size (2–4 mm, or 1–3.5 mm), to prevent segregation during transport and spreading and possibly also of similar density (urea, for example, can create problems through its lightness compared with other fertilizers), and to avoid probable yield reduction.

Possibilities of mixing fertilizers
(limited compatibility is mainly due to hygroscopicity)

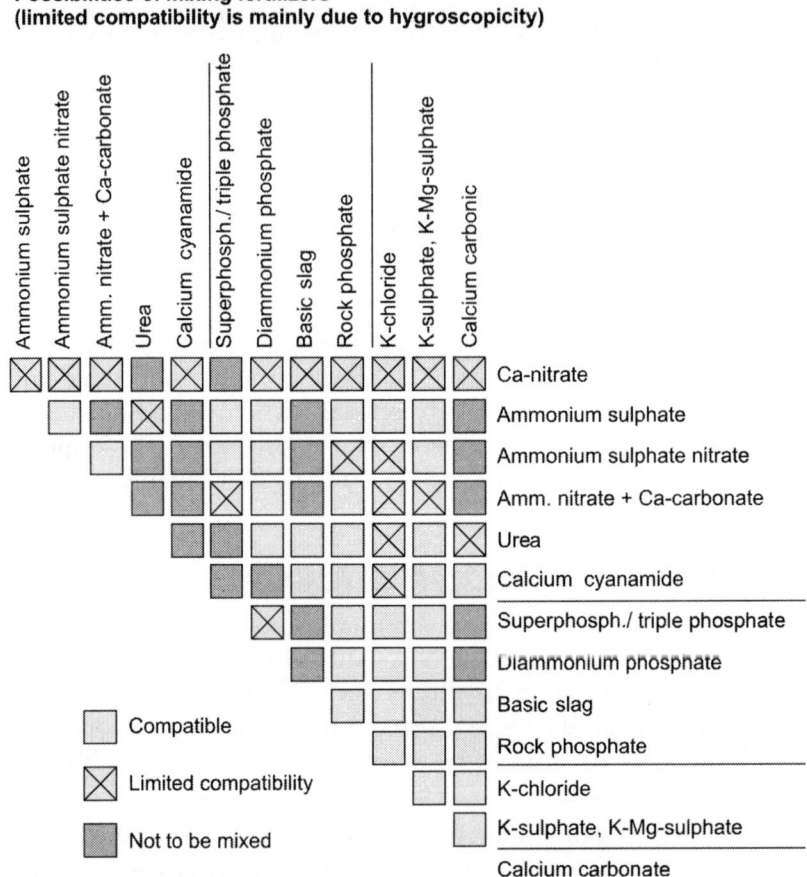

Fig. 1.10: Possibilities of mixing fertilizers (limited compatibility is mainly due to hygroscopicity)
(Courtesy: IFA, Paris)

1.12 FERTILIZER CONTROL ORDER

In order to guarantee the farmer good quality and to exclude hazards, the composition of mineral fertilizers, and the trade in mineral fertilizers are officially controlled in many countries (in Germany since 1918). Recently with the object of obtaining better control of pollution, special regulations have been introduced for the application of certain organic fertilizers and manures (e.g. slurry). In some countries governmental regulations are now being introduced for fertilizer application in general in order to minimize any avoidable fertilizer-induced pollution or food contamination. Many fertilizer products, however, are not yet subjected to legal control though there is an increasing voluntary standardization by producers in order to ensure uniformity of quality, especially for organic and organic-mineral fertilizers. Even so, there still remain a number of "unorthodox" fertilizers (mainly organic) on the market which, in spite of "expert" recommendations, have little real value.

To ensure adequate availability of right quality of fertilizers at right time and at right price to farmers, the fertilizer was declared as an essential commodity and fertilizer control order (FCO) was promulgated under Section 3 of essential commodities Act, 1955 to regulate, trade, price, quality and distribution of fertilizers in India. FCO along with policies regarding the fertilizer industry have been enumerated in the Table 1.10. FCO provides for compulsory registration of fertilizer manufacturers, importers and dealers, specification of all fertilizers manufactured/imported and sold in the country, regulation on manufacture of fertilizer mixtures, packing and marking on the fertilizer bags, appointment of enforcement agencies, setting up of quality control laboratories and prohibition on manufacture/import and sale of non-standard/spurious/adulterated fertilizers. Accordingly there are 67 fertilizer quality control laboratories in the Country which includes 4 set up by Central Government as CFQC&TI, Faridabad and its three Regional Laboratories. The order also provides for cancellation of authorization letter/registration certificates of dealers and mixture manufacturers and also imprisonment from 3 months to 7 years with fine to offenders under ECA. The FCO offence has also been declared as cognizable and non-bailable.

The FCO has been recently amended to make it more user-friendly and ensuing effective enforcement. 5 Urea manufacturers namely; NFL, Sri Ram fertilizers, Indo Gulf fertilizers, Chambal fertilizers & Tata chemicals have been permitted to manufacture Neem coated urea under clause 20A for commercial trials and M/s IFFCO to manufacture fortified NPK complexes with Boron and Zinc. Further, M/s coromandal fertilizers have been allowed to manufacture & sell Bentonite Sulphur for commercial trial. Notification of NPK 16:13:33:0:15 (S) in schedule I part A is also made. For the first time on the consistant demand of State Governments the Bio-fertilizers and organic manures have been brought under the regulatory mechanism. In the Schedule III & IV of FCO, 1985, the specification of important Bio-fertilizers (namely; Phosphate Solublizing Bacteria (PSB), *Azotobactor, Azospirrillium, Rhizobium*) & 3 organic manures (namely Vermi compost, City Compost & Press mud) has been notified besides their tolerance limit, method of sampling and analysis.

The enforcement of this order has primarily been entrusted to State Governments. The Central Government provides training facilities and technical guidance to States and supplements their efforts through random inspection of manufacturing units and their distribution network through the inspectors.

Table 1.10: Overview of policies regarding the fertilizer industry

Period	Policy	Specifics
1957	Fertilizer control order	Price and distribution control
Before 1970	Price control	Control of straight nitrogenous fertilizers including urea, ammonium sulfate and CAN (1966), no or irregular price controls of other fertilizers
Oct. 1970	Review of fertilizer policy	
Around 1970	Common fertilizer pool	Pool used to account for individual cost structure of plants (different retention prices)
1973	Re-introduction of distribution control	Fertiliser movement control order essential commodity Act (ECA): Percentage fertilizer under ECA varied from time to time
1977	Retention price system	Introduction of retention price system for nitrogenous fertilizers
Feb. 1979	Price control	Retention price system (RPS) for phosphatic fertilizers such as DAP and other complex fertilizers (NP and NPK)
June 1980	Price decontrol	Price decontrol of low analysis nitrogenous fertilizers (AS, CAN, ACl)
May 1982	Price control retention	Price system for single superphosphate (SSP)
September 1984	Price control	Price control again for low analysis nitrogenous fertilizers
April 1988	Revision of price control	Reduction of retention prices and subsidies for nitrogenous fertilizer
July 1991	Price decontrol	Price decontrol of low analysis nitrogenous fertilizers
August 1991	Dual pricing policy	30% price increase of fertilizer for big farmers, no price increase for small and marginal farmers
August 1992	Partial decontrol	Decontrol of prices, distribution and movement of phosphatic and potassic fertilizer, recontrol of low analysis nitrogenous fertilizers, 10% price reduction for urea fertilizer
September 1992	Import liberalization	Import of raw material for manufacture of DAP and other complex phosphatic fertilizers (not SSP) allowed at lower official exchange rate (under dual exchange system) with no customs duty

Specifications of some common fertilizer materials as per FCO (2002) have been enlisted below.

1. Urea (46% N) (While free flowing)	
Moisture percent by weight, maximum	1.0
Total nitrogen, percent by weight, (on dry basis) minimum	46.00
Biuret percent by weight, maximum	1.5
Particle size- 90 per cent of the material shall pass through 2.8 mm IS sieve and not less than 80 per cent by weight shall be retained on 1 mm IS sieve	
2. Single superphosphate (16% P_2O- Powdered)	
(i) Moisture per cent by weight, maximum	12.0
(ii) Free phosphoric acid (as P_2O_5) per cent by weight maximum	4.0
(iii) Water-soluble phosphates (as P_2O_5) per cent by weight, minimum	16.0
Particle size- Not less than 90 per cent of the material shall pass through 4 mm IS sieve and shall be retained on 1 mm IS sieve not more than 5 per cent shall pass through 1 mm IS sieve.	
3. Potassium chloride (Muriate of potash)	
(i) Moisture per cent by weight, maximum	0.5
(ii) Water soluble potash content (as K_2) per cent by weight minimum	60.00
(iii) Sodium as NaCl per cent by weight (on dry basis) maximum	3.5
Particle size- 95 per cent of the material shall pass through 1.7 mm IS sieve and be retained on 0.25 mm IS sieve.	
4. Diammonium phosphate (18-46-0)	
(i) Moisture	
(i) Moisture per cent by weight, maximum	1.5
(ii) Total nitrogen per cent by weight, minimum	18.00
(iii) Ammoniacal nitrogen form per cent by weigh, minimum	15.5
(iv) Total nitrogen in the form of urea per cent by weight, maximum	2.5
(v) Neutral ammonium citrate soluble phosphates (as P_2O_5 per cent by weight, minimum	46.0
(vi) Water soluble phosphates (as P_2O_5) per cent by weight minimum	41.0
Particle size- 90 per cent of the material shall pass through 4 mm IS sieve and be retained on 1 mm IS sieve Not more than 5 per cent shall be below than 1 mm size	
5. Nitrophosphate (20-20-0)	
(i) Moisture per cent by weight, maximum	1.5
(ii) Total nitrogen per cent by weight, minimum	20.0
(iii) Nitrogen in ammoniacal form per cent by weight, minimum	10.0
(iv) Nitrogen in nitrate form per cent by weight, maximum	10.0
(v) Neutral ammonium citrate soluble phosphates (as P_2O_5) per cent by weight, minimum	20.0
(vi) Water soluble phosphates (as P_2O_5) per cent by weight, minimum	12.0
(vii) Calcium nitrate, per cent by weight, maximum	1.0
Particle size- 90 per cent of the material shall pass through 4 mm IS sieve and shall be retained on 1 mm sieve. Not more than 5 per cent shall be below 1 mm IS sieve.	

Contd.

Contd.

6. NPK (10-26-26)	
(i) Moisture per cent by weight, maximum	1.0
(ii) Total nitrogen per cent by weight, minimum	10.0
(iii) Ammoniacal nitrogen per cent by weight, minimum	7.5
(iv) Nitrogen in the form of urea per cent by weight, maximum	3.0
(v) Neutral ammonium citrate soluble phosphates (as P_2O_5) per cent by weight, minimum	26.0
(vi) Water soluble potash (as K_2O) per cent by weight minimum	26.0
(vi) Water soluble phosphates (as P_2O_5) per cent by weight minimum	22.1
Particle size- 90 per cent of the material shall pass through 4 mm IS sieve and shall be retained on 1 mm sieve. Not more than 5 per cent shall be below 1 mm IS sieve.	

1.13 FERTILIZER STORAGE

Storage conditions shall ensure that fertilizer is never contaminated with other chemicals or chemical products, and that fertilizer does not escape from the storage facility. Some stores may also need to provide appropriate signage. Fertilizer storage buildings shall be sited to minimise any risk of environmental contamination. In particular, storage sites must not present a risk of direct water contact with stored fertilizer. This includes the entry of storm water or run-off from surrounding areas.

Construction

Fertilizer buildings shall be constructed so that stored fertilizer remains in a useable condition. In particular, fertilizer should stay dry and free from contamination by other fertilizer types or any foreign material. Bulk fertilizer shall be stored in a manner that preserves the physical properties of the fertilizer and allows the fertilizer to be retrieved from storage and used without contamination. The fertilizer shall be stored on an impermeable surface to prevent leaching to groundwater and to prevent the localised accumulation of contaminants in the soil.

1. Fertilizer storage buildings may be subject to approval and issue of the necessary consents from the local government authority.
2. Bagged fertilizer should be protected from direct sunlight, rainfall and contamination by chemical products.

Distribution System

Fertilizers are essential inputs in agriculture and, in particular, production of foodgrains. The marketing system has to carry out the functions of storage, transportation and selling to the farmers spread throughout the country. It includes wholesalers, agents, and retailers. Over time the marketing system for fertilizers has undergone rapid change both in terms of its capacity and mode of operation. Its evolution has been mainly guided by the public policy. Since fertilizer was a new input for the farmers, the spread of know-how and incentives had to accompany the marketing of fertilizers. Initially the demand for fertilizer had to be created. It was to increase agricultural production and not only to sell more fertilizers. Up to the end of the first five year plan (1951–56) the sale of chemical fertilizers was the sole responsibility of co-operative societies and state agriculture departments. Later, the Government allowed the fertilizer production units, which had been licensed before December 31, 1967, to sell 70% of their produce through their own agencies for a period of seven years from the date of commencement of production. The remaining 30% of the production was required to be sold through public or co-operative agencies.

During the early seventies, the proportion of private sector sale points increased at a faster rate but slowed down in the later half of seventies. However, during the eighties and nineties, the private sector fertilizer outlets have expanded at a rate higher than that of the co-operative or the public sector. In order to make available the fertilizers to farmers, the temporary sale points are also provided in some areas.

Constraints in Fertilizer Marketing

- The numbers of sale points are still inadequate farmers in hill and desert areas have to travel long distance to buy the fertilizers.
- The supplies of the fertilizers at many sale points are not sufficient to meet the demand for fertilizers in the area.
- At many sale points, the fertilizers are not stocked at a time when farmers want to purchase. For example, if the supplies to the sale point do not reach before the sowing of crops, the farmers are not able to buy the fertilizer, which they wish to use as basal dose.
- Sometimes the makes and grades of the fertilizers, which the farmers wish to buy, are not available at the nearest sale point.
- Fertilizers are prone to adulteration and several cases of adulteration have been reported.
- Sometimes, the quantity of fertilizers in the bags is less than the specified one.
- When the supply is less than the demand for fertilizers in an area, during a specified season, the dealers charge a price higher than the statutory or normal price.
- Sometimes, the farmers are forced to buy another kind of fertilizer along with the kind desired by them.
- Farmers in many areas do not have cash to pay for the fertilizers. Short-term loan or crop loan from the banks is meant to meet this requirement.
- In many areas, the salesmen do not possess the requisite know-how on the use of fertilizer which farmers wish to seek from them.
- During the last few years, there has been a considerable ad hocism in fertilizer pricing policy, which came in the way of adequate availability of fertilizers to the farmers in time.

Improvement for Fertilizer Marketing

- There is a need to increase the number of sale points specially in hilly, tribal and desert areas so that the farmers have not to travel much distance to buy the fertilizer.
- There is also a need to develop proper distribution arrangements involving a combination of co-operatives, government and private agencies, depending on the potential of the area.
- Sales points should be developed into good agro-service centres. Providing advice to the farmers on different aspects of fertilizer application in addition to making the fertilizer, other inputs and services available.
- Packing material and technology for fertilizers should be improved to minimise the chances of loss during transit and storage as also of pilferage from the bags.
- The procedure of linking credit with fertilizer supply should be simplified.
- Fertilizer should also be made available in smaller packets of 5 to 10 kg.
- There is need to check adulteration and under weighment of bags.
- There is also a need to minimise the number of brand names to avoid confusion among the farmers specially those who are illiterate or have poor educational level.
- The ratio of prices of three nutrients (NPK) should be maintained at levels consistent with the normative use under different cropping patterns and soil conditions.

1.14 DIAGNOSIS OF FERTILIZER REQUIREMENT

The still widely used practice of deciding rates of fertilizer use on the basis of local experience or general data for crop requirements is certainly useful for obtaining at least medium yield levels, but neither very effective nor economic. For obtaining maximum crop yields with maximum benefit to the cultivators, it is most essential that the crop plants should be fed properly with all nutrients. Soils deficient in particular nutrients must be supplied with fertilizers containing those plant nutrients. Thus it is important to know which plant nutrients are lacking in a soil.

Soils differ widely in their capacity for providing nutrients, depending on the amount of total reserves, on mobilization or fixation dynamics, accessability of the chemically available nutrients to the roots, etc. Therefore it remains necessary to assess empirically the nutrient status of soils and plants in order to provide guidelines for effective fertilizer use.

To determine fertilizer needs for crops and soils in any region, the following aspects are important:

1. Which nutrients are needed in the fertilizer?
2. How much of each nutrient is needed to get the highest or optimum yield?

There are several approaches to finding the answers to these questions. Simple and elaborate tests have been developed by the agricultural scientist to estimate the nutritional requirements of soils and crops. These methods are known as diagnostic techniques. The use as a first good indication of the plant nutrient removal at respective yield levels has been commonly used as one of the approach. Other approaches (optical and chemical) are listed and discussed below:

- Nutrient hunger signs on growing crops (deficiency symptoms).
- Soils tests or analyses to determine the fertilizer nutrients and amounts needed.
- Plant and/or plant tissue tests in the field.
- Fertilizer field trials.

Optical Observation in Plants

This is one of the method to know the fertilizer need of plants by means of the hunger signs of plants which can be detected by the eye. The basis of the method is the fact that the plant suffering from severe deficiencies and excess of mineral nutrients usually developed well-defined and typical sign of disorders in various organs, particularly in the leaves. Usually, specific abnormal colours are developed in the leaves due to deficiency of plant nutrients. Although the hunger signs in plants are easily observed, it is not easy to recognise the particular nutrient deficiency in nature due to various field conditions. This requires experience and practice in the field.

If plants do not get enough of a particular nutrient they need, the symptoms can be seen in the general appearance as well as in the colour of the plant. Very typical symptoms are: the nutrient deficient plants are stunted (small), the leaves have a pale green colour or a very dark bluish green colour, are yellowish or have reddish spotting or striping. Identification of nutrient deficiency is easy in some cases, but difficult in others. The reason for this is that deficiency symptoms of two different nutrients can be nearly identical or that the deficiency of one nutrient is hiding the symptoms of another deficiency. The hunger signs may also appear or disappear as the weather changes. It may also be the case that plants are suffering from not yet visible deficiency known as "hidden hunger". Care should also be taken not to confuse hunger signs with disease symptoms or damage caused by insects/animal pests. Clear symptoms will occur only in cases of extreme deficiency of one nutrient. Hunger signs of a deficient nutrient should be verified by soil tests, plant analysis, field tissue tests and/or field trials.

A normal dark green colour characterizes a good nutrient supply, but any change to light green or yellowish tinges, suggests a deficiency, provided other factors such as extreme temperatures, diseases, spray damage, air pollution, etc. are not responsible. The easiest means of diagnosis is by identification from colour photographs showing deficiency symptoms in the particular crop concerned. The precise cause may, however, not be easy to establish from observation alone, particularly in cases of "hidden hunger" for which chemical methods will usually be needed.

Brief Key to Deficiency Symptoms

Symptoms	Deficiency
Symptoms appearing first on older leaves:	
Chlorosis starting from leaf tips	N
Necrosis on leaf margins	K
Chlorosis mainly between veins (which remain green)	Mg
Brownish, greyish, whitish spots (e.g. on cereals)	Mn
Reddish colour on green leaves or stem	P
Symptoms appearing first on younger leaves:	
Mottled yellow-green leaves with yellowish veins	S
Mottled yellow-green leaves with green veins	Fe
Brownish black spots (e.g. on legumes, potatoes)	Mn
Youngest leaf has white tip	Cu
Youngest leaf is brownish or dead (e.g. on beet)	B

General hunger signs for some crops are specified below:

Nitrogen deficiency

- Stunted plants (common to all deficiencies), poor plant health and small plants.
- Loss of green colour yellow discoloration of leaves from tip backward (tip chlorosis), older leaves brown.
- Lower leaves may die prematurely while the top of the plant remains green (sometimes mistaken for lack of moisture).

Phosphorus deficiency

- Stunted growth.
- Leaves dark bluish green, purpling and browning from tip backward (often also at stems).
- Plants slow to ripen, remaining green.
- Fruits may be misshapen, grain is poorly filled.

Potassium deficiency

- Stunted growth.
- Leaves show discoloration along outer margin from tip to base.
- Outer edges of leaves yellow or reddish, becoming brownish or scorched and dead (edge necrosis); leaves wilted.
- Lodging.
- Tree leaves are yellowish, reddish, pinched, cupped or curved.
- Fruit is small, may have lesions or injured spots, poor storage and keeping quality.

Magnesium deficiency

- Yellowish discoloration between green leaf veins (typical stripe chlorosis; Mg is part of chlorophyll, needed for photosynthesis), finally followed by blotching and necrosis (death of tissues), starting at lower old leaves.

Sulphur deficiency

- Whole plant is yellow (similar as N deficiency).
- Yellowing of upper leaves, even on newest growth.
- Delayed crop maturity.

Calcium deficiency

- Young leaves yellowish to black and curved or cupped (brown spots).
- Plants appear to wilt.
- Fruits may appear rotten.
- Roots are malformed.

Boron deficiency

- Leaves frequently misshapen and crinkled, thick and brittle, white, irregular spots between veins.
- Growing tips of buds die, with bushy growth near tips, extension growth inhibited with shortened internodes.
- Water-soaked, necrotic spots or cavities in root crops and in the pith of stems.
- Poorly formed small fruits often with corky nodules and lesions.
- Low seed production due to incomplete fertilization.

Zinc deficiency

- Stunted growth of leaves.
- Fruit trees with typical shortened bushy shoots.
- Chlorotic stripes (white bleached bands) between the leaf veins in lower part of leaf.
- In some cases leaves have an olive green or greyish green colour (very similar to P deficiency).

Iron deficiency

- Young leaves with typical chlorosis between green veins, along the entire length of leaves (usually on calcareous soils).

Hunger signs are useful in giving an indication of nutritional disorders to the farmer, followed by correction through nutrient on an urgent basis. The yield at harvest may still be lower in comparison to crops which are well nourished from planting to harvesting through good agricultural practices. Most helpful methods to reach this aim are soil tests, plant analysis, field tissue tests and field trials.

A direct comparison in the field, sometimes called the "window" technique, may be obtained by using a small control plot without fertilizer which will often reveal an obvious colour difference. If it does not, then chemical methods are necessary.

Soil Tests

Soil testing is one reliable diagnostic tool whose value in evaluating soil-fertility conditions has been recently recognised in India. Soil testing is multipurpose in nature. Its purposes are:

- To group soils into classes relative to the levels of nutrients for suggesting fertilizer practices.
- To predict the probability of getting a profitable response to the application of fertilizers.
- To help evaluate soil profitability.
- To determine specific soil conditions, i.e., alkalinity, salinity, acidity, that limit crop yields and can be improved with soil amendments and other management practices.

Soil testing is used to find out how much of a nutrient will be plant-available from the soil, and how much should be additionally applied in the form of a mineral fertilizer to reach an expected crop yield. The higher the level of a soil test in plant nutrient, the less is the amount needed from fertilizers. Even at high test levels some nutrients should come from fertilizers in order to maintain soil fertility and productivity. There are different kinds of soil tests. However, the main problem is to relate suitable nutrient extraction methods for a given soil with the corresponding yields (calibration). If the concerned experimental station has conducted soil analyses and field experiments and has calibrated the soil tests to crop responses to fertilizers, one should take soil samples there. They will then be able to give a correct interpretation of the soil test result and the corresponding fertilizer recommendation.

How the Soil Test Works

A soil test by a nutrient extraction method chemically extracts and measures the amount of nutrients available to crops from a small sample of soil that is taken to the depth of the arable layer (0–18 cm). The results found are related to fertilizer crop response data from corresponding field experiments. Based on such calibrated data the soil test result can be interpreted and fertilizer recommendations can be given.

How to Take a Soil Sample

A soil test cannot be better than the sample that is tested. Therefore, careful sampling is a mandatory. Of great importance is selecting the area to be sampled. Do not mix different kinds of soil. If any area of soil in a field appears different, or if crop growth is significantly different from the rest, take a separate sample from that area. The tools for taking a sample are a soil borer (auger) or sampling tool or a spade and a knife, and a clean bucket and container. If you use a spade, dig a V-shaped cut to a depth of 15 to 20 cm. With your knife trim-off both edges of the slice leaving a strip (core) of soil on the spade 2 cm wide. Take about 20 spade or borer cores at random over the field 1 hectare plot. Place the cores in the clean bucket and mix them thoroughly. Take a small sample of 0.5 kg of the mixed soil (usually after air drying it on a clean sheet of paper) and place it in a clean paper bag or small box. Record, label and date the sample properly so that you can relate the soil test results correctly to the field.

Problem lies in selecting and calibrating suitable extraction methods for particular soil types, sub-types or units. The value of these methods must be established empirically in the soil area concerned. The choice of a suitable method requires calibration either:

- By field experiments, in which the relative crop yield with and without fertilizer is correlated with the relative extraction data from soil with and without fertilizer (R^2 should be at least 60% and preferably >70%);
- By plant nutrient content, i.e. by correlating the nutrient content in the plant at a particular stage with the nutrient extraction data from the soil or by the appearance of deficiency symptoms, comparing the nutrient extraction data from the soil with the appearance or non-appearance of symptoms.

Plant Testing

Plant analysis

The use of plant analysis as a tool to diagnose fertility status mainly consists of:
1. Plant tissue tests or rapid tests,
2. Total analysis,
3. Bio-chemical methods.

The basis of plant analysis for diagnostic purposes is that the amount of a given nutrient in a plant is an indication of the supply of that particular nutrient and is directly related to the quantity present in the soil. The normal growth of a plant is determined by the supply of the nutrients. However, there is one disadvantage with this method, i.e. while the shortage of one nutrient can limit the growth, other nutrients may show higher contents in the cell sap irrespective of the supply.

The use of plant tissue tests as a means to diagnose soil fertility status has been found to be important. This is a rapid test of the cell sap of the growing plants. The sap from the ruptured cells is tested for unassimilated nitrogen, phosphorus, potash and other nutrients. Tissue tests are getting popular because of the convenience of handling and the small number of equipment needed for the test. The test can be made in a few minutes.

Total analysis is used extensively in research work as this gives a quantitative indication of the level of nutrients in plants. However, it should be remembered that the determination of total analysis gives both the assimilated and unassimilated nutrients. Many nutrients such as N, P, K, Ca, Mg, Mn, Zn, Cu, Fe, Mo and B can be determined by this method. Usually, the mature plants are selected for this testing.

Bio-chemical methods to determine the soil fertility require costly equipments, but offer good opportunities for research work. Two methods are recognised amongst biological tests. They are, use of higher plants, micro-biological methods.

With plant testing the concentration of the different nutrients and their proportion is determined chemically in the plant sap or in the dry matter. If a nutrient is below the minimum concentration (critical value), which is different for each nutrient, it is likely that the application of a fertilizer containing that nutrient will increase yield. It is important that the critical values established are related to the expected yield level. However, the great advantage is that, once properly established, they are applicable to the same crop worldwide. Further this method is advantageous as number of nutrients that can be determined and the accuracy obtained. Plant analysis is particularly valuable in permanent crops and widely used in fruit plantations.

The nutrient content of plants provides reliable information on their nutritional status at the date of sampling, thus giving a guide not only to any supplementary fertilizer needs of the current crop but also to the probable requirements of future crops. Although it is more costly than soil testing and needs more care in the handling of samples, this method is growing in importance. Interpretation is usually based on the total contents of nutrients in leaves, or other suitable plant parts, in comparison with critical nutrient concentrations or "critical values"; but there are more sophisticated methods which either consider the "active" mobile contents (e.g. Ca and Fe), or simple or complex nutrient ratios (e.g. Beaufil's diagnostic and recommendation integrated system = DRIS, which seems to have advantages for more detailed studies). It is essential to ensure that the "critical values" used relate to the expected level of yield (e.g. 80, 90 or 100%); once properly established, they are applicable to the same crop worldwide.

Plant Tissue Testing in the Field

Plant tissue tests are made on green/growing plants in the field. The selected part of the plant, usually the (young, actively functioning) leaves or leaf stalks (petioles), is either cut up and shaken in an extractant, or sap is squeezed onto a test paper and treated with appropriate chemicals (Diphenyl amine sodium cobaltonitrate, etc). The colours which develop, can be compared against known concentrations of nutrients or of healthy productive and well established plants. Plant tissue tests in the field are valuable for verifying deficiency symptoms. Moreover, they help to discover "hidden hunger" which is not indicated by deficiency symptoms. They have the advantage that they can be made rapidly and directly on the growing crop that they are inexpensive and that tests of plants or treatments can be compared directly in the field.

Fertilizer Field Trials

Whereas results from plant analysis and plant tissue tests in the field will indicate nutrient deficiencies, particularly 'hidden hunger' when compared to standards which are developed from well-growing productive plants, soil tests require correlation to crop yields. This correlation or calibration of test methods has to be done through fertilizer field trials. In such trials, fertilizers are applied at known rates of plant nutrients crop responses are observed, and final yields are measured. Field trials have the following advantages:

- Best way to determine the nutrient needs of crops and soils.
- Show how accurate recommendations based on soil and plant testing are in relation to the yield obtained.
- Permit an economic evaluation.
- The growing crops can be photographed which can be used in publicity and demonstrations for many years.
- Demonstrations or simple trials show the benefits of fertilizers to farmers and agricultural workers.

In India, simple field experiments on farmers fields as well as complex field experiments are very popular. In well managed state farms, the level of soil fertility is usually higher than in the farmers fields. This is due to the use of manures, fertilizers, good management practices, etc. Many experiments conducted on farmers fields have revealed the deficiency of nutrients at various levels. These experiment have to be simple in nature with N, P, K, NP, NK, PK, NPK as the treatments. These simple field experiments on farmers fields are very educative and effective for the farmers, as they themselves see the deficiencies and the response of the nutrients. These trials are useful for advising the correct type and amount of fertilizer.

Complex field experiments allow the testing of many factors at a time and permit a study of interaction among various nutrients. Complex fertilizer trials helps in determining the correct kinds of fertilizer, amount and the method of application for each of the soil zone. These experiments are complicated, expensive and can be done only by experienced people.

The experiments may be conducted either in the field or in pots. Although the statistical analysis of the yield results follows standard procedures, great care is needed to ensure that the correct conclusions are drawn concerning cause and effect. A statistically significant yield response to a particular fertilizer treatment might, for example, be due either to an increased supply of a subsidiary nutrient contained in that fertilizer or to an indirect effect on the availability of micronutrients in the soil rather than to the nutrient(s) which the fertilizer was intended to supply. Great care must also be taken in extrapolating the results, which strictly apply only to the soil area of the experimental plots under the conditions then prevailing, not to other areas and other crops in different seasons.

Long-term Field Experiments

General recommendations for a region are available when enough fertilizer trials have been carried out. Examples for your region may be inserted at the end of this booklet. However, nutrient needs for a crop on a given soil cannot be determined once and for all, because conditions change rapidly. When only one nutrient is applied (unbalanced fertilization), another may become limiting. Not enough or too much of one nutrient may reduce yield or lower the profitability of fertilizer use to the farmer. Unbalanced nutrient supply may also result in increased susceptibility to disease, lodging or late maturity. Therefore, continuing studies are necessary, i.e. long-term field experiments should be conducted to find out the amounts and ratio of nutrients required. The earliest long-term field experiment was started at the Rothamsted Experiment station, Harpenden, England in 1843. In India permanent manual experiments were started at Kanpur (UP), Pusa (Bihar), and Coimbatore (TN) in 1885, 1908 and 1909.

Other Factors Limiting Crop Yields

Fertilizer use is one of the most important factors which contributes to increased productivity and sustainable agriculture. But it will not solve all the problems of crop production. Several other factors or practices which can limit and affect crop yields and reduce fertilizer use efficiency. In applying good agricultural practices the farmer should pay particular attention to:

- Proper and timely preparation of the seed bed;
- Crop varieties (preferably high yielding varieties (HYV));
- Correct seeding rate:
    a. Plants per hectare,
    b. Spacing between plants or rows,
- Optimal seeding time;
- Sufficient moisture (use irrigation where available, a bare field should be covered with mulch to avoid erosion and conserve soil moisture);
- Adequate drainage (remove excess water by surface or tile drainage);
- Control weeds (use hoeing, cultivation or chemical treatments);
- Control crop diseases (use resistant crops or approved chemical treatments);
- Control pests (use recommended and approved control measures);
- Use crop rotations that reduce crop diseases, weeds and pests;
- Improve the soil structure (through crop rotation, amendment or manure/green manuring); and
- Maintain soil organic matter (through crop rotation, bulky manure or organic matter supply). It is, of course, difficult to estimate the losses caused

through other factors affecting plant growth and crop yield precisely. Some
calculations have been made for weed control and crop protection.

1.15 FERTILIZERS AND AGRICULTURAL SUSTAINABILITY

In many parts of the country industrial agriculture using chemical fertilizer and
other "modern" methods have yielded bumper harvests. However, it also has
severely damaged the environment and impoverished the land. The use of heavy
machinery in soil preparation has led to compaction and other detrimental changes
in soil structure. Chemical fertilizers also have affected the ability of crops to
adequately absorb nutrients. The chemicals have contaminated groundwater,
rendering it unfit for human consumption.

The transfer of high-input agricultural technology to our country, in the mistaken
belief that it could bring the same benefits everywhere, has, in many cases, hurt
more than it has helped. Not only was the technology often entirely inappropriate,
but the lack of follow-up money and inadequate maintenance often rendered it
unproductive within months. Under such conditions, agricultural production ceases
to be economically and ecologically sustainable.

Many farmers and entrepreneurs are attracted to the dramatic increase in yields
promised by modern agricultural systems. The results, however, decrease as the
organic matter in the soil declines and the soil itself becomes lifeless and prone to
erosion. Increasing quantities of fertilizer are then needed to maintain production,
thus raising production costs. Moreover, since crops that are grown with the use of
chemicals lack natural health and resistance, ever-increasing quantities of pesticides
are needed to protect them, polluting both soil and atmosphere and undermining
the health of farm workers. Such a system achieves only temporary gains and is
not sustainable in the long-run.

Soil is a rich but fragile eco-system. It is also living. One handful of good soil is
home to millions of micro-organisms, which ensure and sustain fertility. Under a
given set of normal conditions even a centimetre of soil can take centuries to develop.
But it can be lost for ever-blown away by wind, washed-off deforested slopes by
rain, sterilized by salts, poisoned by chemicals, bled dry of nutrients or buried
under swamps or buildings.

Through the mismanagement of land resources, farmers are losing valuable
topsoil to wind and rain. In tropical areas, what is referred to as "slash-and-burn"
agriculture eliminates rain forests to create farm land. After the harvest is complete,
fields are often left barren, exposed to drought and flood. Valuable topsoil is lost,
and in many areas desertification results.

1.16 FERTILIZERS AND ENVIRONMENTAL ISSUES: LONG-TERM EFFECT ON ATMOSPHERE, HYDROSPHERE AND LITHOSPHERE

Fertilizers are relatively safer than pesticides which exhibit toxic properties on living
systems. However, all the quantities of fertilizers applied to the soil are not fully

utilized by plants. About 50 per cent of fertilizers applied to crops are left behind as residues. Whereas positive effects of fertilizer use on the environment are often overlooked, attention nowadays is focussed on negative aspects. Mineral and organic fertilizers are accused of:

- Accumulation of dangerous or even toxic substances in soil from fertilizer constituents, e.g. Cd from mineral phosphate fertilizers or from town or industrial waste products;
- Eutrophication of surface water, with its negative effect on oxygen supply (damaging to fish and other forms of animal life);
- Nitrate accumulation in ground water, thus diminishing the quality of drinking water;
- Unwanted enrichment of the atmosphere with ammonia from organic manures and mineral fertilizers, and with N_2O from denitrification of excessive or wrongly placed N fertilizer.

As to contamination of soils with toxic heavy metals, it can easily be shown that mineral fertilizers (SSP,TSP,RP,AS) make only a rather small contribution in comparison with, for example, town wastes. However, as soil fertility must be considered in the very long-term and not only in decades or centuries, the annual addition should be kept at such a low level that the enrichment is negligible. Industrial waste products should always be carefully checked to determine whether they contain potentially toxic substances, and appropriate critical limits should be established.

Nutrient losses from the soil into surface and ground water (mainly nitrate by leaching and phosphate by erosion) occur even when fertilizers are not used, but they are increased slightly but unavoidably even by correct fertilizer use and are increased substantially by excessive or unbalanced use, which can be avoided.

Considerable leaching of nitrate is caused, for example, by:

- Excessive application of nitrogenous fertilizer;
- Intensively fertilized speciality crops;
- Ploughing of cropland;
- Fertilizer application for over-optimistic yield expectations which fail to materialize;
- Part of the correctly estimated N requirement remaining unused because of other limiting factors not being taken into account, e.g. deficiencies of secondary or micronutrients.

In other words, N losses are mainly due to mistakes in fertilizer use or crop management, not to fertilizer use itself. Moreover, counter-measures can be taken to prevent loss of nitrate residues after harvesting and to prevent soil erosion.

N loss by leaching seems to range from 10 to more than 100, in extreme cases more than 150 kg/ha N depending on the accuracy of fertilizer use and the extent of the preventive methods used. From a scientific point of view, much more attention needs to be given to the enigma of N balance sheets before drawing premature conclusions on N losses. Loss of phosphate by leaching (< 1 kg/ha P) is negligible, while loss by erosion is due to bad soil management rather than fertilizer use. In an extensive survey by ICAR, New Delhi it was found that many streams and more than 20% of wells contain 10 to 50 mg or even more of nitrates per litre of water. The contamination is caused by domestic sewage leaking to the ground water. The nitrates in drinking water can lead to several ailments. *Blue - baby syndrome* in infants and gastric and other forms of cancer have been related with nitrates in drinking water or diet.

Algae blooms occur when the nutrient load is high, and these smother other aquatic vegetation and also interfere with the oxygen regulation in the water bodies. This phenomena may lead to loss of fish. Among the major synthetic plant nutrients, nitrogenous fertilizers cause most harm. Contamination of the environment arises because not all the fertilizer applied is taken up by the crop and removed at harvest. In tropical climate (Temp >37 °C) the maximum recovery in dry land crops is 50 to 60 per cent and 40 per cent in rice because much of nitrogen is lost as ammonia into the atmosphere through volatalization process.

Among the mineral fertilizers, only urea and ammonium sulphate might cause significant NH_3 volatilization losses, especially if not incorporated. To minimize these losses, incorporation into the soil or application before rain or irrigation is recommended.

Another hazard associated with excessive use of fertilizers is the gaseous loss of nitrogen, into the atmosphere. High doses of carbon dioxide and ammonia that escape into the atmosphere both from fertilizer manufacturing plants and soils affect human health. Further the oxides of nitrogen have been reported to adversely affect the ozone layer, which protects the earth from UV radiation and heating up of earth.

The contention that agriculture contributes considerably to N_2O production via denitrification, as a result of excessive or wrongly applied fertilizer N, is a serious problem, because this gas contributes to the destruction of the ozone layer in the stratosphere which protects against ultra-violet radiation. Official estimates, derived mainly under artificial conditions or by the difference method, showing losses of approximately 15% or more of the applied N, are not really substantiated; total denitrification losses in the range of 5–10% of the applied N, of which only about 10% is as N_2O, seem to be more realistic, especially for soils under normal moisture conditions.

The oxides of nitrogen cause respiratory diseases like asthma, lung cancer and bronchitis. Arsenic, ammonia are waste stream components of nitrogen manufacturing plants while fluoride, cadmium, chromium, copper, lead and manganese are waste stream components of phosphatic fertilizer industry. If these waste stream of components are not properly disposed they cause harm to human beings and animals with contamination of air and water.

Though, inorganic fertilizers are not directly toxic to man and other life forms, they have been found to upset the existing ecological balance. Since pollution of the environment should be minimized, governments are trying to control the avoidable negative influences by special laws.

Fertilizers and Climate Change

Both at the point of production and at end user site to stimulate crop growth, fertilizers have an impact on greenhouse gas emissions and other aspects of climate change. Taken in isolation, fertilizer production leads to inevitable emissions of some greenhouse gases, but these can be minimized, and the fertilizer industry has taken great strides to improve its performance in this area during recent years. Depending on management practices, crop fertilization can either produce a positive, negative or neutral impact on climate change. This is true regardless of whether farmers are using fertilizers, other sources of crop nutrients or a mix thereof.

Before the 20th century, limited supplies of plant-available nutrients were a major factor holding back agricultural production and slowing population growth. In the 19th century, two figures stand out as the founders of modern fertilization. In England, JB Lawes with Gilbert, Student of Justos von Liebig created the world's first fertilizer factory to produce superphosphate and established an agricultural research station that still carries on some of the original experiments started in 1843. In Germany, Justus von Liebig studied the importance of minerals and atmospheric nitrogen to nourish plants, resulting in his famous 'Law of the Minimum', which states that a deficiency in any growth-limiting factor will impair plant development.

Unlike other nutrients, mineral sources of nitrogen for fertilization have been rare and largely unavailable. For this reason, nitrogen remained the single most important limiting factor for crop production and stable food supplies until well into the 20th century. In 1909, Fritz Haber discovered how to synthesize ammonia from air under high pressure and temperatures, which led him to receive the 1918 Nobel Prize in Chemistry. Carl Bosch subsequently made the breakthroughs necessary to bring the process to an industrial scale, thus ushering in the modern nitrogen fertilizer industry. In 1931, Bosch was Nobel Chemistry Laureate for this accomplishment. Industrial nitrogen fixation is the only achievement to date to be recognized by two Nobel Prizes.

Following the privations of World War II, many countries made food security a top priority. In the following years, policies were put in place to encourage farmers to use fertilizers and other modern farming technologies. Fertilizer consumption grew rapidly, largely in parallel with an accelerating expansion of the world population.

It has been estimated that some 40 per cent of the protein consumed by humans depends on the Haber-Bosch process. More than 99 per cent of all nitrogen fertilizers are derived from ammonia, which is both an intermediate and a final product. The vast majority of the energy consumed by the fertilizer industry is used for ammonia synthesis (~ 94%).

There are environmental concerns that need to be taken into consideration when using fertilizer. Elements such as nitrogen and phosphorus can get washed into our surface waters and cause algae blooms and excess plant growth. This excess growth in plant material can cause numerous problems, namely the reduction of oxygen which can lead to fish kills. Nitrogen leaching into our ground waters and drinking water supplies is a concern because excess nitrogen (>45 ppm NO_3–N) in drinking water can contribute to the "blue-baby" syndrome in infants under one year of age. Excesses of minor elements in the soil, such as copper and zinc, can cause problems in crop production. Any fertilizer in any form, whether it is organic or synthetic, can harm the environment if misused.

How can Fertilizer be used Properly and Still Protect the Environment?

There are several things to keep in mind to protect the environment when using fertilizer:

1. *Regular soil testing*: Soil testing is the only way that you will know what nutrients are in the soil. If you have sufficient amounts of elements such as phosphorus, then there is no need in applying extra phosphorus. The only way that you will know this is by testing the soil.

2. *Knowledge of nutrient requirement of crop*: If your crop only needs 5 kg of nitrogen per thousand square meter, then only apply 5 kg of nitrogen per thousand square feet. Any more than this will not do any good and will most likely not be used. Unused fertilizer can be washed away into lakes, rivers and streams or leached into ground water. Study the crop you're growing and learn about it's nutrient needs. Use this knowledge plus information from your soil test to determine the amount of fertilizer to apply.

3. *Application at proper time*: Know when your crop needs to be ferilized. There is no need to apply fertilizer when the crop will not use it. Again, this unused fertilizer can be washed away or leached before the plant can use it.

4. *Necessary precautions*: Applying fertilizers on slopes can lead to the washing away of nutrients. This is how most of these nutrients wind up into our surface waters. Take precautions to control your run-off from your property. Do not allow your fertilizer to drift onto the streets because this fertilizer will certainly make its way into the storm drains. Above all, control soil erosion. Elements that are tightly held by the soil, make their way into the surface waters on soil that is washed away. Phosphorus is an example of this type of element.

5. *Testing of used organic fertilizer*: Like the soil, the only way that you can know what is in your organic fertilizer source is to have it tested and the only way to know how much organic fertilizer to apply is to know what is in it. The nutrient contents of organic materials vary considerably from lot to lot, therefore information on average contents of individual materials are not

always reliable. Be sure of what you are applying, have your organic materials tested.

6. *Application of fertilizer as per plant health*: An unhealthy plant or in the case of a crop, poor plant stand, is not going to use as much nutrient as a healthy crop. Applying the same amount of fertilizer to an unhealthy plant can lead to unused fertilizer and can also harm the plant. Find out what is causing the problem. Fertilizer may not be the solution and if applied, could lead to polluting the environment.

7. *Proper storage of fertilizer*: Keep your fertilizer sources from being washed away by rains. Keep them under a shelter and off of the ground so the nutrients want get caught in rain water run-off.

8. *Plant residue as an alternative source*: Remember that your crop residue left over from last year, mulch and compost contain plant nutrients. These nutrients can also get into the environment as well. When deciding the amount of fertilizer to apply, take into consideration the nutrients from these sources and reduce the amount of fertilizer that you apply.

9. *Split application of fertilizer*: Nutrients leach very readily on sandy soils. If you apply more than the plant can use at the time, one good rain or irrigation can leach the nutrients down below the plant roots before it can use them. On sandy soils, break up fertilizer applications into several smaller applications instead of a few larger applications.

10. *Light irrigation followed by fertilizer application*: A light irrigation is good to activate the fertilizer, but a heavy rain or irrigation can leach or wash away nutrients. Keep this in mind when applying fertilizer.

Protecting the environment concerns all of us.

Minimising Risks

Being intimately involved with the farm, knowing its history and having observed how it reacts to varying circumstances and trials, the farmer is the person most suited to judge environmental risks. Here are some general package of practices to reduce risk to the environment:

- Annual soil testing: Take several samples spread over the farm at recurring spots and in the same month each time. Take advice from an agricultural expert. Remember that the tests measure immediately available nutrients, whereas soil organisms release 'unavailable' nutrients slowly. Good soils may have high pools of 'unavailable' nutrients.
- Analysis of plant tissues for actual nutrient take up.
- Keeping a record of soil and tissue tests, fertilizer application and crop yields. Also rainfall.
- Fertilizer application in calm wind conditions, less than 5 km/hr. Spread/apply evenly. Avoid open water.

- Don't fertilise when the soil is saturated with water (is at field capacity). Apply when tile drains are not running.
- Soil temperatures should exced 5 °C. Time applications with the season of fastest growth.
- Slow-release fertiliers application in preference to fast-release, or a mix of both to meet expected demand.
- Application of smaller quantities more frequently if possible and affordable.
- Be present during fertilisation, and check their result.
- Make sure that the land is suitable for your type of use of the land (soil, slope).
- Keep an eye on plant growth in surrounding open waters. Test open water and aquifer water for nutrients.

Fertilizers and Health

Although the fertilizer-induced increase in the content of essential food constituents does not confirm the fact that fertilizers improve health. Before the advent of fertilizer use, deficiency diseases in farm animals and humans were widespread: bone weaknesses due to lack of P, Ca vitamin deficiencies due to inadequate plant nutrition, diseases in grazing livestock due to deficiencies of Cu, Mo and Co, for example. Furthermore, some virus and bacterial diseases seem to have diminished in their infective capacity as a result of improved nutrition. The considerable increase in human life expectancy must also be attributed in part at least to having more and better food, stemming in turn from fertilizer, etc.

1.17 ECONOMICS OF FERTILIZER USE

Use of fertilizer by the farmer for increased crop production depends almost entirely on its economics. This is usually done by presenting response per unit area or per unit nutrient applied. With a view to convince the farmer about the profitability of fertilizer use, cost benefit ratio is also worked out. Almost all such calculations are based on evaluating the extra produce at the support/market price and deducting the cost of fertilizer only at the statutory prevailing rates.

Economic optimum levels of fertilizer use can be calculated using yield response curve under field condition (Fig. 1.11). The main problem is that such ideal response curves for a single nutrient often assume that there is no deficiency in any other nutrient, which is rarely the case in farmers' fields. Economic interpretation of response curves therefore needs to be undertaken with considerable caution. A further difficulty is that, in soils well supplied with nutrients such as P and K, unless the results of long-term field experiments extending over several years are available, it may not be possible to produce any yield response curve at all to these nutrients. In this case the practical solution is simply to apply fertilizer on the basis of nutrient removal, which is generally economic in the high yield range.

In cases, where yields are lower, a simple thumb rule is provided by the value: cost ratio (VCR the ratio between the value of the extra yield obtained by using fertilizer and the cost of the fertilizer applied) which has been found to range from 1 to 10. It is recommended that VCR should be at least 2, i.e. the value of the extra output obtained should be at least double the cost of the input. Here too, a measure of caution is needed. Unless the field experiments from which the ratio is derived were carried out on typically managed farmers' fields, there is always a danger that the economic value of the response may be slightly exaggerated, so that a purported ratio of 2 may perhaps in reality be only 1.5. This, of course, is one of the reasons why it is recommended that the VCR should be at least 2.

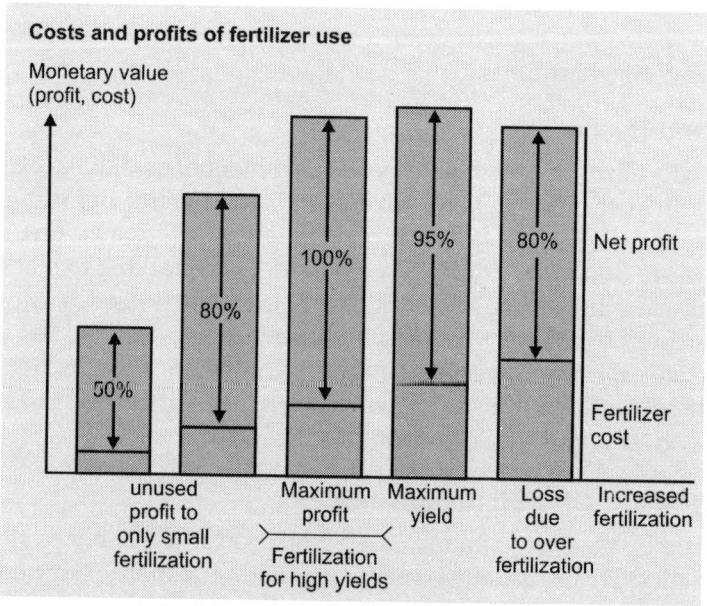

Fig. 1.11: Costs and profits of fertilizer use (Courtesy: IFA, Paris)

Due to high cost of commercial fertilizer marketed in India, the question of economics of fertilizer use has assumed great importance. The fertilizer association of India (FAI), New Delhi, therefore, organised series of group discussions on "Economics of Fertilizer use" during 1975. The recommendations of these group discussions are listed below:

1. Uniformity of approach in studying the economics of fertilizer is essential.
2. The fertilizer recommendations should be based on soil test values.
3. Balanced use of fertilizer should be advocated for better economic returns.
4. Use of nitrogenous fertilizer in split doses economises fertilizer use.
5. Micronutrient deficiencies should be corrected as and when needed.
6. Fertilizer schedule should be adopted for the whole crop sequence instead of a single crop.

To get the maximum benefit from the applied fertilizers, crops should be irrigated at the critical growth stages.

1.18 NUTRIENT REMOVAL BY CROPS

The values presented in Table 1.11 are estimates of nutrient removal or the quantity of nutrients removed in the harvested portion of the crop. They should not be confused with nutrient uptake which refers to the total nutrients absorbed by the growing crop. Actual nutrient removal may vary by 30% or more depending on the specific growing conditions of the crop such as soil fertility level, yield, soil moisture, crop vigor, and limiting nutrients as well as the actual crop variety and fertilizer package. Changes to soil fertility may differ from the amount removed by the crop. In some instances, weathering of soil minerals and organic matter may compensate for part of the nutrient removal by crops. In other instances, nutrients may be chemically fixed by the soil or lost by leaching, and the loss of nutrients will exceed crop removal.

Table 1.11: Nutrient removal by different crops

Field crops	Unit	N	P_2O_5	K_2O
Barley (spring)	lb/bu	1.10	0.40	0.35
Canola	lb/bu	1.88	0.91	0.46
Corn (grain)	lb/bu	0.75	0.44	0.29
Corn (grain)	lb/cwt	1.34	0.79	0.52
Corn (silage, 67% water)	lb/ton	8.30	3.60	8.30
Cotton (lint)	lb/bale	32.00	14.00	19.00
Flax	lb/bu	2.00	1.10	0.65
Lentils	lb/bu	2.00	0.62	1.10
Oats	lb/bu	0.80	0.25	0.20
Peanuts	lb/ton	70.00	11.00	17.00
Peas (field)	lb/bu	2.40	1.20	0.71
Rice	lb/bu	0.57	0.30	0.16
Rice	lb/cwt	1.27	0.67	0.35
Safflower	lb/cwt	5.00	1.20	3.80
Sorghum (grain)	lb/cwt	1.50	0.75	0.38
Soybeans	lb/bu	4.00	0.80	1.40
Sugarbeets	lb/ton	4.00	1.50	6.60
Sugarcane	lb/ton	2.00	1.25	3.50
Sunflower	lb/cwt	2.80	1.10	0.60
Tobacco (flue)	lb/cwt	2.80	0.50	5.20

Contd.

Table 1.11: Nutrient removal by different crops *(Contd.)*

Field crops	Unit	N	P_2O_5	K_2O
Tobacco (burley)	lb/cwt	4.30	0.43	4.70
Wheat: 10% protein	lb/bu	1.10	0.50	0.35
Forage crops	**Unit**	**N**	**P_2O_5**	**K_2O**
Alfalfa	lb/ton	56	15	60
Bahiagrass	lb/ton	43	12	35
Bermudagrass	lb/ton	46	12	50
Bromegrass	lb/ton	36	13	59
Clover-grass	lb/ton	50	15	60
Fescue	lb/ton	38	18	52
Orchardgrass	lb/ton	50	17	62
Sorghum-sudan	lb/ton	40	15	58
Timothy	lb/ton	38	14	62
Vetch	lb/ton	56	15	46
Vegetable crops	**Unit**	**N**	**P_2O_5**	**K_2O**
Broccoli	lb/cwt	0.44	0.17	0.42
Cabbage	lb/cwt	0.39	0.09	0.36
Celery	lb/cwt	0.19	0.11	0.50
Lettuce	lb/cwt	0.24	0.08	0.50
Potatoes	lb/cwt	0.35	0.15	0.56
Squash	lb/cwt	0.42	0.10	0.60
Sweet potatoes	lb/cwt	0.52	0.23	1.00
Tomatoes	lb/ton	2.50	0.92	5.70
Fruit and Nut Crops	**Unit**	**N**	**P_2O_5**	**K_2O**
Almonds (in shell)	lb/ton	130	50	170
Apples	lb/ton	6.0	3.6	16.8
Cantaloupe	lb/ton	7.3	2.3	13.0
Grapes (table)	lb/ton	8.3	3.0	13.0
Oranges	lb/ton	8.8	1.8	11.0
Peaches	lb/ton	6.3	2.7	8.0
Pears	lb/ton	5.7	1.7	6.3
Prunes	lb/ton	6.0	2.0	8.7

Source: PPI-PPIC

1.19 FERTILIZER REQUIREMENTS/SUPPLEMENTATION RELATED CALCULATIONS: PERCENTAGE PLANT FOOD IN FERTILIZER MIXTURES; CALCULATION OF THE UNIT VALUE OF A FERTILIZER

The following simple calculations will allow you to accurately determine how much fertilizer to put on your soil. Before applying fertilizers of any type, you should assess the nutrient content of your soil, and understand that other factors i.e. soil type, soil depth, current crop type and previous cropping history need to be considered as well.

Units

Often a recommendation talks about units of a nutrient (e.g. phosphorus). A unit is the same as kilograms of that nutrient (e.g. 1 unit P is 1 kg P). But this is not the same as a kilogram of a fertilizer.

N:P:K:S

Fertilizers contain different amounts of nutrients, affecting the amount of the fertilizer you need. The nutrients are often written on the bag or packing slip as percentages, or as N:P:K:S (nitrogen:phosphorus:potassium:sulfur).

Example: Single superphosphate is 0:16:0:12. This means that in 100 kg, there is 16 kg phosphorus, 12 kg sulfur. There is no nitrogen or potassium.

Calculating the Amount of Fertilizer Required

This information can be used to calculate the amount of a fertilizer needed for a given amount of a nutrient:

Calculation A: Amount of fertilizer kg/ha = kg/ha nutrient ÷ % nutrient in fertilizer × 100.

Example: You need 20 units (kg) /ha of phosphorus (P) and you plan to use single superphosphate with 16% P.

Apply Calculation A: Amount of superphosphate required (kg/ha) = 20 kg/ha P ÷ 16 P × 100 = 250 kg/ha

Calculating the Amount of Nutrient Applied

You can reverse this calculation to work out how much of a nutrient you are applying.

Calculation B: Amount of nutrient (kg/ha) = Amount of fertilizer (kg/ha) × % nutrient in fertilizer ÷100

Example: You plan to apply 125 kg/ha of single superphosphate (approx 1 bag/acre).

Apply Calculation B: Amount of P applied (kg/ha) = 125 kg/ha × 16 P ÷ 100 = 20 kg/ha P

Calculating the cost per single nutrient: You should select fertilizers for the nutrients they supply, what your soils lack and what your plants require. If only one nutrient is deficient, compare fertilizers on the cost of that nutrient. Use the following calculation to compare the price of that nutrient.

Calculation C: Price per kg nutrient = Price per tonne ÷ 10 ÷ % nutrient

Calculating the Cost for More than One Nutrient

You can use a range of fertilizers, including blends, to apply the same amount of nutrients. For the fertilizers you are considering, work out the rate you would have to apply to get the nutrients required (calculation A), then use calculation D to work out the cost per hectare. When a fertilizer has two or more of the desired nutrients, use the nutrient in least supply in the fertilizer for the calculation of rate.

Calculation D: Cost per ha = cost/tonne × rate kg/ha (from A) ÷ 1000

Other Questions to Consider

Choosing the fertilizer to use should not just depend on price. You should also consider:

- **Response to fertilizer:** Do you need fertilizer? For example, legumes fixes its own nitrogen so does not need N application; native pastures are adapted to low phosphorus and may not respond to fertilizer application.
- **Availability:** Is the fertilizer you are considering available in your area, or at the time of year you want? Factor in freight costs.
- **Availability of nutrient:** Consider if the nutrients in the fertilizer are slow-release or rapidly available.
- **Handling:** Can your machinery apply the necessary rates? Can you handle small bags or 1 tonne bags? Blends, while often more expensive, can be easier to handle. If hiring someone to spread the fertilizer, what are the associated extra costs? Does that affect the fertilizer choice?
- **Timing and placement:** Fertilizers should be applied so the nutrients are available during the plants' main growth period. But do you have the time? Plan for spreading! How much of a nutrient is safe when placed with the seed? Does this fertilizer need to be incorporated? How long before sowing?
- **Side effects:** Some fertilizers are more acidifying than others and should be used sparingly on low pH soils. Some fertilizers may contain heavy metals or salts; how much is safe? Is the fertilizer highly leachable? What precautions should be taken? What is the risk of erosion, and of fertilizer and soil contaminating waterways? Use buffer zones around waterways. Are there any animal health risks (for example, nitrate poisoning with excessive nitrogen application)?

More Calculations on Fertilizer Rates

The amount of fertilizer to be applied per hectare or on a given field is determined through the amount of nutrients needed and the types and grades of fertilizers available. Usually mineral fertilizers are delivered in 50 kg bags. Therefore, the farmer has to know the quantity of nutrients contained in a 50 kg bag. The easiest way to calculate the weight of nutrients in a 50 kg bag is to divide the number printed on the bag by 2.

Example: How many bags of ammonium sulphate (AS) (with 21% N and 24% S) are needed to supply 60 kg/ha of N?

21 divided by 2 gives 10.5. Thus approximately six bags of AS are needed to give (a little more than) 60 kg/ha N. In addition, six bags of AS will supply 72 kg/ha of sulphur.

If the area of the field is only 500 m² (square metres), the required amount of fertilizer would be one-twentieth of that for one hectare: 1 hectare: 10000 m² divided by 500 m² = 20, i.e. for an area of 500 m², 300/20 = 15 kg of ammonium sulphate are necessary to apply the amount of nitrogen corresponding to 60 kg/ha N.

If the recommendation is 60-60-60, the easiest option for the farmer is to buy a multinutrient fertilizer grade 15-15-15. One 50 kg bag contains 7.5-7.5-7.5. 60 divided by 7.5 gives 8. Thus eight 50 kg bags of 15-15-15 are needed to apply the recommended rate of 60 kg/ha N, 60 kg/ha P_2O_5 and 60 kg/ha K_2O.

When the recommendation per hectare is 60-30-30, with eight 50 kg bags of a 15-15-15 grade the farmer would apply double the amount of phosphate and potassium needed. In this case he should apply only four 50 kg bags per hectare, giving half of the recommended rate of nitrogen and the full rate of phosphate and potassium as basal dressing. The remaining 30 kg/ha N should be applied in the form of a straight nitrogen fertilizer as one or two top-dressings in line with good agricultural practices.

The situation is more complicated if the recommendation per hectare is 60 kg N, 30 kg P_2O_5 and 50 kg K_2O and there is no grade with the required ratio of 2:1:1.7 available (or 1:1:1.7 plus straight N). In this situation the farmer has three possibilities:

1. He can try to combine available multinutrient grades with straight (primarily nitrogen) fertilizers, splitting the nitrogen fertilizer rate recommended.
2. He makes a fertilizer use plan to cover the whole crop rotation, applying nitrogen every year exactly at the recommended rate for the individual crop, and phosphate and potash independently of the individual crop. However the P_2O_5 and K_2O should be applied in such amounts that finally the total quantity recommended for all crops in the crop rotation is given.
3. He can apply straight fertilizers separately, or he can mix straight fertilizers to produce his own multinutrient fertilizer mixture or blend according to the necessary nutrient ratio.

The recommended rate of 60-30-50 could be a mix of ammonium sulphate (21% N), where also sulphur is necessary, or of urea (45% N), triple superphosphate (46% P_2O_5) or diammonium phosphate (18% N and 46% P_2O_5) and muriate of potash (60% K_2O).

To obtain the corresponding mixture/blend the following quantities of fertilizer material are needed:

60 kg/ha × 100 Urea ÷ 45 = 133 kg/ha
30 kg/ha × 100 Triple superphosphate ÷ 46 = 65 kg/ha
50 kg/ha × 100 Muriate of potash ÷ 60 = 83 kg/ha

The resulting mixture of urea, triple superphosphate and muriate of potash should be spread on the field as soon as possible after mixing. When ammonium sulphate is used instead of urea, the farmer needs the following quantity of ammonium sulphate:

60 kg/ha × 100 Ammonium sulphate ÷ 21 = 286 kg/ha

In addition to 60 kg N, 30 kg P_2O_5 and 50 kg K_2O this blend would also contain 69 kg/ha sulphur.

If diammonium phosphate is used instead of triple superphosphate the quantity necessary should be based on the recommended rate for phosphate:

30 kg/ha × 100 Diammonium phosphate ÷ 46 = 65 kg/ha

This would also supply 12 kg/ha of N. The remaining 48 kg/ha of N might be incorporated into the mixture or directly applied in one or two split applications in the form of a straight nitrogen fertilizer.

However, not all fertilizers can be mixed together. Fertilizers, which are mixed together must be compatible both chemically and physically.They have to be chemically compatible to avoid caking due to increased hygroscopicity or gaseous losses of ammonia. When fertilizers containing ammonia are mixed with basic slag, rock phosphate or lime, evaporation losses of ammonia will occur. Similarly, water soluble phosphate fertilizers (single and triple superphosphate, ammonium- and nitro-phosphates) should not be mixed with fertilizers containing calcium (e.g. calcium nitrate), since the calcium will revert the water-soluble phosphate into insoluble form. Mixtures of urea and superphosphates or ammonium phosphates and superphosphates should also be avoided. To prevent an increase in hygroscopicity, as a general rule mixtures or blends should always be spread as soon as possible after mixing.

Fertilizers that are to be mixed should also be physically compatible, i.e. they should be of similar granule size and possibly also of similar density to prevent segregation during handling, storing and spreading. This is of particular importance when centrifugal spreading equipment is used. However, segregation is also possible when the mixture is broadcasted by hand.

To avoid mixing errors when preparing the necessary mixture on the farm, the farmer may avail himself of the services of his local fertilizer retailer with a mixing unit (the investment for a mixing or bulk blending installation is usually relatively low). The retailer can prepare individual blends with nutrient ratios tailored to the needs of the farmer's soils and crops. He will know which types of fertilizers can be mixed with each other and which cannot. However, because the farmer is normally unable to check the nutrient content and quality, particularly with fertilizer mixtures or blends, the retailer preparing the blend should be known as trustworthy and reliable.

For determining the quantities of fertilizers from the recommended rates of application N, P or K, or *vice versa*, the following conversion factors (Table 1.12) may be used:

Table 1.12: Conversion factors determining quantities of fertilizers

Quantity	Multiplied by	Gives corresponding quantity of
Nitrogen	4.854	Ammonium sulphate
Nitrogen	2.222	Urea
Nitrogen	3.846	Ammonium sulphate nitrate
Nitrogen	4.000	Ammonium chloride
Nitrogen	3.030	Ammonium nitrate
Phosphoric acid (P_2O_5)	6.250	Superphosphate, single
Phosphoric acid (P_2O_5)	12.222	Superphosphate, double
Phosphoric acid (P_2O_5)	2.857	Dicalcium phosphate
Phosphoric acid (P_2O_5)	5.000	Bonemeal, raw
Potash (K_2O)	1.666	Muriate of potash
Potash (K_2O)	2.000	Sulphate of potash
Ammonium sulphate	0.206	Nitrogen
Sodium nitrate	0.155	Nitrogen
Urea	0.450	Nitrogen
Ammonium sulphate nitrate	0.260	Nitrogen
Ammonium chloride	0.250	Nitrogen
Ammonium nitrate	0.330	Nitrogen
Superphosphate, double	0.450	Phosphoric acid (P_2O_5)
Dicalcium phosphate	0.350	Phosphoric acid (P_2O_5)
Bonemeal, raw	0.200	Phosphoric acid (P_2O_5)
Muriate of potash	0.600	Potash (K_2O)
Sulphate of potash	0.500	Potash (K_2O)

1.20 PRACTICAL RECOMMENDATIONS FOR DIFFERENT CROPS UNDER DIFFERENT SOIL CONDITIONS — CONVENTIONAL AND RECENT ADVANCEMENT BASED ON STCR AND LEAF TISSUE ANALYSIS

Soil Test Crop Response (STCR) Correlation Studies

Interpreted soil test data is the best basis for fertilizer recommendation. But the response of the crop depends on other factor like plant population, crop variety, soil moisture, etc. – many methods were suggested to improve ST interpretations. The all India co-ordinated project for investigation on ST-crop response – started in 1967. The studies have indicated significant regression equation for different soil types for predicting crop response and for preparing suitable fertilizer schedules based on ST data. The purpose of ST crop response studies is securing and selecting the best ST method and the calibration of ST values for fertilizer recommendation – the studies enable to know the type of response curve operating in a set of soil-crop-agro-climaric condition, e.g. of each curves - linear, mitscherlich-bray, sigmoid, etc. – curves are useful to determine fertilizer does to obtain economic yield – different approaches – critical level approach, percentage yield approach, targeted yield/prescription method.

Leaf Tissue Analysis

Of the many factors affecting crop quality and yield, fertility is one of the most important. It is fortunate that producers can control fertility by managing the plant's nutritional status. Nutrient status is an unseen factor in plant growth, except when imbalance become so severe that visual symptoms appear on the plant. The only way to know whether a crop is adequately nourished is to have the plant tissue analyzed during the growing season. Plant tissue analysis shows the nutrient status of plants at the time of sampling. This in turn shows whether soil nutrient supplies are adequate. In addition, plant tissue analysis will detect unseen deficiencies and may confirm visual symptoms of deficiencies. Toxic levels also may be detected. Though usually used as a diagnostic tool for future correction of nutrient problems, plant tissue analysis from young plants will allow a corrective fertilizer application for that same season. Not all abnormal appearances are due to a deficiency. Some may be due to too much of certain elements. Also, symptoms of one deficiency may look like those of another. A plant tissue analysis can pinpoint the cause, if it is nutritional. A plant analysis is of little value if the plants come from fields that are infested with weeds, insects, disease organisms; if the plants are stressed for moisture; or if plants have some mechanical injury. The most important use of plant analysis is as a monitoring tool for determining the adequacy of current fertilization practices. Sampling a crop periodically during the season or once each year provides a record of its nutrient content that can be used through the growing season or from year to year. Corrective measures can be applied during the season or, if the crop is perennial, during the next year. Combined with data from a soil analysis, a tissue analysis is an important tool in determining nutrient requirements of a crop. The elements which can be determined in a plant sample are nitrogen, sulfur, boron, phosphorus, iron, sodium, potassium, copper, chlorine, calcium, zinc, molybdenum, magnesium and manganese. Levels of elements such as cadmium, lead, arsenic, and selenium also can be examined. The most important factor is selection and collection of samples for analysis.

1.21 FERTILIZER EFFICIENCY

At present, India is producing about 250 million tonnes (mt) of foodgrain and the fertilizer consumption has reached an all time high of 30 mt. The one billion plus population in India is increasing at a rate of 2.2%, while the population growth is expected to stabilize only around 2050. Until the population stabilizes, India has to keep producing enough food and other crops matching the population growth rate. Obviously, further increase in fertilizer use will be, among others, a mainstay to reach our target in the next fifty years. Moving productivity upward through fertilizer remains a wide-open option, since current intensity of fertilizer use is relatively low in India as compared to even several developing countries. At the same time, it is imperative that we evolve an efficient, economic and integrated nutrient management system to sustain the productivity of different crops and cropping systems. An efficient nutrient management would minimize loss of nutrients, saving unnecessary input costs. It is appropriate here to mention that efficient nutrient use is essentially an offspring of balanced fertilizer use and sound management practices and decisions. Balanced fertilizer use is not only the first requirement; it is rather a pre-requisite since no amount of agronomic manipulation can produce high efficiency out of an imbalanced fertilizer dose. In contrast, when balanced fertilization is practiced, one nutrient increases the efficiency of others through a synergistic effect.

Nutrient use efficiency can be expressed several ways. Commonly four agronomic indices commonly used to describe nutrient use efficiency: Partial Factor Productivity (PFP, kg crop yield per kg nutrient applied); Agronomic Efficiency (AE, kg crop yield increase per kg nutrient applied); Apparent Recovery Efficiency (RE, kg nutrient taken up per kg nutrient applied); and Physiological Efficiency (PE, kg yield increase per kg nutrient taken up). Crop removal efficiency (removal of nutrient in harvested crop as % of nutrient applied) is also commonly used to explain nutrient efficiency. Available data and objectives determine which term best describes nutrient use efficiency.

Causes for Low and Declining Crop Response to Fertilizers: Crop response to fertilizer during the different five year plan have been presented in Table 1.13.

Table 1.13: Declining crop response to fertilizer

Period	kg food grains per kg nutrients (NPK)	Reasons
5th Plan (1974-79)	15.0	Inadequate and imbalanced fertiliser use, increasing multinutrient deficiency, Lack of farmers awareness about balanced plant nutrition, lack of varietal breakthrough, poor crop management (Excess fertilizer dose not be the substitute of poor management).
8th Plan (1992-97)	7.5	
11th Plan (2007-12)	6.0	
9th Plan (1997-02)	7.0	
10th Plan (2002-07)	6.5	

Nutrient Supply and Soil Fertility

- Continuous use of fertilizer N alone or with inadequate P and K application leading to mining of native soil P and K.
- Continued practice of intensive cropping systems like 'rice-wheat' with high-yielding varieties even under recommended NPK use, impoverishing soils of secondary and micronutrients specially S, Zn, Mn, B and Fe.
- Use of high analysis fertilizers and inadequate addition of organic manures resulting in widespread deficiencies of S and micronutrients.
- Fertilizer application mostly not based on soil-test values.
- Inappropriate time and method of fertilizer application.
- Excessive use of irrigation in rice-wheat cropping system, sugarcane and others.
- Heavily fertilized crops leading to leaching of nitrogen and other plant nutrients.
- Inadequate availability of appropriate kind of fertilizers at the right time.
- Antagonistic reaction between some plant nutrients.
- Low status of soil organic carbon.
- Subsoil impedance to plant root system restricting nutrient uptake.
- Soil degradation due to high salinity/sodicity/acidity/waterlogging, affecting nutrient availability.
- Lack of adequate and quality soil testing facilities and meager availability of fertilizer recommendations under aberrant weather conditions.
- Environmental degradation, having negative impact on below ground biodiversity, especially agriculturally important microorganisms.

Seed

- Non-availability of sufficient seeds of high-yielding varieties of crops at affordable price and at the appropriate time.
- Lack of more efficient nutrient using genotypes.

Agronomic Practices

- Delayed sowings/plantings.
- Low seed rates resulting in poor crop stands.
- Poor weed management.
- Inefficient tillage.
- Inefficient irrigation and rainwater management.
- Large scale monoculture.
- Lack of consideration of previous cropping in the same field.
- Lack of capturing water-nutrient synergic interaction.
- Inadequate plant protection.

Weather Aberrations

- High intensity rain leading to nutrient loss.
- Abnormal high/low temperature.

Measures to Increase the Efficiency of Fertilizer Use

Soil testing: It is critical to test the soil to determine the level of soil nutrients. Soil testing also provides information about the soil's pH and organic matter content. Knowledge of the soil characteristics will help optimize the use of fertilizers. Once the nutrient level of the soil is known, only use the amount of soil additives necessary to amend the soil to the required level. If some fields associated with a given farm have low fertility, while others have high fertility, only fertilize the fields with low fertility, rather than fertilizing all fields equally. It is typically recommended that soil testing be done in one to four-year intervals on all crops.

Maintenance of soil pH: The pH of a soil is a determining factor for the availability of plant nutrients. In most cases, a fairly neutral soil pH in the range of 6.0 to 7.5 is desirable for maximum nutrient availability, particularly for the primary nutrients of nitrogen, phosphorus, and potassium. However, different nutrients have greater availability at different pH levels. For example, minor nutrients such as iron, copper, and zinc are more available in acidic soils, whereas those such as calcium and magnesium are more available in moderately alkaline soils. The pH of acidic soils can be raised to the neutral level by liming with minerals such as dolomite and calcite. Basic soils can be made more acidic by adding iron and sulfur fertilizers, or acidic organic materials such as pine needles. It is generally more cost-effective to raise the pH than to reduce it.

Use of high-analysis fertilizers: It is less energy-intensive to use high-analysis fertilizers. These fertilizers contain a larger fraction of nutrients per volume, resulting in lower transportation, storage, and handling requirements than for fertilizers that are not as nutrient rich. This applies both to individual chemical compounds and to formulated fertilizers. For example, some compounds are more nutrient-rich than their alternatives (e.g. ammonium nitrate contains about 60% more nitrogen than ammonium sulfate). In addition, some formulated fertilizers use less filler material to achieve a given ratio of ingredients. Therefore, per unit weight, high-analysis fertilizers contain more energy.

Using known and reliable products: New fertilizer products are constantly coming to the market. It is prudent to avoid the use of newer products until they become well established. Instead of rushing to purchase the latest innovation, conduct research to find out what products and practices are proven and recommended for the particular soil type and crop, and then implement the proven technologies.

Application of fertilizers efficiently: One of the most important methods for increasing fertilization efficiency is to apply the appropriate amount of nutrients in the required location. Efficient fertilizer application is accomplished by distributing the fertilizer uniformly in the needed area. Too much fertilizer in a given area results in waste. If feasible, consider band application of fertilizer in place of broadcasting. This will lower fertilizer requirements. In addition, if possible, combine the application of fertilizer with other tillage tasks to reduce the number of passes on the field. For example, it is more efficient to apply starter fertilizer during the planting or drilling stage than it is to apply it by broadcasting. It is also very important to make sure fertilizers are applied so that they are incorporated in the rooting zone.

Application of fertilizers at the appropriate time: Plants will utilize nutrients more efficiently if the nutrients are applied at the correct point in the plants' growing cycle. In particular, phosphorus should be applied early on as a nutrient for seedling development, and nitrogen application should be timed so that the nitrogen enters the rooting zone at the optimum time for the specific crop. Proper timing will increase yields and reduce fertilizer energy use. Another benefit of proper timing is that the plants will more likely be able to assimilate the nutrients before nutrient leaching and volatilization occur.

Application of fertilizers through irrigation system: In some cases it may be feasible to add nutrients to irrigation water. This will hasten the transport of nutrients to the root zone, but over-irrigation could result in the loss of nutrients to leaching.

Mulching: If cost-effective, the use of mulch provides many benefits to crops. In addition to keeping the ground temperature cooler and reducing evaporation, it can lessen nutrient volatilization. The application of plastic, or similar, mulch will also reduce nutrient leaching in times of heavy rainfall.

Crop rotation: Legume crops are capable of nitrogen fixation, and therefore they can restore the nitrogen level in the soil if their waste products are tilled back into the ground. It is very effective to rotate non-legume crops (which depend heavily on nitrogen) with legume crops to reduce the requirement for nitrogen fertilizer amendment. Generally, annual legumes do not leave behind as much nitrogen as biennial or perennial varieties. It is also important to note that more nitrogen is added to the soil for unharvested legume crops; nevertheless a benefit is still achieved from harvested crops. For farmers who do not want to lose a cash crop, a good legume choice might be soybeans, as the soybeans can be sold, and the residual plant material can be incorporated into the soil for a lesser nitrogen benefit. Another alternative is 'interplanting', in which alternate rows of legumes and the cash crop are planted. In this scenario the benefits of a cash crop and legume crop are combined. However, interplanting is more labor-intensive and complicated. Legumes are also useful as cover crops. They can be planted in summer, and then tilled in during the spring to serve as a nitrogen source for a subsequent crop. One limitation of cover crops is that the timing for the second crop may not be optimal.

Utilization of organic residues and waste: Animal and other types of organic wastes can provide a very good source for soil nutrients. In addition to their nutritional benefits, organic waste fertilizers also improve the soil's quality by increasing its water-holding capacity, filtration, aeration, and soil aggregation. One downside of organic fertilizers is that they contain fewer nutrients per unit weight than inorganic fertilizer, and the nutritional content is often less characterized.

Depending on their source, they may also contain heavy metals, soluble salts, weed seeds, and other undesirable contents. In many cases the use of organic fertilizers, augmented with inorganic nutrients as needed, is an energy-efficient and cost-effective alternative. However, if the distances between the source of organic material, the composting plant, and the end-use location are large, the costs associated with transporting and applying the wastes may outweigh the benefits of reduced chemical fertilizer use.

A number of nutrient management practices are used to enhance fertilizer use efficiency and reduce nutrient losses into the environment. These practices include:

- Assessing nutrient need through annual or regular soil and plant tissue testing before applying nutrients, in contrast to limited or no testing before applying nutrients. Soil testing identifies the amount of nutrients already available for plant uptake, and is used to identify the additional amounts of nutrients needed to meet a realistic yield goal. A plant tissue nitrogen test uses chlorophyll (or greenness) sensing to detect nitrogen deficiency during the growing season to assist in assessing the need for additional commercial fertilizer applications. Correction of any nitrogen deficiency is then made through chemigation or other foliar application.

- Timing nutrient application to tailor feeding to plant-growth needs, for example, split application of nitrogen fertilizer into at planting and after planting, in contrast to fall and early spring applications of nitrogen before planting.

- Applying nutrients close to the root zone so they are more readily accessible to the plant, through banded and injected applications and chemigation, in contrast to ground and air broadcast and application in the furrow. With side-dressing or banded application, granule or liquid nitrogen fertilizer is placed to one side of the plant or placed every other row at planting or during the growing season.

- Selecting the nutrient product according to the chemical stability in the soil, in order to minimize nutrient loss to the environment. For example, use an ammonia-based fertilizer on fields with high leaching soils, and a nitrate-based fertilizer on fields where ammonia volatilization is a problem.

- Rotating nitrogen-using with nitrogen-fixing crops. Cover crops are planted between crop seasons to tie up and preserve nutrients, in contrast to continuous planting of the same nitrogen-using crop and not planting any cover crops.

- Applying manure and organic waste based on manure and waste test results and nutrient management plan. Adequate storage is available for manure so that applications will mesh with plant nutrient needs and applications are injected or incorporated into the soil.

- Using nitrogen inhibitors and other products to slow the release of nitrates from ammonium fertilizers until later in the growing season, by delaying the conversion of ammonium nitrogen into nitrate nitrogen, which is susceptible to leaching. N-inhibitors can also be used with manure and other forms of organic nitrogen fertilizer.

- Urease inhibitors—Chemical compounds that can be added to urea to slow the conversion of urea to ammonium and therefore to slow nitrate leaching.
- Slow-release nitrogen fertilizer—Fertilizer coated with chemicals that can retard release of nitrogen from applied fertilizer and prolong the supply of nitrogen for plant uptake.
- Refraining from broadcasting nitrogen fertilizer, or if broadcast, incorporating the product into the soil, which reduces the losses of nitrogen to the atmosphere. Certain nitrogen products, especially urea, are subject to extensive volatilization when broadcast. Certain nitrogen products are injected or knifed-in, usually 12–24 cm below the soil surface. Nitrogen can also be incorporated into the soil by tillage. High-pressure liquid nitrogen such as anhydrous ammonia is the most common form of nitrogen injected into the soil. Nitrogen solutions in low-pressure liquid form are also injected into the soil.
- Applying all nitrogen at and/or after planting, when the demand by the crop is greatest, which reduces the risk of nitrogen loss through leaching. Conversely, applying all nitrogen in the fall can increase the risk of leaching, under certain soil and weather conditions.

Role of Enhanced Efficiency (EE) Fertilizers to Improve Fertilizer use Efficiency by Crops

Fertilizer products with characteristics that minimize the potential of nutrient losses to the environment, as compared to reference soluble products. These products have traditionally been used in specialty horticulture applications (e.g. turf, ornamentals, etc.). Over the past few years these products have been gaining in use and popularity in production agriculture.

Enhanced N Efficiency

- Synthetic organic compounds containing N: These can be further divided into biologically decomposing compounds usually based on urea-aldehyde condensation products, such as urea-formaldehyde (UF), and chemically (mainly) decomposing compounds, such as isobutyledenediurea (IBDU).
- Physical coating or barrier around soluble N fertilizer, such as SCU, NCU, LCU, PCU.
- Mechanisms of N release
- Pin holes, cracks
- Microbial degradation
- Is the result of the average behavior of many particles
- Factors affecting N release
- Coating thickness and uniformity
- Effective coating thickness is equal to thinnest area of coating

- Temperature
- Moisture
- Stabilized materials
- Nitrification inhibitors interfere with activity of *Nitrosomonas* bacteria, slowing the nitrification process.This leaves more N in ammoniacal form, thus reducing the chance of leaching and denitrification
  - e.g. nitrification and urease inhibitors

Some patented nitrification inhibitors are:

Chemical name	Common name	Inhibition by day 14 %
2-chloro-6-(trichloromethyl) pyridine	ATC N Serve	82
4-Amino-1, 2, 4, 6-triazole-HCl	CL-1580	78
2, 4-Diamino-6-trichloromethyltriazine	DCD	65
Dicyandiamide	TU	53
Thiourea	MT	41
1-Mercapto-1, 2, 4-triazole	AM	32
2-Amino-4-chloror-6-methylpyrimidine	AM	31

- Urease inhibitors interfere with the process of urea hydrolysis. The slowing of conversion of urea to ammoniacal N can significantly reduce the potential for NH_3 volatilization.

Potential benefits of EE fertilizers include:
- Match the kinetics of nutrient release with the kinetics of plant growth.
- Improved yields.
- More applied nutrient used by plant.
- Reduction in nutrient loss (leaching, atmospheric, soil reactions, etc.).
- Reduced application frequency.
- More uniform plant growth.

Future Prospects

India's foodgrain requirement to feed the estimated population of 1400 million by 2025 will be 300 million tonnes. There will be a corresponding increase in requirement of other crops such as cotton, sugarcane, fruits and vegetables. The country will require about 45 million tonne of nutrients (30 million tonnes for foodgrains and 15 million tonnes of nutrients for other crops) from various sources of plant nutrients, i.e. fertilizers, organic manures and biofertilizers. The further increase in crop production will have to come from an increase in yields as there is limited scope for increasing cultivated area. The yields of the majority of the crops are relatively low and there is great potential for increasing them through the increased use of inputs such as fertilizers. Fertilizer use will remain key to the future development of agriculture. The handling of increasing quantities of fertilizers will put pressure on storage and handling facilities and transport. Products and practices that improve fertilizer-use efficiency will need special encouragement and enthusiasm. Fertilizer promotion from both private and public sector will have to include activities that promote not only increased rates of use but also better balances between the nutrients and higher efficiency. Attention also needs to focus on the availability of credit, an essential factor in ensuring the availability of fertilizers to farmers. India will continue to be a major importer of raw materials, intermediates as well as finished products. The fertilizer product pattern is unlikely to change in the near future, and urea and DAP will continue to dominate fertilizer production. Attention will need to focus on ensuring the availability of good-quality micronutrient fertilizers and availability of macronutrient fetilizers at government fixed rate during the main crop season.

2

Organic Manures

2.1 HISTORY

The Roman literature 'Ruralium commodorum libri duodecim' compiled by a senator of Bologna, Petrus Crescentius about the year 1240 was one of the most popular treaties on agriculture of any time (Augsburg, 1471). The Roman literature is considered as the foundation to the large standard European treatises of the sixteenth and seventeenth centuries. It had been a maxim with the older agricultural chemist that 'Corruption is the mother of vegetation'. van Helmont (1577–1644) regarded water as the sole nutrient for plants. Glauber JR (1656) set up the hypothesis that saltpeter is the 'Principle of vegetation'. The early investigators (1630–1750) sought for the Principle of vegetation to account soil fertility and plant growth phenomenon. Many of the agricultural writings of the seventeenth and eighteenth centuries reflected the idea that plants were composed of one substance, and most of the workers during this period were searching for this principle of vegetation.

Great interest in the search for plant nutrients was taken in agriculture in Europe during the latter half of the eighteenth century (the Phologistic period, 1750–1800). Some of the important treatises during this period are 'Horse Hoeing Husbandry', London 1731 and 'The Principle of agriculture and vegetation, Edinburgh, 1757. Theodore de Saussure's 'Researches Chimiques sur la vegetation' Paris, 1804 on quantitative experimental methods was the basis of subsequent modern agricultural chemistry work by Boussingault, Liebig, Lawes and Gilbert. The middle of the nineteenth to the twentieth century was a time during which much progress was made in the understanding of plant nutrition and crop fertilization. Among the men of this period who made significant contribution are JB Boussingault and J Von Liebig. JB Boussingault was the first to introduce field experiments methods (1834), which was the foundation of agricultural science. Liebig is considered as the father of the mineral nutrition theory of plants. In 1840, Liebig's famous report 'Chemistry in its Application to Agriculture and Physiology' was published, which afterwards (1843) became known as the Law of the Minimum. The essence of the law is, by the deficiency or absence of one necessary constituent, all the others being present, the soil is rendered barren for all those crop to the life of which that one constituent is indispensable. Liebig's two laws – the law of minimum and the law of complete return can be considered as the origin of soil fertility, plant nutrition and fertilizer use in agriculture. The first law states the yields of field crops reduce or increase in the exact proportion to the reduction or increment in the quantity of minerals applied to the soil in the form of fertilizer. The essence of the *law of complete return* reveals that the soil must get back everything that has been taken away from it.

Meanwhile the great field experiments at Rothamsted had been started by Lawes and Gilbert in 1843. During the 1860s and 1870s great advances were being made in the field of bacteriology. Warrington (1878) had been investigating the role of nitrates in the soil process and found that there were two stages and two distinct organisms: the ammonia was first converted into nitrite and then to nitrate. But he failed to obtain the organisms responsible for the process. Winogradsky (1890), however, isolated these two groups of organism showing they were bacteria. Beijerinck (1888) was successful in isolating *Bacillus radicicola*, now known as *Rhizobium*. The physical, chemical and biological factors that control the fertility of soils have advanced greatly in twentieth century. The application of this knowledge has resulted increases in crop productivity.

Important advances made in twentieth century have resulted from the application of new methodologies like X-ray analysis for understanding crystalline structures of layered aluminosilicate minerals, spectrographic analyses on the distribution of micronutrients. The forms of nutrient reserves on soils, their mobility and availabilities, dynamics of nutrients applied through fertilizers, radioisotopes study, thermodynamic concepts and kinetics to the solubility of nutrient ions has continued through 20th century. Schofield's ratio law (1947), the use of Quantity (Q) and intensity (I) factors further advanced our understanding on ion exchange relationship in soil-plant system. The identification of nutrient deficiencies and the need for fertilizers were considerably advanced by studies of deficiency symptoms in plants. The management of soil has been much improved as a result of scientific work in the last century.

Manure: It is organic matter used as fertilizer in agriculture. Manures contribute to the fertility of the soil by adding organic matter and essential nutrients, such as nitrogen, phosphorus, potash and micronutrients that are required for growth and development of plants in the soil.

The word *manure* came from Middle English *"manuren"* meaning "to cultivate land", and initially from French word *"main-oeuvre"* meaning "hand work" addressing to the work which involved manuring land. Ronald Fisher seems to have used the word manure systematically for what we would call fertilizer today.

There are two main classes of manures in soil management: green manures and animal manures. Compost is distinguished from manure in that it is the decomposed remnants of organic materials (which may, nevertheless, include manure).

Most animal manure is feces — excrement of plant-eating mammals (herbivores) and poultry — or plant material (often straw) which has been used as bedding for animals and thus is heavily contaminated with their feces and urine.

Green manures are crops grown for the express purpose of plowing them under the soil. In doing so, the fertility of the soil is increased through the addition of nutrients and organic matter of the green plant that are added to the soil. Leguminous crops, such as peas and beans, also "fix" nitrogen through *rhizobia* bacteria in specialized nodes in the root structure.

Uses of Manure

Manure has been used for centuries as a fertilizer for farming, as it is rich in nitrogen and other nutrients which facilitate the growth of plants. Liquid manure from pig/and other animals are usually buried (applied) directly into the soil to reduce the unpleasant odors. Due to the relatively lower level of proteins in grasses, which herbivores eat, cattle manure has a milder smell than the dung of carnivores — for example, elephant dung is practically odorless. However, due to the quantity of manure applied to fields, odor can be a problem in some agricultural regions. Poultry droppings are harmful to plants when added fresh but after a period of time are valuable fertilizers. The dried manure of animals has been used as fuel throughout history. Dried manure (usually known as dung) of cow was, and still is, an important fuel source in countries such as India, while camel dung may be used in treeless regions such as deserts. It has been used for many purposes, in cooking fires and to combat the cold desert nights. Another use of manure is to make paper, this has been done with dung from elephants where it is a small industry in Africa and Asia, and also horses, llamas, and kangaroos. Other than the llama, these animals are not ruminants and thus tend to pass plant fibres undigested in their dung. Livestock manure is traditionally a key fertilizer in organic and sustainable soil management. It is most effectively used in combination with other sustainable practices. These include crop rotation, cover cropping, green manuring, liming, and the addition of other natural or biologically friendly fertilizers and amendments. In organic production, manure is commonly applied to the field in either a raw (fresh or dried) or composted state. There are clear restrictions on the use of raw manure in organic farming. These restrictions are detailed in the national organic program (NOP) regulations, which constitute the federal standard for organic production.

2.2 RAW MATERIALS

2.2.1 Crop Residues

There is no published data on straw/stover yield of different crops at National level. The department of economics and statistics, Ministry of agriculture, Govt. of India only reports district-wise grain yield of crops. Therefore, grain: straw ratios of different crops have been used to compute straw and stover yields of crops. The availability of crop residues have been estimated to be 355.7 million tonnes (based on 1995–96 crop yield data) by the project directorate of cropping systems research, Modipuram (PDCSR, 1996).

- Three-fourth of total residues is produced by rice, wheat and oilseed crops. The remaining one-fourth are sugarcane and sorghum.
- A sizeable portion of crop residues, i.e. about two third is fed to animals in India only remaining one third is available for incorporation into the soils.
- Out of the available residues for incorporation, 53% are available in kharif and rest 47% in rabi season.
- In kharif, half of residues are available from rice followed by groundnut (18%), soyabean (7%), pearl millet (6%) and maize(6%). Likewise in rabi, wheat contributed 42% followed by sugarcane (30%) and rapeseed and mustard (15%).
- The availability of crop residues in India would be 300, 343 and 496 million tonnes in 2000, 2010 and 2025, respectively, as per the projection. The possible nutrients (N+P₂O₅+K₂O) would be of the order of 2.05, 2.34 and 3.39 million tonnes in the respective periods.
- Out of the total organic residues produced, crop residues comprised about 70%, animal residues about 23%, logging and wood manufacturing wastes about 5% and each of other groups less than 1%.

Composition of plant residues: –

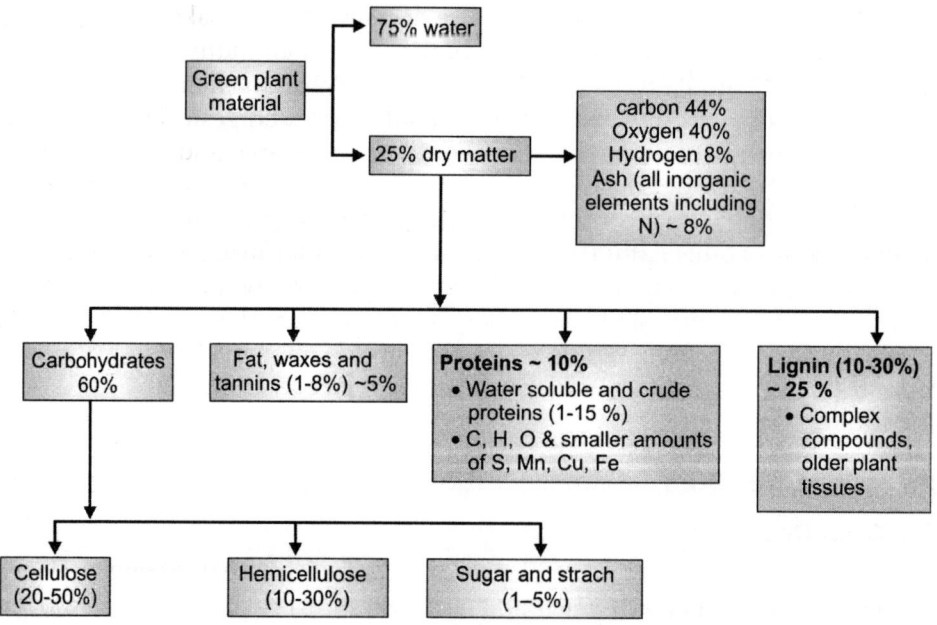

Fig. 2.1: Schematic presentation of composition of green plant materials added to soils

The moisture content of plant residues is high, varying from 60 to 90% with 75% on an average, the schematic is shown in Fig. 2.1. On the weight basis, the dry matter is mostly carbon and oxygen, with less than 10% each of hydrogen and inorganic elements (ash); however, on an elemental basis (number of atoms of the elements), hydrogen predominates. In representative plant residues, there are 8 H atoms for every 3.7 C and 2.5 O atoms. These 3 elements dominate the bulk of organic tissue in soil.

Composition of animal residues:

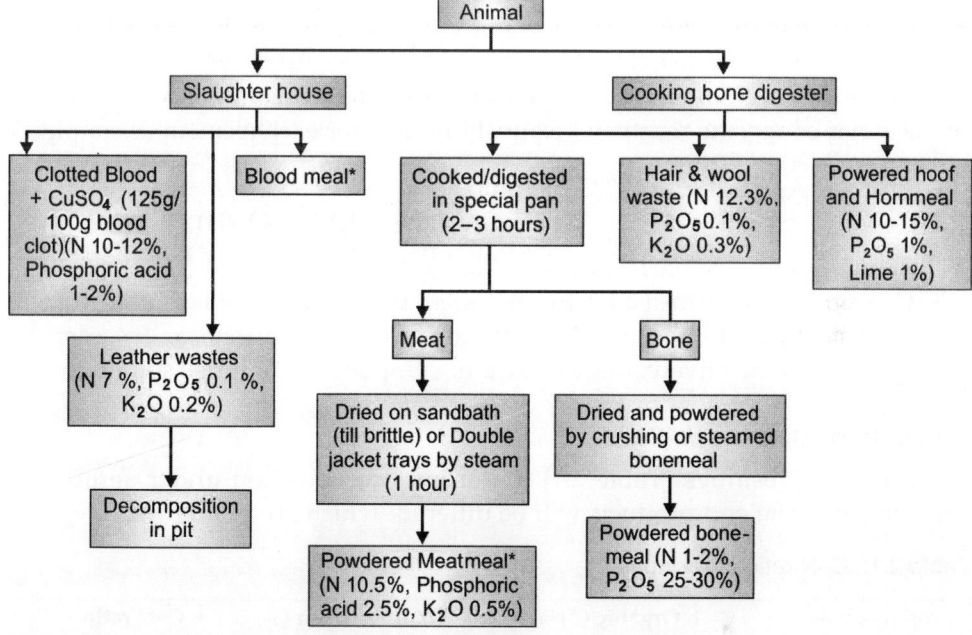

* Quick acting manure and effective for all the crops in all soil types

Fig. 2.2. Schematic presentation of elemental composition of animal residues

Animal residues (Fig. 2.2) have relatively higher amount of nutrient element (nitrogen, phosphorus, sulphur etc.). Besides these, it is quick acting when incorported in soils.

2.3 DECOMPOSITION OF PLANT RESIDUES

Organic compounds in crop residues vary greatly in their rate of decomposition. They may be listed in terms of ease of decomposition as follows:

Components	Order of decomposition
1. Sugar, starch and simple proteins	Rapid decomposition
2. Crude protein	
3. Hemicellulose	
4. Cellulose	
5. Fats, waxes, etc.	
6. Lignin	Very slow decomposition

When organic tissue of green plant materials are added to the soils, three general reactions take place:

1. The bulk of the material undergoes enzymatic oxidation with carbon dioxide, water, energy and heat as the major products

$$(C, 4H) + 2O_2 \xrightarrow{\text{Enzymatic oxidation}} CO_2 + 2H_2O + energy$$

(in well-aerated soil)   (more than 2/3 of the residues, 60–80% oxidizes to carbon dioxide)

2. The essential elements such as N, P and S are released and/or immobilized by a series of specific reactions relatively unique for each element. Example:

Protein $\xrightarrow{\text{Enzymatic reaction}}$ Amino acids $\longrightarrow$ NH_4^+

e.g. Glycine (CH_2NH_2COOH) NO_3^-

Cysteine ($CH_2HSCHNH_2COOH$) SO_4^-

3. Compounds very resistant to microbial actions are formed either through modification of compounds in the original plant tissue or by microbial synthesis. Collectively, theses resistant compounds comprise soil humus.

Products of Decomposition

When organic residues (Table 2.1) undergo decomposition under aerobic and anaerobic soil, the end products will be different which are as follows:

Table 2.1: C–N ratio of residues

Crop residues	Organic C (%)	Total nitrogen (%)	C–N ratio
Alfalfa (very young)	40	3	13:1
Corn stalks	40	1	40:1
Straw	40	0.5	80:1
Sawdust	45	0.2	225:1
Paddy straw	–	–	22.8:1

Well aerated soil (aerobic condition)	Waterlogged soil (anaerobic condition)
CO_2	CH_4 (swamp gas), CS_2 (carbon bisulfide)
NH_4^+, NO_3^-	Organic acid (R-COOH) e.g. butyric acid
$H_2PO_4^-$	NH_4^+
SO_4^-	Amine residues (R-NH_2)
H_2O	H_2S (toxic hydrogen sulfide)
Numerous other essential plant nutrient elements in small quantities	Ethylene ($H_2C{=}CH_2$)
Resistant residues	Resistant humus residues

2.4 TECHNIQUES OF FARM RESIDUE UTILIZATION

2.4.1 Farm Yard Manure

- Commonly used organic manure
- Readily available
- Important agricultural by-products

Advantages

- Ability to improve the soil, tilts and aeration.
- Increases the water-holding capacity of the soil.
- Stimulate activity of microorganisms that made plant food elements in the soil readily to crops.

This is the traditional manure and is mostly readily available to the farmers. Farm yard manure is a decomposed mixture of cattle dung and urine with straw and litter used as bedding material and residues from the fodder fed to the cattle. The waste material of cattle shed consisting of dung and urine soaked in the refuse of the shade is collected daily and placed in trenches about 6–7 m long, 1.5–2 m broad and 1 m deep. Each trench is filled upto a height of about 0.5 m above the ground level. The top of the heap is to be made dome-shaped and plastered over with cow dung earth slurry. It becomes ready to apply after 3–4 months. By this process it is possible to prepare 7–8.5 cubic meter of manure (5–6 tonnes or 10–12 cart loads) per year per head of cattle. Well-rotten farm yard manure contains 0.4 to 1.5 per cent N, 0.3–0.9 % P_2O_5 and 0.3–1.9% K_2O. Animal and cow dung from biogas are also used in similar manner.

2.4.2 Composts

There are two groups of compost:

- Rural Compost
- Town or Urban Compost

Composting is a process of reducing vegetable and animal waste to a quickly utilizable condition for improving and maintaining soil fertility. These are produced through the action of microorganisms on wastes. Wastes may be leaves, roots and stubbles, crop residues, straw, hedge clippings, weeds, water hyacinth, saw dust, kitchen wastes and human habitation wastes.

The waste materials undergo intensive decomposition under medium-high temperatures in heaps or pits with adequate moisture. There are two types of composting process, that are discussed below:

Time required: 3–6 months

Finished Product (Compost): An amorphous, brown to dark brown humified material.

Optimum value of different parameters for compost (based on analysis) is given below:

Parameters	Optimum Value
C–N ratio of feed	25 to 35
Particle size	10 mm for agitated systems and forced aeration, 50 mm for long heaps and natural aeration.
Moisture content	50 to 60%
Temperature	55 to 60 °C held for 3 days
Agitation	No agitation to periodic turning in simple systems and short burst of vigorous agitation in mechanized system.
pH control	Normally not necessary
Heap size	Any length, 1.5 m high and 2.5 m wide for heaps using natural aeration. With forced aeration heap size depends on need to avoid overheating.
Activator	Use of efficient cellulolyotic, fungi and bio-fertilizers

Types of Composting

Aerobic

The used bedding, the sweeping from cattle shed and some urine soaked earth from the stable floor are removed every day, mixed with cattle dung and two or three handfuls of wood ash are deposited on a well drained site to gradually build up a low pile, about 30 to 45 cm in height, about 5 cm in width and of any convenient length. The pile is built up before the start of the rainy season. After the first heavy showers, the welted material in a 1.2 m strip of each side of the long heap is tuned with a rake on to a 2.4 m wide strip in the middle, thus raising the height of the heap to nearly 1 meter. This process prevents a loss of moisture and ensures a quick start of decomposition. When the heap sinks appreciably and such a sinking takes about three to four weeks, it is given a turning and made into a fresh heap, thus mixing outside material with that from inside. After about a month or more, depending on the incidence of rains the heap is given a final turning on a cloudy or modernity rainy day & rebuilt with in vacant parts of original position. The compost becomes ready for use in about four months.

Anaerobic

The mixed farm residues are collected in pits of a convenient size, say, and 4.5 m × 1.5 m × 1 m. Each day's collection is spread in a thin layer, sprinkled with a mixture of fresh cow dung (4.5 kg), ash (140 to 170 g) and water (18 to 22 liters) and compacted. The pit is filled till the raw material stands 30 to 46 cm above its edge and is then plastered with a 2.5 cm layer of a mixture of mud and cow dung. Under such conditions decomposition is anaerobic and high temperature does not develop. Insoluble nitrogen compound gradually become soluble and carbonaceous matter is broken down into carbon dioxide and water. The loss of ammonia is negligible, because of high concentration of carbon dioxide. The plastered pit also prevents the fly nuisance. The compacted, moist materials become compost in about four to five months without any further attention. The well made compost contains 0.8% to 1% nitrogen and holds all good property of FYM.

2.4.2.1 Factors Affecting the Rate of Composting

1. **Availability of air:** Two composting procedures are available. Anaerobic (lack of oxygen) composting is slow but requires very little management input. Manure piled outside will compost over a period of time. The procedure will require a year or more, and the results may not be uniform. Aerobic composting requires that the material be exposed to air on a regular basis. This is accomplished by turning the material 1 to 3 times per week. Aerobic composting is much faster than anaerobic composting and may require 30 to 60 days to complete. Equipment alternatives for aerating the material include a front-end loader, rototiller or mechanical aerator.

2. **Moisture level:** Composting material should be 40 to 60% moisture. The material will feel wet but not soggy. Care must be taken to not add too much water as soluble nutrients will be lost and surface and ground water contamination could occur. If properly managed, composting can be done outdoors on well drained sandy soil, on a concrete slab or on a concrete floor under a roof.

3. **Particle size:** The smaller the particle size, the more efficient the composting procedure will be. Therefore, grinding may be appropriate for some types of materials. However, more frequent aeration may be necessary for smaller particle sizes.

4. **Temperature:** Microbial metabolic activity will generate considerable heat. The center of the pile may reach 130 °C to 160 °C. This heat is advantageous to the rate of composting and will destroy many life forms present in the material including plant seeds, parasite larvae and eggs, and some bacteria. Heat must be controlled since low moisture materials could ignite if they are in contact with hot compost.

5. **Carbon/nitrogen ratio:** Organisms require nitrogen for multiplication. Since some bedding materials are very low in nitrogen, additional nitrogen should be added to maximize decomposition rate. A C–N ratio of 15 to 30 will allow maximum fermentation rates. Organic nitrogen sources such as cottonseed meal grass clippings or additional manure can be added as a nitrogen source or inorganic nitrogen sources such as urea can be used.

6. **pH:** The composting of some materials may produce acids that lower the pH and stop the process. This is normally not a problem with livestock wastes, unless an unusual bedding material is used. The addition of ground limestone as a buffering agent will correct the problem. Composting systems that are part of a horse farm or a nursery are generally considered to be an agricultural activity. If composting is a primary business, it is usually considered to be a manufacturing activity and appropriate land use regulations must be followed.

Regardless of the type of operation, the site selected should minimize the possibility of ground or surface water contamination. Properly managed, a composting site should not produce fly or odor problems. However, visual impact may not be very favorable, so it should be screened from public view.

2.4.3 GREEN MANURING

- Improves soil fertility.
- Supply a part of nutrient requirement of crops (particularly N).
- Green manure refers to fresh matter added to the soil largely for supplying the nutrient contained in the bio-mass.
- This can either be grown in sites and incorporated or grown else where and brought in for incorporation in the field to be manured.
- Any plant cannot be used as a green manure in practical farming.
- Leguminous plant are largely used as green manure due to their symbiotic N fixing capacity, some non-leguminous plants are also used due to local availability, drought tolerance, quick growth and adaptation to adverse conditions.

An ideal green manure should possess the following traits:

- Show early establishment, high seedling vigor.
- Tolerant to drought, shade, flood and adverse temperature.
- Possesses early onset of N fixation and its efficient sustenance.
- Ability to accumulate large biomass and N in 4–6 weeks.
- Easy to incorporate.
- Quickly decomposable.
- Tolerant to pest and diseases.

It is the practice for enriching the soil by ploughing or burying into soil undecomposed green plant tissues for the purpose of improving structure and fertility of the soil. Generally sunhemp (*Crotalaria juncea*), dhaincha (*Sesbania aculeata*), guar (*Cyamopsis tetragonoloba*), glyricidia (*Glyricidia maculata*), karanj (*Pongamia pinnata*), etc. are used as green manures. Legume crops, leaves of bushes and trees is buried in the soil and allowed to decompose in the field. Macro and microorganisms decompose the organic matter and develop a well-balanced soil biota which fixed minerals in soil matrix. It increases water-holding capacity and organic colloids in soil.

1. Green manuring is the practice in which leguminous plants are grown, particularly in the monsoon, before sowing of crops and the succulent tender plants are ploughed into the soil and allowed to decompose *in situ* under favorable soil moisture conditions.
2. In this process, some organic matter and nitrogen are added to the soil.

3. The most commonly grown green manure crops are *Sesbania aculeate* (Dhaincha) and *Crotalaria juncea* (Sunhemp).

4. The common green manuring crops have potential to provide 4–5 t/ha dry biomass and 80–100 kg of N/ha within 50–60 days of plant growth.

5. Green manuring also helps in accelerating the decomposition of high C–N ratio residues (e.g. straws along with green manuring has been shown to produce rice yield similar or higher than that obtained with application of 150 kg N/ha).

6. Nitrogen supplied through green manure crops is readily available to the subsequent crops because of its low C–N ratio and easy mineralization. Apparent recovery of green manure N in different crops varies from 30 to 58%.

7. There are three possible ways of green manuring practice
   a. Sowing green manuring crop before main crop e.g. Rice - Dhaincha – Wheat.
   b. Inter-space green manuring, e.g. Caster (long duration crop): inter-space, 90 cm. Cowpea (40–45 days): leguminous crop in interspaces and then turned into soil.
   c. Green leaf manuring: e.g. as agro-forestry system.

Annual crop (Sorghum) - Annual crop - Perennial tree (*Leucaena leucocephala*)

When loppings, approximating 9.45 tonnes/ha green biomass of *Leucaena leucocephala* is green manured, around 75.1, 2.9 and 2.6 kg of N, P and K per hectare soil is replenished per annum respectively.

For *in situ* decomposition, adequate soil moisture, either rainfall or by irrigation is essential. Water is a valuable input in Indian agriculture. Thus, availability of water turns out to be the limiting factor in green manuring.

2.5 BIOWASTE

2.5.1 Agricultural Wastes

Waste generated during processing of agricultural products can be advantageously recycled to soil for improving nutrient availability. These bio-solids and liquid wastes can be converted to valuable manures for supplementing the nutrients and organic matter requirements of the crops.

2.5.1.1 Sugar Industry Waste

- Sugar industry is one of the largest agro-based industries in India.
- The release of *bagasse* as a by-product from the sugar industry is about 30% of the weight of cane crushed. From the sugar factories alone, there is possibility of collecting about 45 Mt of *bagasse*. It can be recycled as nutrient for plant and also can be utilized for the paper/pulp industries, manufacture of particle board, used as fuel in high pressure boilers and also for power generation in India.

- The other type of waste material obtained from sugarcane is *sugarcane trash*. Instead of burning the sugarcane trash in the field, it can be efficiently composted using *Trichoderma viride* and *Pleurotus sojar – caju* by adopting bio-conversion technology and used as organic manure.

- Processing of cane in sugar mills result into production of solid waste known as *press mud*. The press mud has potential to supply nutrients particularly S and Ca and organic matter provided technology of co-composting is utilized for their conversion into valuable manures.

- Fermentation of molasses in distillery industry result into production of liquid waste known as *spent wash*. The molasses are used in the distillery industry for every litre of alcohol produced about 15 liters of spent wash is released as waste water. There is a possibility of getting about 10–11 billion liters of waste water from distillery industries alone. About 700 million liters of alcohol is produced annually from the molasses obtained from sugar industries. All such waste materials are to be processed systematically and scientifically for profitable utilization and resource sustainability.

2.5.1.2   Plantation Crops Waste

Plantation and spices crops are important commercial crops (coconut, areca nut, cocoa, cardamom, cashew, tea, coffee, shade trees in tea, coffee), etc. grown in Assam, Kerala, Karnataka, Tamil Nadu and other parts of India. Large quantities of bio-degradable waste, viz. coir pith, coir dust, husk, dried leaves, pruning twigs, coffee husk, tea waste, oil-palm waste, etc., are available for recycling of organic matter through composting and to replenish nutrients. Recycling of these wastes after composting (inoculate: spawn of *Pleurotus sojar – caju*, available as bottle form (250 g bottle) has potential to supplement the nutrient requirements of crops.

2.5.1.3   Fruits and Vegetables Waste

- India produces around 33 million tones of fruits and 50 million tones of vegetables annually. It is estimated that roughly 10 to 15% of total produce in available either as residues or bio-degradable wastes for recycling in agriculture.

- Processing of fruits and vegetables results in the production of around 5 millions tones of solid wastes.

- Most of these wastes are ligno-cellulose in nature and contain macro and micronutrients.

- Mushroom production in India has registered a phenomenal growth during the last decade with current production ranging between 30,000 to 35,000 tonnes. Spent mushroom waste is half decomposed material having high nutrient concentration. These wastes provide good quality manure for agriculture.

2.5.1.4 Poultry Waste

It is also valuable organic manure. It contains about 0.5 to 0.7% N, 0.4 to 0.6% P_2O_5 and 0.3–1.0% K_2O. It is effective to all types of crops.

- Poultry industry has achieved significant growth in the last two decades. Presently there are about 60,000 poultry farms producing 450 millions broilers and 30 billion eggs.
- Poultry sector also generates poultry manures and hatchery wastes of high economic value. It is estimated that the fertilizers value of poultry manure from 3 birds on deep tiller is superior in terms of nutrients content value compared to manure from one cow.
- Average daily fresh manure production from broilers ranges between 70–80 kg/1000 kg live weights.
- Poultry manure and litter contain high amounts of N<P and other nutrients (N, 3.5%, P 1.6%, K 1.8%).
- Disadvantage of direct application of deep (or poultry dropping) litters:
  1. When it is used as fresh manure, it affects the land/crops by creating local alkalinity.
  2. Major fraction of N present in poultry manure is in the form of uric acid, which is rapidly converted to NH_4-N and lost through volatilization (NH_3) during storage and handling. Poultry manure application directly to fields often results into significant losses of nitrogen (>50–60% N).
- Co-composting of poultry litter/manure with crop residues or other biodegradable wastes (e.g. coir pith, water hyacinth chopping or vegetable/fruits waste) is effective method (using *Pleurotus* and *Trichoderma* mixed culture) of not only eliminating the pathogens from poultry wastes, but also to conserve the nutrients.

2.5.1.5 Biogas Slurry

Biogas is one of the potential renewable sources of energy. Instead of directly using the animal dung for composting it can be used for production of biogas by feeding through biogas plant. From the 1800 Mt of animal dung per annum in India even if two-third of the dung is used for biogas generation, it is expected to yield biogas (anaerobic decomposition leading to CH_4 and other hydrocarbon gases) not less than 120 million m³/day. In addition the manure (in the form slurry) produced would be about 440 Mt per year, which is equivalent to 2.90 Mt of N, 2.75 Mt of P_2O_5 and 1.89 Mt of K_2O.

2.5.1.6 Fermentation Industry Waste

- India has made rapid progress in the production of drugs and other chemicals through fermentation processes of different substrates.
- After production of useful products, the left out materials contain large amount of organic matter and minerals in solid and liquid form.

- It is estimated that with one kg of antibiotic produced through fermentation, there is a generation of around 7000–8000 liters of waste water with solid content ranging between 40–50 g/L (BOD load of about 30,000–60,000 mg/L). This wastewater also contains around 2–6% N.
- There could be more judicious use of fermentation industry waste in enriching the composts prepared from other bio-solids like crop residues and agro-industry wastes.

2.5.1.7 Saw Mill or Forest Mill Wastes

- The total of sawdust waste in the country from sawmills and plywood manufacture is estimated about 2.5 million tones. It is a wide C/N ratio material (500:1) low in nitrogen (0.11%) and also low in phosphate (0.20%).
- It has limited scope to use as such as fertilizers, but it can be used as organic manure in tropical soils.
- Dried sawdust has good liquid absorbing capacity and absorbs 2–4 times more moisture than cereal straw.
- Thus, it can be used as good absorbent for soaking in cattle sheds and as bedding materials for cattle which can be composted and converted in valuable organic manure.

2.5.1.8 Oilseed Industry

Oil cakes

There are many varieties of oil cakes which contains not only nitrogen but also some P and K along with large percentage of organic matter. These oil cakes are of two types:

   i. Edible oil cakes– suitable for feeding cattle.
  ii. Non-edible oil cakes– not suitable for feeding cattle.

Oil cakes are quick-acting organic manure. Though they are insoluble in water, their nitrogen became quickly available to plants in about a week or in 10 days after application. Oil cakes should be well powdered before application, so that they can be spread evenly and are easily decomposed by microorganisms. Depending on crops, oil cakes are applied as broadcast, drilled or placed near root zone while earthing up.

- Major oilseeds occupy an important position in the agricultural economy and groundnut in most important crop followed by rape, mustard, sesame, linseed and castor.
- Oilcakes obtained as by product (after the extraction of oil from oilseed/nut) are mostly as cattle feed and manure.
- Non-edible oilcakes, such as neem, karang, mahua, cotton seed, castor, etc.
- A large variety of oilcakes produced in the country can be grouped into classes, viz. (a) edible cakes–suitable for feeding to cattle and (b) non-edible oilcakes–

not suitable for feeding to cattle. Both the types of oilcakes are utilized as concentrated organic manures.

- The nitrogen content varies from 3–9% depending on the nature of oilcakes. All the oilcakes contain small percentage of P_2O_5 (0.8 to 2.9%) and K_2O (1.2 to 2.2%).
- Because of low C–N ratio, the decomposition rate of oilcakes is faster as compared to cereal and legume residues.
- This nitrifies very quickly and about 60–80% of N is converted in available form within 2–3 months time.
- Mahua cake is poor in nitrogen and takes longer time to nitrify. It is better to apply mahua cakes about 2 months in advance to soil before sowing of the crop.

2.5.2 Animal Feedlots

2.5.2.1 Bonemeal

Bones from slaughter houses, carcasses of all animals and from meat industry constitute bonemeal, which is the oldest phosphatic fertilizer used. It also contains some amount of nitrogen. Various types of bone meal are:

i. **Raw or untreated bonemeal:** Bones collected from city slaughter houses and from countryside are dried and powdered without any treatment. It contains 2.4% N and 20.0 to 25.0% P_2O_5.

ii. **Steamed bonemeal:** Bones are soaked in water and caustic soda. They are sterilized with steam and then they are dried in warm rotating oven and powdered. It contains about 27.0% P_2O_5 and 1.0% N. It is well-suited fertilizer for acidic soil and also for long duration crops like sugarcane and banana.

2.5.2.2 Fish Meal

Fish manure or meal is processed by drying non-edible fish, carcasses of fish and wastes from fish industry. It contains 4.0–10.0% N, 3.0–9.0% P_2O_5 and 0.3 to 1.5% K_2O. It has an offensive smell. It is available either as a dried fish or as fish meal or powder. The fish is dried, crushed or powered and filled in bags. Fish meal is quick acting organic manure and is suitable for application to all crops on all soils.

2.5.3 Urban Solid Waste

Sewage and Sludge

The liquid wastes like sewage and sludge contains large quantities of essential plant nutrients and are used for growing vegetables, sugarcane, and fodder crops near large towns or at peri-urban interface. Use of raw sewage is a danger to health. Sewage is allowed to stand in a septic tank to undergo a preliminary fermentation. Then it is aerated in the setting tank by blowing air through it. The sludge that settles at the bottom in this process is called as 'activated sludge'. It brings about rapid oxidation of matter present in fresh sewage. It contains 3.0 to 6.0% of N, about 2.0% P_2O_5, and 1.0% K_2O in forms that can become readily available to plant when applied in soil. However, produce grown on a sewage farm may have problems of heavy metal toxicity, therefore, proper amelioration techniques should be followed to reduce the metal concentration in the produce.

Solid waste

- The municipal solid waste is the solid matter discarded as waste by the citizen. The solid waste is a mixture of several items having different physical properties with a daily generation rate of about 500 g per individual.
- The waste includes combustible, recyclable and inert materials.
- The solid waste generated daily from Mumbai, Delhi, Kolkata and Chennai are 6050, 4000, 3500 and 2500 tonnes respectively.
- The mixed Indian waste has a large proportion of biodegradable material of 30–57% containing 0.56–0.71% N, 0.52–0.82% P_2O_5 and 0.52–0.83% K_2O. Obviously, the waste after composting could be an invaluable source of organic material/manure and plant nutrients.
- The municipalities find it difficult to collect and dispose such solid wastes, while disposing itself at source power. If the wastes are segregated then the handling problem can be solved. Paper, cloth, wrapper, sheets and board can be kept separately for recycling. The perishables, vegetable crop/food residues, waste fruit, animal wastes of organic nature can be placed separately in each colony for collection and composting.
- By following appropriate bio-conversion technology the period of composting can be reduced considerably.
- The value of compost, however, is questioned when it has prohibitive levels of heavy metals threatening human and animal health.

The contamination of urban solid waste compost with the heavy metals could be avoided by segregating the industrial waste containing heavy metals and toxic chemicals from the bio-degradable waste.

2.5.4 Composting Farm Wastes

Compost

Compost is well-rotted organic manure prepared by decomposition of organic matter. Composting is largely a biological process in which microorganisms of both types, aerobic (require oxygen for deep development) and anaerobic (functions in absence of air or free oxygen), decompose the organic matter and lower down the C:N ratio of refuse. The final product of composting is well-rotted manure known as compost. It contains relatively higher quantity of major nutrients than that of FYM. Compost is prepared from waste materials like vegetable refuse, farm litter such as weeds, bhusa, sugarcane trash, sewage sludge and animal wastes. The waste material is collected and stored in a trench of 5 m long, 1.6 m wide and 1 m deep. Collected waste material is mixed well and spread in thin layers of 30 cm thick on the floor of the trench. The layers are moistened by sprinkling slurry of cow dung and earth mixture. The process is repeated till the heap rises to height of 0.5 m above the ground level. The top is covered by thin layer of earth and dung and left undisturbed for rotting (anaerobic decomposition) for 3–4 months. Well-rotten compost is used in the same way as FYM.

Composting is the microbial decomposition of piled organic materials into partially decomposed residues, which are called compost or humus. Composting is carried out in pits of 4 m × 2 m × 1 m (depth).

- The crop residues of farm wastes are filled to a thickness of about 15 cm in the pits uniformly over this layer cow dung slurry is sprinkled to a thickness of about 5 cm. above this layer, bone meal/rock phosphate at the rate of 1kg is spread.
- The process of residue cow dung slurry and bone meal is repeated till the height reaches 0.5 m above the ground level.
- The material is covered with mud plasters to prevent entry of rain water.
- The temperature within the compost pit will be 65–75 °C within a few weeks and most of the hazardous pathogens will be destroyed in such high temperature.
- After 4–5 weeks, the material is turned and then it becomes an anaerobic process.
- The compost will be ready within five months.
- Application of cow dung slurry enhances the rate of biodegradation.
- The application of bone meal/rock phosphate helps to conserve N loss from composting pit and at the same time adds P to composting material.

The macronutrient (NPK) contents of some of the commonly used organic manures are given in Table 2.2. In practice manures are evaluated on the basis of their N content.

Table 2.2: Nutrient ingredients (%) of organic manures

S. No.	Name of Manure	N	P_2O_5	K_2O
1.	Farm Yard Manure	0.4–1.5	0.3–0.9	0.3–1.9
2.	Compost a. Rural b. Urban	0.5–1.0 0.7–2.0	0.4–0.8 0.9–0.3	0.8–1.2 1.0–2.0
3.	Green Manures	0.3–0.85	0.12–0.2	0.5–0.6
4.	Fish Meal	4.0–10.0	3.0–9.0	0.3–1.5
5.	Sewage and sludge a. Dry b. Activated dry	2.0–3.5 4.0–7.0	1.0–5.0 2.1–4.2	0.2–0.5 0.5–0.7
6.	Oil-cakes a. Edible b. Non-edible	4.0–7.9 4.3–5.2	1.4–2.9 0.5–1.8	1.2–2.2 1.2–1.8
7.	Bonemeal	2.4	20.0–25.0	–
8.	Sheep and goat droppings	0.5–0.7	0.4–0.6	0.3–1.0

Compost is the traditional source for the crops. The special merit lies in its capacity to supply large number of essential nutrients, which are becoming eficient in the intensively cultivated areas. The supply of micronutrients particularly satisfies the hidden hunger in plants and even safeguards against toxicity in soil plant system. It improves soil physico-chemical and biological properties like soil structure, water holding capacity, nutrient supply and the beneficial soil microbial population in soil. Some improved form of composts have been developed recently and discussed below:

- In order to encourage soil biological properties, regular use of *Cow Pat Pit (CPP)* and *Cow Horn Manure (BD-500)* is beneficial.
- Use of liquid manure prepared from cow dung; cow urine, leguminous leaves or *vermi-wash* is also effective in promotion of growth and fruiting.
- Biodynamic compost is an effective soil conditioner and is an immediate source of nutrient for a crop. Biodynamic compost can be prepared by using green leaves (nitrogenous material) and dry leaves (carbonaceous material) in 8–12 weeks.
- Use of cow dung slurry enhances the decomposition process of composting. The compost becomes ready in 75–100 days depending upon the prevailing temperature.
- NADEP compost is the most effective one for organic agriculture and is being used commercially.

Cow dung

Since ancient times, human beings have recognized the importance of cows and their contribution to the society. Cow dung and cow urine are the important component in composting.

Vermicompost

Vermiculture is a branch which deals with rearing and maintaining of earthworms for vermicompost preparation. Earthworms decompose waste organic materials and given out in a granular form which is known as vermicompost. It also includes cocoons and young stages of earthworms. It includes different organic waste material like crop residues, straws, leaves, animal waste, residues of green manuring crops, household waste material, etc.

Generally there are 3200 species of earthworms occurring in nature. Out of these *Eisenia fetida* and *Eudrelis eugina* are commonly used for preparing vermicompost.

Two common methods are used for vermicompost preparation.

- Heap method
- Trench method

Benefits of Vermiculture

- The earthworms play a vital role in the process of ploughing and fertilizing the soil and providing the needed nutrition to the plants.

- The earthworms have contributed to improve the soil structure, soil fertility, promote soil aggregation, encourage favorable soil reactions and enrich the nutrient status of the soil and in the process promoting the plant growth and improving the quality of the produce.
- Earthworms churn the soil and make it porous.
- They improve the soil by helping it achieve proper air, water and solids in the required ratio for maximum plant growth.
- Earthworms improve the water infiltration rate. Its made of tunnels increases the soil's ability to absorb water.
- Earthworms bring up minerals and make plant nutrients more available.
- Earthworms also neutralize soil pH. Analysis of earthworm castings or manure shows that the soil in the castings has neutral pH (7) regardless of whether the existing soil is above or below pH (7).
- Earthworms compost plant residues.
- Earthworms stimulate microbial population. Free-living nitrogen fixing bacteria are more numerous around the sides of the earthworm's burrows.

Steps to be followed for Vermicompost Preparation

- The basin of the tree itself can be used as a vermibed.
- Vermicastings at the rate of about 5–10 kg should be applied per tree depending on the size and age of the tree.
- About 25 kg of any farm yard manure (FYM) should be applied evenly on the top of the vermicastings.
- This is then mulched with organic litter. Slashed weeds available on the farm can be used for this purpose.
- Watering should be done as per the regular applications itself, ensuring that proper moisture is maintained.
- When all the above steps are followed, a conducive atmosphere is created for triggering the vermicastings and starting the vermiculture process.
- Once the earthworms have the suitable environment for existence, they start consuming the organic matter and turning it into rich vermicompost.
- This vermicompost is a bio-fertilizer enriched with beneficial soil micro-organisms.
- The vermicastings are highly stable and do not disintegrate thus preventing soil erosion.
- The vermicompost contains all the essential plant nutrients like N, P, K and micronutrients, thus eliminating usage of any further chemical inputs.

Vermicomposting using Paddy Straw

Vermicomposting is an appropriate technique for efficient recycling of animal wastes, crop residues and agro-industrial wastes. Paddy straw is a wide C–N (80:1) organic material, low in nitrogen and phosphorus but fairly rich in potassium. In conventional method of composting, paddy straw takes 6–8 months for decomposition resulting in a poor quality of compost. The process of conversion of organic materials into manure is chiefly microbiological and greatly influenced by the proportion of carbonaceous and nitrogenous materials present in organic wastes.

Microorganisms need carbon for cell structure formation and nitrogen for cellular protein synthesis. It was found that C–N ratio of 30:1 or lower for raw material was desirable for efficient composting. The C–N ratio of organic materials poor in nitrogen should be made narrow by adding nitrogen in the form of any nitrogenous fertilizer to it for better decomposition. Superphosphate is generally added to fortify the phosphorous content of the compost.

Earthworm activities are important in adding faster decomposition process mainly done by microbial actions. An experiment was conducted taking red earthworm (*Eisenia foetida*) for the decomposition of paddy straw in presence of fertilizer sources to add N and P. Dried and chopped (3–4 cm) paddy straw, after thorough mixing with fresh cow dung slurry was introduced into pots. Nitrogen in the form of calcium ammonium nitrate was applied to raise the N level of the straw to 2% N and phosphorus as single super phosphate to raise the total P_2O_5 content to 0.2%. Watering was done to pots to maintain the moisture content to 40–50%. After 2 weeks of preliminary decomposition, red earthworms were released at 10 adults per pot. The experimental results showed neutral reaction of the compost masses indicating their suitability for soil application. The straw decomposition was 91% by vermiculture in presence of fertilizer N and P which was greater than the control. The C–N ratio decreased to 10:1 due to earthworm activity alone and further decreased to 8–1 when inoculated in presence of N+P, showing better influence for the decomposition of a wide C:N ratio material like paddy straw. The earthworm population was increased by 16–20 times.

Vermi-wash

Vermi-wash is prepared from the heavy population of earthworms reared in earthen pots or plastic drums. The extract contains major micronutrients, vitamins (such as B_{12}) and hormones (gibberellins) secreted by the earthworms. Earthworms produce bacteriostatic substances found in the vermi-wash which can protect the bacterial infections. Vermi-wash can be sprayed on crops and trees for better growth, yield and quality.

2.6   RAW MANURE USE: PROBLEMS AND SOLUTIONS

Raw manure is an excellent resource for organic crop production. It supplies nutrients and organic matter, stimulating the biological processes in the soil that help to build fertility. Still, a number of cautions and restrictions are in order, based on concerns about produce quality, food contamination, soil fertility imbalance, weed problems, and pollution hazards. Some manure may contain contaminants such as residual hormones, antibiotics, pesticides, disease organisms, and other undesirable substances. Since many of these can be eliminated through high temperature aerobic composting, this practice is recommended where low levels of organic contaminants may be present. The recent research, however, has demonstrated that *Salmonella* and *E. coli* bacteria survive in the composting process, therefore, the possibility of transmitting human diseases discourages the use of fresh manures (and even some compost) especially for the crops that are commonly eaten raw. Unlike conventional farmers, who have only safety guidelines regarding manure use, certified organic farmers must follow stringent protocols. Raw manure may not be applied to food crops within 120 days of harvest where edible portions have soil contact (i.e. most vegetables, strawberries, etc.); it may not be applied to food crops within 90 days of harvest where edible portions do not have soil contact (i.e. grain crops, most tree fruits). Such restrictions do not apply to feed and fiber crops. Organic substances are not the only contaminants found in livestock manures. Heavy metals can be a problem, especially where industrial scale production systems are used. Concerns over heavy-metal and other chemical contamination have dogged the use of poultry litter as an organically acceptable fertilizer, where it's readily and cheaply available. Heavy-metal contamination is also a concern with composted sewage sludge (bio-solids) — a major reason for its being prohibited from certified organic production.

Under federal organic standards, certifiers may require testing of manure or compost if there is reason to suspect high levels of contamination. It has long been acknowledged that improper use of raw manure can adversely affect the quality of raw vegetable crops such as potatoes, cucumbers, squash, turnips, cauliflower, cabbage, broccoli, and kale. As it breaks down in the soil, manure releases chemical compounds such as skatole, indole, and other phenols. When absorbed by the growing plants, these compounds can impart off-flavors and odors to the vegetables. For this reason, raw manure should not be directly applied to vegetable crops; it should instead be spread on cover crops planted in the previous season.

Precautions

Manure generates heat as it decomposes, and it is not unheard of for manure to ignite spontaneously should it be stored in a massive pile. Once such a large pile of manure is burning, it will foul the air over a very large area and require considerable effort to extinguish. Large feedlots must therefore take care to ensure that piles of fresh manure (faeces) do not get excessively large. There is no serious risk of spontaneous combustion in smaller operations. There is also a risk of insects carrying feces to food and water supplies, making them unsuitable for human consumption.

Fertility Imbalance

Raw manure use has often been associated with imbalances in soil fertility. There are several causal factors:

• Manure is often rich in specific nutrients like phosphate or potash. While these nutrients are of great benefit to crops, repeated applications of manure can result in their building to detrimental levels. Nutrient excesses also "tie up" other minerals. Excessive phosphate interferes with plant uptake of both copper and zinc; excessive potash can restrict boron, manganese, and even magnesium.

- Continual manure use tends to acidify soil. As manure breaks down it releases various organic acids that assist in making soil minerals available—a benefit of manure that is often unrecognized. Over time, however, this process depletes the soil of calcium and causes pH levels to fall below the optimum for most crops. Manures do supply some calcium, but not enough to counterbalance the tendency toward increased acidity.

- When fresh manure containing large amounts of nitrogen and salts is applied in excessive amounts to a crop, it can burn seedling roots, reduce immunity to pests, and shorten produce shelf life.

2.7 IMPACT OF MANURE ON SOIL-PLANT SYSTEM

Long-term applications of farm yard manure influence organic matter as well as other soil-quality parameters, but the magnitude of change depends on prevailing soil-climatic and hydrological conditions.

Climate

The most important climatic characteristics affecting processes such as emission, leaching and decomposition of organic material are temperature, precipitation and evapo-transpiration. Temperature strongly influences all microbiological processes. Higher temperatures, therefore, lead to higher rates of nitrification, denitrification and decomposition of organic material, but also to faster crop growth and the associated uptake of nutrients from manure. Nitrates are formed faster and are therefore more susceptible to leaching, but are also taken up faster by plants if a crop or vegetation is present. At higher temperatures and under reduced conditions NO_3^- will, be denitrified more rapidly and N_2O, (harmful to the ozone layer), will be formed more quickly. The extent of nutrients leaching to the ground water is largely determined by the balance of precipitation and evapotranspiration. Potential evapo-transpiration (PET) also strongly influences the rate of NH_3 volatilization; high PET leading to high rates of volatilization.

Soil

Of the soil characteristics, only texture and pH is more pertinent. The water and nutrient holding capacity of clay soils is higher than that of sandy and silty soils, therefore leaching of NO_3^-, P, other nutrients and organo-chlorines is dependent on soil texture. Conversely the risk of accumulation of harmful components in the root zone following repeated application of large doses of manure is higher in heavier textured soils than in light soils. Clay soils become more easily waterlogged after heavy rainfall because of a lower hydraulic conductivity, i.e. the possible rate of water transport through the soil. Under waterlogged conditions, denitrification can occur and harmful N_2O may be formed. Under extreme acid or alkaline conditions (pH<4 or>9), soils tend to deflocculate, the structure is destroyed and leaching of many organic and inorganic components becomes inevitable. Volatilization of NH_3 from soils with higher pH values (pH>9).

Hydrological Conditions

The hydrological conditions strongly influence the leaching process, for example, faults or sinks in karst zones can cause leaching into deep, ground water-carrying layers. Pollutant containing top soil can come into contact with deep aquifers via old ground water wells. The flow from ground water to surface water is usually direct in areas with a shallow ground water level. In this way, leached nutrients/pollutants can flow rapidly from the soil via the ground water to the surface water and cause eutrophication and toxicity problems.

Manure application to agricultural land involves the addition of all the components of the manure to the soil. An appropriate balance should be maintained between agronomic requirements and negative environmental impacts. Negative impacts, that could be defined as soil pollution, have to do with the addition of heavy metals, organo-chlorines and too many salts. Also, weed seeds could be spread through manuring the land. On the other hand, manuring almost always has a positive influence on the build up of soil organic matter and thus improves the "intrinsic" fertility of the soil, as well as the soil structure.

After application of manure, decomposition by microorganisms of the organic material will start into carbon dioxide (CO_2), water (H_2O) and minerals of plant nutrients such as N, P, S and metals. The transformation of organically bound elements into plant available nutrients during microbiological decomposition is called mineralization. Organic matter that remains one year after application is assumed to be part of the soil organic matter and will decompose gradually over the years, releasing plant nutrients in a way that resembles a slow release fertilizer. A more fertile soil, consequently, has less need for mineral fertilizers. A small fraction of the added organic material is transformed into organic matter that is resistant to microbiological breakdown, the so-called humus or stable organic matter. Humus contributes to soil fertility by retaining plant nutrients through adsorption. It also acts as binding material in the soil, improving soil structure and is responsible for making clay soil less susceptible to compaction caused by heavy traffic, or a silty soil less susceptible to erosion. In addition, humus increases the water-holding capacity and the cation exchange capacity (CEC) of any type of soil.

The heavy metals Cu and Zn have been mentioned as major contaminants from the heavy application of pig slurry. Repeated application of large doses of pig slurry to the same plot may lead to Cu and Zn levels in the soil that are toxic, for instance, to soil fauna and sheep. There is a danger of incomplete degradation of organo-chlorines by microorganisms. Through manuring, they could be taken up by crops and pose a threat to humans by accumulating somewhere in the food chain. Many countries have replaced organo-chlorines with organo-phosphates, but residues from insecticides still continue to be the main source of organo-chlorines in feed. Organo-chlorines originating from substances used against ecto-parasites can also be found. Manure contains much dissolved potassium chloride (KCl) and sodium chloride (NaCl). Repeated application of large amounts of manure in arid or semi-arid climates may easily lead to salinisation of the soil, making it unsuitable for many crops.

Manure is applied to agricultural land chiefly because of its fertilizing value. Animal manure supplies all major nutrients (N, P, K, Ca, Mg, S,) necessary for plant growth, as well as micronutrients (trace elements), hence it acts as a mixed fertilizer. The fertilizing effect on crops can be compared to the effect of mineral fertilizers, and expressed in working coefficients. If, for example, the N in pig slurry on maize is half as effective in terms of yield increase as the N from ammonium nitrate (which is the reference chemical fertilizer), the working coefficient is 0.5. Manure application in a given year will influence not only crops grown that year, but also crops in subsequent years, because decomposition of the organic matter is not completed within one year. Working coefficients for subsequent years could be determined as well. Therefore, the application of manure, thus, saves mineral fertilizers for various nutrients. This illustrates that nutrients from animal manure can be substituted for mineral fertilizers and which is far better for the environment.

A disadvantageous aspect of the uptake of components from manure by the crop is over-dosage, which can lead to the absorption by plants of non-degradable components such as heavy metals (Cu, Zn) and organo-chlorines. These components can accumulate in the food chain and become a health hazard.

3 Beneficial Microorganisms in Agriculture

3.1 BIOFERTILIZERS

Biofertilizers are the preparations containing live or latent cells of efficient strains of nitrogen fixing, phosphate solubilizing or cellulolyotic microorganisms used for application to seed or composting areas with the objective of increasing the numbers of such microorganisms and accelerating those microbial processes which augment the availability of nutrients that can be easily assimilated by plants. Biofertilizers harness atmospheric nitrogen with the help of specialized microorganisms which may be free living in soil or symbiotic with plants. 'Microbial inoculants' are carrier-based preparations containing beneficial microorganisms in a viable state, intended for seed or soil application, designed to improve soil fertility and help plant growth by increasing the number of desired microorganisms in plant rhizosphere.

Microbial Inoculants: In soil the activities of nitrogen fixation, mobilization of plant nutrients and degradation of ligno-cellulotic wastes are being carried out by a large number of microorganisms. Artificially multiplied cultures of selected microorganisms augment the natural recycling of organic resources. There are different types of microbial inoculants:

A. Nitrogen fixers

1. Symbiotic: *Rhizobium* inoculants for legumes
2. Non-symbiotic: For cereals, millets, and vegetables
   a. Bacteria:
      i. Aerobic: *Azotobacter, Azospirillum, Azomonas*
      ii. Anaerobic: *Closteridium, Chlorobium*
      iii. Facultative anaerobes: *Bacillus, Escherichia*
   b. Blue green algae: *Anabaena, Anabaenopsis and Nostoc*
      i. Phosphate solubilizing microorganisms
      ii. Cellulolytic and lignolytic microorganisms
      iii. Sulphur dissolving bacteria
      iv. *Azolla*

Rhizobium Inoculants

Inoculation: Carrier-based inoculants are mixed with little water to form slurry (sugar or gum added to enhance survival of *Rhizobia*) and seeds are uniformly coated with the inoculants, dried and sown immediately. Other specialized methods include–pelleted seed (for acidic soils), per-inoculated seeds, liquid and frozen concentrates, granular soil inoculants, porous gypsum granules and natural peat granule.

Agronomic importance: Response to *Rhizobium* inoculation has been amply demonstrated with most of the legumes-arhar, urad, mung, gram, soybean, etc. Besides, legume cultivation also leaves behind a naturally nitrogen enriched soil for subsequent crops.

Azotobacter Inoculants

Inoculation: Slurry of the carrier-based inoculants is made with minimum amount of water and seeds are mixed with the slurry, dried in shade and sown; seedling dip (10–13 min) in slurry is done for transplanted crops and planted immediately. For sugarcane etc., secondary inoculation with slurry near the root zone in early stages of plant growth are also recommended. The inoculants can also be mixed with FYM and broadcast near the root zone.

Crop response: *Azotobacter* inoculants on onion, wheat, rice, brinjal, tomato, cabbage, sugarcane, oat, barely, maize, potato can increase 7–12% crop yields. *Azotobacter* spp. increase plant yield primarily by fixing molecular nitrogen in soil, but it is also reported to synthesize auxins, vitamins, growth substances and antifungal antibiotics, which have beneficial effects of this bacterium on seed germination and other metabolic processes.

Azospirillum Inoculants

Occurrence in soil: Soil pH in range of 5.6–7.2 registers *Azospirillum* activity with optimum at 6.7 to 7.0; below pH 5.6 the soil is devoid of *Azospirillum* and presence of organic matter in soil generally favours multiplication of this bacterium. Powdered and sterilized FYM+soil, FYM alone or FYM+charcoal are used as carriers.

Blue Green Algal Inoculants

The inoculants are specially recommended for paddy crop grown in wet land conditions which also favour the growth of blue green algae. These algae also possess photosynthetic activity. Besides they excrete vitamin B_{12}, auxins and ascorbic acid which contribute to growth of rice plants.

Azolla– an Organic Manure

Methods of application: It is applied as green manure prior to rice planting and as dual cropping with rice, when fern grows side by side with paddy.

Crop response: Soil application is more beneficial than dual culture method; 10 tonnes fresh *Azolla*/ha is equivalent to 25–30 kg N/ha and increasing application rate from 5–20 tonnes/ha has direct response in grain yield of paddy.

3.1.1 *Rhizobium*

It is known that legumes enrich the soil by contributing nitrogen through symbiotic nitrogen fixation by *Rhizobium* through centuries. However, scientific demonstration of value of legumes in contributing nitrogen nutrition of plants was only done in 19th Century. This was established by the facts that nodules on legume roots are responsible for fixing atmospheric nitrogen through bacterium *Rhizobium*. Due to new technological development a substantial contribution in increasing production of legumes besides improving fertility of soil, is made.

How to Separate *Rhizobium* from Nodules?

Different types of legumes form various sizes and shapes of nodules on their roots. Differences have been even found within the same species of legumes. Hence, nodules are collected when plants are in flowering stage and one can make out an effective nodule which is large in size and red in colour. Such nodules are used for separation of *Rhizobium* in the laboratory. An isolation of *Rhizobium* is made by following usual techniques. Yeast mannitol agar is the special medium used to grow *Rhizobium*. Colonies grown on a medium may not be only of *Rhizobium* they can be even of Agro bacterium. For definite conclusion one has to inoculate seeds of particular sequence and wait for formation of nodules on such plants. How to recognize *Rhizobium*? In order to confirm whether isolated colonies are of *Rhizobium* for this purpose one has to see that inoculated plants form effective nodules on roots. For further combination following tests are performed in the laboratory:

 i. Growth on yeast monitol agar.

 ii. Examination under microscope.

 iii. Congo red test.

 iv. Alkaline mixture test of Hoffer.

 v. Lactose agar test.

Besides there are several tests of nodule formation on roots of legume, of which following are most important:

 i. Complete plant cover test.

 ii. Hecnard jar test.

 iii. Test in earthen pots.

 iv. Separation of root and their testing.

 v. Tissue culture test.

 vi. Field experiment.

Estimation of nitrogen fixation: In order to estimate biological nitrogen fixation generally Kjeldhal's method is used. However, if the difference between two treatments is higher than some other methods are used, viz. Label nitrogen N^{15}. For this method, Mass-spectrometer and label nitrogen (N^{15}) are must. One can estimate the nitrogen fixed by the organism by observing the N^{15} taken up by the plant.

At field level nitrogen estimation can be done by calculating the difference between nitrogen found in nodules of legume plant and the nitrogen found in non-nodulating legume plant variety. For legume a small amount of chemical nitrogen is applied and hence biological nitrogen fixation is found efficiently whereas for cereals higher doses of chemical nitrogen are applied. For cereals nitrogen from soil is only available. On the other hand for legumes nitrogen from soil as well as from nodules is made available. Difference between the two is the nitrogen fixed by the legumes.

During the nitrogen fixation nitrogenous enzyme converts nitrogen into ammonia, and then acetylene into ethylene. This method is most efficiently used to estimate the nitrogen fixed by plants. This method is simple, accurate and used on a large scale.

Cross innoculation groups: Nubbe (1891) described cross innoculation groups as a new concept that is separate rhizobium species only nodulate specific related legumes. For example, *Braddyrhizobium japonicum* – nodulating soyabean crop cannot infect groundnut plants and *vice versa*. The cross innoculation groups have waterbigul compartment and no exceptions are found. From the published information so far it is not known what are the reasons for existence of cross innoculation groups in the nature. Fred and his associates (1932) recognized eight cross innoculation group in legumes as mentioned below:

S. No	Group	*Rhizobium* species	Crop infected
1.	Chavali	*Rhizobium sp.*	Mung, Groundnut, Dhaincha, Guar, Chavali, etc.
2.	Chickpea	*Rhizobium sp.*	Chick pea
3.	Peas	*Rhizobium sp.*	Peas, Masoor
4.	Beans	*Rhizobium phaseoli*	All types of beans
5.	Soyabean	*Braddyrhizobium japonicum*	Soybean
6.	Alfalfa	*Rhizobium milileti*	Methi, Alfalfa
7.	Barseem	*Rhizobium trifoli*	Barseem
8.	Lupin	*Rhizobium lupini*	Lupin

Above cross inoculation groups are recognized everywhere and accordingly *Rhizobium* species is selected to inoculate a particular crop.

How *Rhizobium* enter the roots of legumes?

Rhizobium enters the roots of the legumes either through root hair or directly at the point of emergence of lateral roots. Curling or controlled growth and branching of root hairs is the first visible plant response to *Rhizobium*. Although, legume nodules generally seem to harbour only one strain of *Rhizobium* a given root can certainly form nodules with more than one strain.

It is reported that *Rhizobium* strains capable of infecting a legume releases a specific polysaccharides that induces more pectolytic activity by the root that accounts for cross inoculation specificities. It is not known how *Rhizobium* initiates the infection thread. Some suggested mechanical rupture with *Rhizobium* entering a break in root hair wall. *Rhizobium* may also get trapped within the fold of growing deformed hair.

How a nodule is formed?

The infection thread enters and penetrates the context of the root from cell to cell. Finally the thread bursts and liberates the rod-shaped bacteria into a critical cell. This cell divides to form nodular tissue in which bacteria divide and multiply. Eventually, a demarcation develops, a centrally located bacteria containing, the tissue called the bacterial zone is marked out in the nodule from the surrounding bacteria-free tissue called the nodule cortex. The nodular tissue grown in a size pushes itself through the root and then emerges as an appendage on the root system. Its size and shape depends on the species and legume.

There are two types of nodules–effective and ineffective ones.

- **Effective** nodules are formed by effective strains of *Rhizobium*. They are well developed, pink colour due to the presence of pigment posses' leghaemoglobin. The bacterium tissue is well developed and well organized with plenty of bacteriods. On the contrary **ineffective** strains of *Rhizobium* form ineffective nodules which are generally small and contain poorly developed bacterium tissue showing accumulation of starch in host cells which don't contain *Rhizobium*. The bacteria of ineffective nodule contain glycogen.

Red Pigment – Leghaemoglobin: A cross-section of a mature nodule reveals a pink or red coloured central-bacteriod zone surrounded by thin-walled cells. The red colour is caused by the presence of a pigment called "leghaemoglobin". Similar to the one found in human blood, the prefix "leg" indicates its unique presence in root nodules of leguminous plants. The amount of red pigment in nodules is directly proportional to the amount of nitrogen fixed by nodules.

The red pigment in the nodules acts as a biological value in regulating the supply of oxygen into the bacteriod tissue. The supply of oxygen at an optimum rate to help the maximum activity of the enzyme "nitrogenase" which is key factor in the mechanism of nitrogen fixation.

Mechanism of N-fixation: The nodules are simply, a protective structure and bacteriods are the seats of N-fixation. Reduction of N_2 to NH_3 is mediated through enzyme 'nitrogenase'. Nitrogenase is made up of two components – one with iron and molybdenum and the second without molybdenum. N-fixation is essentially anaerobic process. The oxygen supply to bacteriod is excluded due to presence of leg haemoglobin around it. This pigments limits oxygen supply and helps in providing low oxygen conditions near the bacteriods and thus protects the oxygen sensitive nitrogenous from damage. The enough oxygen is made available at the site for generation of ATP. The quantum of N-fixed is closely related to the amount of leg haemoglobin and the extent of bacteriod tissues in nodules. The first stable intermediate in N-fixation is ammonia. This nitrogen is then converted into amino acids and proteins, thereby plants are benefited.

3.1.2 *Azotobacter*

Introduction: The worldwide spread of inflation, initiated by several fold rises in petroleum price thereby depicting its striking influence on the prices of chemical nitrogenous fertilizers, have nearly doubled during the last 3–4 years. This has necessiated to search for cheaper source of nitrogen to meet the needs of crops. This has rejuvenation of soil microbiology to tap out the biological fixation of nitrogen.

Azotobacter **spp:** These are free-living bacteria which grow well on a nitrogen-free medium. These bacteria utilize atmospheric nitrogen gas for their cell protein synthesis. This cell protein is then mineralised in soil after the death of *Azotobacter* cells thereby contributing towards the nitrogen availability of the crop plants.

Characteristics of *Azotobacter*: *Azotobacter* is gram negative and polymorphic i.e. they are of different sizes and shapes. Their size ranges from 2–10 × 1–2.5 m, young cell possess *Peritrichous flegella* and are used as locomotive organs. Old population of bacteria includes encapsulated forms and have enhanced resistant to heat, desiccation and adverse conditions. The cyst germinates under favourable conditions to give vegetative cells. They also produce polysaccharides. *Azotobacter spp*. is sensitive to acidic pH, high salts, and temperature above 35 °C.

There are four important species of *Azotobacter* viz. *A. chroococcum, A. agilis, A. paspali* and *A. vinelandii* of which *A. chroococcum* is most commonly found in our soils.

Nitrogen fixation by *Azotobacter*: The species of *Azotobacter* are known to fix on an average 10 mg of N/g of sugar in pure culture on a nitrogen free medium. A maximum of 30 mg N fixed per gram of sugar was reported by Lopatina. However, *Azotobacter* is a poor competitor for nutrients in soil. Most efficient strains of *Azotobacter* would need to oxidise about 1000 kg of organic matter for fixing 30 kg of N/ha. This does not sound realistic for our soils which have very low-active carbon status. Besides, soil is inhabited by a large variety of other microbes, all of which compete for the active carbon.

Azotobacter **in soil:** In Indian soils, the population of *Azotobacter* is not more than 10 thousand to 1 lakh/g of soil. The population of *Azotobacter* is mostly influenced by other microorganisms present in soil. There is some microorganism which stimulates the *Azotobacter* population in soil thereby increasing the nitrogen fixation by *Azotobacter*. On the other hand there are some microorganisms which adversely affect the *Azotobacter* population and hence nitrogen fixation process is hampered. For example *Cephallosporium* is most commonly found organisms in soil which restricts the growth of *Azotobacter*.

Azotobacter also produces some substances which check the plant pathogens such as *Alternaria, Fusarium* and *Helminthosporium*. Hence, *Azotobacter* also acts as a biological control agent.

Functions of *Azotobacter*: *Azotobacter* naturally fixes atmospheric nitrogen in the rhizosphere. There are different strains of *Azotobacter* each has varied chemical, biological and other characters. However, some strains have higher nitrogen fixing ability than others. *Azotobacter* uses carbon for its metabolism from simple or compound substances of carbonaceous in nature. Besides carbon, *Azotobacter* also requires calcium for nitrogen fixation. Similarly, a medium used for growth of *Azotobacter* is required to have presence of organic nitrogen, micro-nutrients and salt in order to enhance the nitrogen fixing ability of *Azotobacter*.

Besides, nitrogen fixation, *Azotobacter* also produces, thiomin, riboflavin, nicotin, indol acitic acid and giberalin. When *Azotobacter* is applied to seeds, seed germination is improved to a considerable extent, so also it controls plant diseases due to above substances produced by *Azotobacter*.

Selection of *Azotobacter* strains: After isolation of *Azotobacter* from soil its purity is tested in the laboratory in a pure form. In fertile soil spp. *A. chroococcum* is found, commonly. The organism is aerobic in nature, requires oxygen for its growth. In old culture malinin chemical is formed which gives the blackish colour to the culture. The organism is prominently found in alkaline or neutral soils. Strains of *Azotobacter* vary in their nitrogen fixing ability which depends upon pH of soil, crop and atmosphere of soil. Therefore nitrogen fixing capacity of strains is tested frequently. In order to obtain most efficient strains of *Azotobacter*, one has to conduct different tests or experiments in glass house, earthern pots and field under the guidance of micro-biologists, some of them are explained below:

1. **Acetylene reduction test:** Different strains of *Azotobacter* in pure form are grown in the laboratory in separate conical flasks. These flasks are then kept on shaker for about 72–50 hours so as to obtain full growth of bacteria in the medium of which 10–15 ml, of both is transferred to a bottle, to this bottle 10 ml of acetylene gas is added and bottle is closed with cork borer and allowed to stand in the shed for 2–4 hours to have reaction of enzyme nitrogenase with acetylene gas. During this period, acetylene is converted to ethylene. Percentage of both the gases is measured chromatographically. The strain which has more nitrogenase enzyme forms more ethylene gas. Naturally, this strain with more nitrogen actvity will be selected for further use.

2. **Pot culture experiment:** After having tested different strains in the laboratory and selected efficient strains, next test comes the pot culture experiment. In this test, earthern pots are cleaned properly and disinfected with some common laboratory disinfectent and filled in with uniform amount of garden soil already sterilized.

Strain found efficient in acetylene reduction test are selected and multiplied in a pure form. The broth is mixed with liquid and inoculant so prepared is used to inoculate the seeds. Seeds are then dried in shed and sown in pots. Suitable inoculated control plants are kept for comparision. Plants are watered as and when required and allowed to grow for about 45–60 days. Differences between inoculated and uninoculated plants in respect of height, nitrogen content of plant and soil, dry weight of plants are noted. Efficient strains are used for field tests.

3. **Field test:** Strains found efficient under glass house conditions are required to undergo field test which is most important test from the farmer's point of view. Strains found efficient in glass house and acetylent tests when used in field are required to compete with native flora for their nutrition. Efficient strains of *Azotobacter* are applied to seeds of particular and sown. An adequate control is kept for comparision. All other factors are kept similar except seed inoculation with efficient strains of *Azotobacter*.

After maturity yield figures are noted and comparision is made. Such experiments are repeated for 3 to 4 years at different places. From this data an efficient strain is selected and used for the production of *Azotobacter* on a large-scale. Such strains are stored under cold storage conditions or in refrigerator. For production of bio-fertilizer, it is always advisable to use more than one strain on safer side. Field experiments conducted in Russia with *Azotobacter* as a biofertilizer for wheat, barley, oat, maize, sugarcane, etc. revealed that the performance of *Azotobacter* was medium to poor. Experiments on the use of *Azotobacter* for seed inoculation of various crops have also been conducted in other countries including India. The results of these experiments indicate that benefits obtained from inoculation of seeds with biofertilizer were marginal in soil with poor organic matter content. While in rich soils results were quite encouraging. The field soils are inhabited by a very large number of microbial species. The co-existence of the relative populations of each one of the species is determined by ecological factors prevailing in the soil. These various species survive in soil while maintaining a balance of population is between various microbial species within certain limits.

a. **Growth of *Azotobacter*:** Usually *Azotobacter* is grown on a solid medium free of nitrogen. After some time (6 months) old growth of *Azotobacter* is transferred to a fresh solid medium to renew the growth. This procedure is repeated periodically so that the culture can be maintained in good condition.

b. Production:

i. Mother culture: A pure growth of any organism on a small-scale is called as a mother culture. Mother culture is always prepared in a conical flask of 500 or 1000 ml. capacity and then this mother culture is used for further production.

For this purpose, one litre conical flasks are taken to which 500 ml of broth of nitrogen free medium is added and these flasks are then plugged with non-absorbent cotton, sterilized in an autoclave for 15–20 minutes at 75 lbs pressure for 15 minutes. Flasks are then inoculated with mother culture with the help of inoculating needle aseptically. The flasks are transferred to shaker and shaking is done for 72–90 hours so as to get optimum growth of bacteria in broth. Bacteria are multiplied by binary method i.e. cell division. After about 90 days, the number of per milliliters comes to about 100 crores. Total growth of bacteria in this broth means starter culture or mother culture, which should carefully be done, since further purity of biofertilizer or quality of biofertilizer depends upon how mother culture is prepared.

ii. Production on a large scale: *Azotobacter* is multiplied on a large-scale by two ways viz. Fermenter and Shaker. The fermenter is most automatic and accurate method of multiplication of any microorganism. In this method, the medium is taken in a fermenter and then sterilized. After this pH of the medium is adjusted and 1% mother culture is added. In order to get an optimum growth of the *Azotobacter* required temperature and oxygen supply is adjusted so that concentrated broth is made. This concentrated broth of the culture is then mixed with a carrier previously sterilized and bio-fertilizers is prepared. Depending upon the demand and supply suitable fermenter is selected.

In the 2nd method, i.e. shaker method, a suitable medium is prepared transferred to conical flask of suitable capacity. These flasks are then sterilized in an autoclave at 15 lbs pressure for 15 minutes. Each flasks is inoculated with 10 ml mother culture and they are transferred to shaker for multiplication where they are kept for 72–90 hours. This broth is mixed with a suitable carrier previously sterilized. Thus biofertilizer is prepared, filled in plastic bags and stored in cool place.

Selection of Carrier

A carrier is nothing but a substance which has high organic matter, higher water holding capacity and supports the growth of organism in order to transport the biofertilizer and becomes easy to use the suitable carrier selected. Generally lignite cool, compost and peat soil are suitable carriers for *Azotobacter*. Out of these carriers lignite is most suitable for this organism, since it is cheaper, keeps organism living for longer period and does not lower the quality of bio-fertilizers.

The lignite comes in clouds and hence it is ground in fine powder by grinding machine. Its finesses should be 250–300 mesh. The pH of the carrier is adjusted to neutral by adding $CaCO_3$. The lignite naturally has a variety of microorganism and hence it is sterilized in autoclave at 30 lbs pressure for 30 minutes. After this the broth is mixed with lignite 1:2 proportion by following method.

Galvanized trays are sterilized and used. To these trays, previously sterilized lignite is transferred and broth is then added (lignite:broth = 1:2) and mixed properly. Trays are then kept one above the other for 10–12 hours for allowing the organism to multiply in the carrier. This mixture is then filled in plastic bags of 250 g or 500 g capacity. Plastic bags are properly sealed. All the required information such as name of biofertilizer, method of use, expiry date, etc. is printed on plastic bags. In this way, biofertilizer is ready to sell or use. If biofertilizer is used immediately then bags are stored in cool place otherwise they should be stored in cold storage in order to keep biofertilizer in good quality.

As per ISI standards, one gram of biofertilizer immediately after it is prepared should have one crore cells of bacteria and 15 days before expiry date one gram of biofertilizer should have 10 lakh bacteria. If biofertilizer is stored at 15–20 °C then it will remain effective for 6 months. However, at 0 to 4 °C (cold storage) the bacteria will remain active for 2 years. The storage period is decided after testing the biofertilizer for that particular storage condition, such temperature and humidity.

Use of Biofertilizer

Plant needs nitrogen for its growth and *Azotobacter* fixes atmospheric nitrogen non-symbiotically. Therefore, all plants, trees, vegetables get benefited. However, especially cereals, vegetables, fruits, trees, sugarcane, cotton, grapes, banana, etc., are known to get additional nitrogen requirements from *Azotobacter*. *Azotobacter* also increases germination of seeds. Seeds having less germinating per cent if inoculated can increase germination by 20–30%.

How to apply bio-fertilizer?

a. **Seed inoculation:** The required quantity of fresh biofertilizer is secured and slurry is made by adding adequate quantity of water approximately 10–20 litre of water with 250–500 g sticker and 1 kg of finely grim garden soil. Seed inoculation is the most economic at the same time equally efective option for application of biofertilizer in soil-plant system. Depending on the basis of efficiency of inoculum, inherent microorganism present in the soil and type of crop, the rate of biofertilizer application varies. Generally, 500 g to 1 kg biofertilizer is used for inculating seeds require for sowing in one and were of cultivates law. This slurry is uniformly applied to seed; seed is then dried in shed and sown. Some stickers are used in order to adhere biofertilizer to seeds, viz. Jaggery or gum Acacia arabia.

b. **Seedling inoculation:** This method of inoculation is tranplanted where seedlings are used to grow the crop. In this method, seedlings required for one acre of cultivation are inoculated with 4–5 packets of biofertilizers approximately 2–2.5 kg of inoculum. For this, in a bucket adequate quantity of water is taken and biofertilizer 2 packets (1 kg) dipper is added to bucket and mixed properly with 250 g jaggery and 1 kg of finelly grim garden soil. Roots or seedlings are then dipped in this mixture so as to enable roots to get inoculums. These seedlings are then transplanted preferbly in the evening, e.g. tomato, rice, onion, cole, crops, flowers.

c. **Self inoculation or tuber inoculation:** In this method 50 liters of water is taken in a drum and 4–5 kg of *Azotobacter* biofertilizer is added and mixed properly. Sets required for one acre of land are dipped in this mixture. Potato tubers are dipped in the mixture of biofertilizer and planting is done.

d. **Soil application:** This method is mostly used for fruit crops, sugarcane, and trees. At the time of planting fruit tree, 20 g of biofertilizer mixed with compost is to be added per sapling, when trees became matured the same quantity of biofertilizer is applied.

In sugarcane after two to three months of planting i.e. before earthing up 5–6 kg of biofertilizer per acre is applied by mixing with compost or soil. Although, *Azotobacter* fixes nitrogen non-symbiotically, it also fixes atmospheric nitrogen in the rhizosphere region i.e. soil around the seedlings or trees. Biofertilizer applied to seed or seedlings bacteria remain around seeds or seedlings and use organic carbon for their metabolism. When seeds are germinated or seedlings set in soil they leave or exude root exudates which become food of these bacteria. They grow on these substances which include sugars, organic acids, amino acids and fix atmospheric nitrogen most efficiently. Nitrogen so fixed by these bacteria becomes available to plants after dead and degradation of bacterial cells.

Salient features of *Azotobactor*:

1. *Azotobacter* contributes moderate benefits.
2. *Azotobacter* is heaviest breathing organism and requires a large amount of organic carbon for its growth.
3. It is poor competitor for nutrients in soil and helps inducing its growth promoting substances, fungistatic substances.
4. *Azotobacter* is less effective in soils with poor organic matter content.
5. It improves seed germination and plant growth
6. *Azotobacters* are tolerant to high salts and thrives even in alkaline soils.

3.1.3 Blue Green Algae

Introduction: The global energy crisis and dwindling mineral oil reserves have widened the gap between supply and demand of nitrogenous fertilizers. An introduction of fertilizer responsive high-yielding crop varieties has further increased the demand of this important crop nutrient. This has resulted in further burden on small and marginal farmers, especially in developing countries. This has become necessary to look for alternative sources to meet atleast a part of nitrogen requirement of crop production.

In India, rice is cultivated on about 40 million hectares of area, which constitutes about 37–40% of total area under cereals. Though, rice cultivation is an age-old practice in our country, the average production is only about 1.7 t/ha. This is because more than 85% of the total area of rice is owned by small and marginal farmers. These farmers cannot afford to use various inputs needed to harvest maximum yield of rice. They do not get full returns/unit nitrogenous fertilizers in their fields because of high nitrogen losses in the ecosystem.

The past few decades have widened remarkable advancement in harnessing some of the potentially useful microorganisms to build up the fertility of the soil to increase the crop yield. In recent years, blue-green algae, a group of soil microorganisms have been shown to be agriculturally important, particularly in tropical rice field soils. This is because of capacity of some of the algae to synthesize organic substances and also to fix atmospheric nitrogen.

Submerged conditions of a rice field provide congenial habitat for blue-green algae where they form most efficient system providing biologically fixed nitrogen to the crop. The importance of blue-green algae was first recognized by De (1936) who reported that these microorganisms are responsible for spontaneous fertility of tropical rice field soils. Since then series of reports have been appeared emphasizing their role in nitrogen cycle in general and rice field in particular. The propagation of blue-green algae will not only enrich the nitrogen status of the soil by their fixation process but also provide organic matter and biologically potent substances for plant growth. These algae form a living constituent of the soil biotype and continue their activity year after year. Besides they release oxygen for the paddy roots and increase soil phosphate. Some of them prevent the loss of soil ammonia and leaching out of nitrates by converting them into organic nitrogen. Blue-green algae also produce surface humus after death and exert a solvent action on certain minerals – maintaining a reserve supply of elements in a semi-available form for higher plants either by secretion or upon death and decomposition.

a. **Distribution of blue green algae in rice field soils:** Blue-green algae have been found in almost all the conceivable habitats. They are widely distributed throughout the tropical, subtropical and temperate regions. However, the frequency of their occurrence was more prominent in Southern than in Northern regions. Tropical soils harbour comparatively higher population of blue-green algae.

In Southeast Asia including Japan the presence of species *Tolypothrix, Nostoc, Cylindrospermum, Calothrix, Anabaena, Plectonema* and *Anabaenopsis* was found prominent. In Senegal, the dominant species reported were *Nostoc* and *Anabaena*, whereas, *Scytonema* and *Calothrix* were respectively found in 50 and 15 per cent area. In Indonesia *Cylindrospermum, Anabaenopsis, Nostoc* and *Nodularia* were found to be common. In North Australia blue-green algae flora was dominated by *Nostoc* and *Anabaena*. The dominant species in Philippines were *Nostoc* and *Anabaena*. In Russia, *Nostoc* and *Anabaena* were found most common.

In India, a general predominance of blue green algae except in acidic soils of Kerala, Assam and parts of Tamil Nadu forms like *Anabaena, Nostoc* and *Calothrix* were found to be widely distributed throughout rice growing tracts of India.

Other forms like *Cylindrosporum, Tolypothrix, Scytonema* and *Aulosira* had localised distribution. The distribution of soils harbouring blue-green algae in India varies from as low as 7 to as high as 80 per cent in different States. Uttar Pradesh soils are rich in *Aulosira* and *Mastigocladae* is found in Gujarat. *Westiella* is found very dominant in Maharashtra and *Cylindrospermum* in Karnataka and *Calothrix* in Punjab, soils of Vidharbha and Konkan of Maharashtra are dominated by blue green algae.

During recent years, quantitative studies showed consistent presence of N_2 fixing blue green algae at high densities in soils under rice cultivation in countries like India, Malaysia, Philippines and Portugal. *Nostoc* sp. was dominant followed by *Anabaena* and *Calothrix*. Blue green algae occurred at densities from 1.0×10^{-2} to 8.0×10^{-6} CFU/cm^{-2} and their abundance was correlated to pH and available 'P' content of soil.

b. **Strain variation:** Biological N_2 fixation in nature or agricultural ecosystem is rarely limited by a lack of N_2 fixing microorganisms. Nevertheless, very little nitrogen is fixed in nature. Apart from the ecological stresses the efficiency of strains themselves may play an important role. A great differences in the amount of nitrogen fixed by various genera and sometimes by the same species from different localities are observed. The need for wide collection, culturing and testing for the relative efficiency of different strains is, therefore, obvious. The possible reasons for the reported differences in their efficiency in fixing nitrogen may be due to variations in the cultural conditions like light, temperature, nutrient deficiencies, etc. It is also known that the secret of increasing nitrogen fixing capacity lies in the adequate supply of trace elements like molybdenum (Mo) and iron (Fe),which induces formation of AzoFerMo and AzoFer protein resposible for lingner nitrogenase in soil - plant system.

Likewise, the influence of genetic constitution might also play a vital part in determining the capacity to fix nitrogen. Apart from the natural inherent variations, combined nitrogen and various agro-chemicals play a vital role in determining the nitrogen contribution by the added blue-green algae in field. This offers an opportunity to select strains for specific ecosystem.

c. **Strain competition:** The successful induction of a microorganism in an ecosystem depends upon its ability to adopt and compete with the indigenous biotypes. For the positive introduction of an effective blue-green algae strain in an area depends upon its ability to survive and compete with the native flora for establishment, growth and effective nitrogen fixation.

Prior to seeding, the paddy field water may be sprinkled with lime powder, which will be effective in suppressing the growth of other algae and at the same time will lower the acidity of water to a favourable level. It is possible that antagonistic effects of other organisms may affect the successful survival of particular algae strain. Similarly, possibilities for the presence of algo-phages cannot be ruled out. There is a great deal of indirect evidence to show that some algae can liberate antibiotic substances. There are reports that there was no marked difference in the total amount of nitrogen fixed and bacteria under water-logged conditions. Thus nitrogen fixation is essentially an algae process and the part played by bacteria is relatively unimportant. The decomposition of blue green algae is enhanced by the presence of bacteria in an adequate quantity. Besides fertilizing action of nitrogen fixing blue green algae in the field is considerably improved by bacterial flora.

d. **Strain selection:** The production of strains, likely to be superior, in nature to those which already exist is daaunting challenge. **First** it is essential to select N_2 fixing strains capable of rapid growth. Well studied *Cyanobacteria* such as *Anabaena cylindrica* are relatively slow growing with a generation time of 16–24 hours. *Anacystis nidulans*, which was doubling time of 2 hours does not fix nitrogen. However, with improved culture media and methods of obtaining axenic cultures, the selection of rapidly growing N_2 fixing strains has a reality.

Second, Cyanobacteria should be selected which can fix N_2 equally well under aerobic, micro-aerobic and anaerobic conditions, so that they can tolerate the very wide range of oxygen tension found in rice fields. The heterocystous and certain unicellular forms satisfy these conditions. However, N_2 fixing unicellular forms which can tolerate oxygen extremes and high light intensities and grow rapidly are not yet available. Heterocystous forms are currently better alternatives.

Third, it is important to choose *Cyanobacteria* that fix N_2 under photoautotrophic, phoheterotrophic and chemoheterotrophic conditions. These *Cyanobacteria* include species of *Anabaena, Anabaenopsis, Nostoc* and *Tolypothrix*.

Fourth, strain that show little or no H_2 evolution should be selected. The extent of H_2 production varies in different N_2 fixing *Cyanbacteria* and it is important to select strains that little showlittre H_2 such production and ATP wastage.

Fifth, the selection of strains that possess non-repressible nitrogenase could possibly be important nitrogenase is inhibited by high level of N_2 –N and it is thus important to obtain cynobacteria strain in which this does not occur.

Sixth, strains should be selected that not only liberate extracellular nitrogen but liberate it in substantial amounts, exceeding the requirement of *Cyanobacteria* for optimal growth and is released in a form that can be readily assimilated.

Seventh, the way in which glutamine synthetase is regulated is of importance in nitrogen fixing Cyanobacteria.

Blue-green algae, biofertilizer has been proved to be most efficient source of organic nitrogen in low-land paddy.

N_2 from blue green algae

Nitrogen constitutes in general 1–2 per cent of total dry weight of plants and in unfertilized soils this often limits crop production. Use of chemical fertilizers during 1960–1970 was preferred by farmers due to its cheapness and easiness of application. Later on these fertilizers become most expensive and hence farmers were unable to use these fertilizers as required by crops. The production of N-fertilizer is the energy intensive process and this energy is provided from fossil fuels to convert N_2 to NH_3, however, with the energy crisis of the late 1970s the cost of chemical fertilizer was escalated. Hence it was necessary to search for alternative source to maintain the production level of grains to feed the increasing population.

The most inexhaustible energy source is the solar radiation. Thus there is particular interest in those organisms which can use this energy within their protoplasm to produce ammonia from nitrogen. There are two groups of microorganisms viz. Cyanobacteria (blue-green algae) and photosynthetic bacteria.

Blue green algae (BGA) are photosynthetic procaryotic microorganisms. Their main photosynthetic pigments are chlorophyll-a, carotenes, xanthophylls, together with phycobiliproteins, c-phycocyanin (blue) and e-phycoerythrin (red). Due to the presence of these latter pigments and mucilage, the colour of BGA in nature ranges from dirty yellow, through various shades of blue-green to brown or black.

Some blue green algae can fix atmospheric nitrogen because they contain an O_2 sensitive enzyme nitrogenase. The term *algal* biofertilizer was coined in early sixties to embody such blue green algae which have the capacity to metabolize the molecular nitrogen and bring about an addition to the nitrogen content of the soil. The conversion of elemental nitrogen to ammonia was the monopoly of heterocystous blue green algae till the findings of Whyatt and Silvey in 1961 who reported nitrogen fixation by a unicellular algae *Gloeocapsa*. Since then more than a dozen non-heterocystous genera of blue-green algae have been found to fix air nitrogen.

Heterocysts

Some blue green algae have empty looking thick-walled structures in their trichomes, known as *heterocysts*. These specialised cells lack pigment system-II and as such there is no endogenous evolution of oxygen. The oxygen from air cannot diffuse through their thick walls. The anaerobic conditions are so created inside the heterocysts that keep nitrogenase active in them. Thus, under aerobic conditions only the heterocysts blue green algae can fix nitrogen.

The nitrogenase in the vegetative cells also can become active if the entire trichome is transferred to microgerobic or anaerobic conditions. The non-heterocysts blue green algae find such an environment in the subsoil region and soil water interphase in a rice field where they add substantial amount of nitrogen through nitrogen fixation.

Growth promoting effects of blue-green algae

In addition to contributing about 30 kg N/ha/season, blue green algae helps in maintaining the soil fertility by way of liberating growth promoting substances like auxin, vitamins. They add organic matter because of their photolithotrophic nature. They also solubilize insoluble phosphate and improve physical and chemical properties of soil.

Blue green algae have been found to synthesize and liberate biologically potent substances into the medium. The liberation of auxins, vitamin B_{12} and amino acids has been found to be maximum during the stationary phase of the growth. The substances benefit the crop growth and enable plants to utilize more of the applied nitrogen.

Photosynthesis by blue-green algae

Blue green algae possess permanent property of metabolizing both elemental nitrogen and carbon dioxide from the atmosphere simultaneously. The process of photosynthesis in these organisms meets the entire energy requirement including the power needed for reducing nitrogen to ammonia. As such these algae form a completely independent system and they don't dwell upon soil organic matter for energy supply. As a consequence of algal growth, organic matter is added to the soil. But because of high nitrogen content and high rate of decomposition in the water-logged conditions no appreciable addition to the organic matter content in soil is observed. The presence of organic matter in the soil has been found to favour the growth of the blue green algae. This is attributed to the increased availability of carbon dioxide for the process of photosynthesis.

The polysaccharidic sheath present around the trichomes of these algae binds the soil particles and increases the particle size. This improvement in soil aggregates formation increases aeration and water holding capacity. Some saprophytic algae like *Calothrix, Tolypothrix* and *Scytonema* grow on moist soil surface forming a velvety growth and protect the soil from erosion.

Iron toxicity

Algae have been found to grow in the subsoil zone upto a depth of about 20 cm. Being photosynthetic in nature they liberate oxygen in this zone which helps in bringing down utilizable organic matter content of soil. This has an important implication in areas where 2 to 3 crops of rice are taken in one year. In these areas continuous water-logging conditions create reducing conditions which results in iron toxicity. The oxygen liberated by the blue green algae in the micro-aerobic or anaerobic zones of a rice field converts Fe^2 to Fe^3. The latter being insoluble gets participated and iron content of the water is reduced. Iron, if present beyond 5 ppm, is known to adversely affect the cell permeability.

Phosphate solubilization

Many algae have been found to solubilize the insoluble phosphate to the extent of 2.27 mg P_2O_5/ml/15 days. This attains importance in view of the fact that most of the phosphatic fertilizer, when applied to soil, is immediately converted into insoluble calcium phosphate and becomes unavailable to the plants.

Response of BGA to various external stresses

Algae when introduced in the field are subjected to physical, chemical and biotic stresses. The physical stress is exerted by soil texture, temperature and moisture. Chemical properties of the soil, pH, fertilizers and various agricultural chemicals constitute the chemical stresses. Varieties of microorganisms present in soil exert antagonistic and synergistic effects on the introduced algae.

Physical stresses

Heavy soils rich in organic matter and with higher water-holding capacity support good algal growth. Saline alkali soils with higher water table and poor drainage harbour rich flora of blue green algae. Conversely, sandy soils have a poor algal growth. Blue green algae can grow at temperature range of 30 to 45 °C. Blue green algae are essentially true hydrophytes, although many of them exist in sub-aerial and terrestrial habitats. Although water-logged conditions favour the growth of BGA, quite a few of them grow as true saprophytes. In such forms no significant reduction in growth and nitrogen fixation was observed even when water was present upto 50% of the total water holding capacity of soil. Increased humidity coupled with high temperature and shade favour luxurious growth of algae in rice fields.

Chemical stresses

Soil pH plays an important role in distribution and predominance of algae. Acidic soils show a higher incidence of green algae while neutral to slightly alkaline soils support a rich blue green algae flora. The ideal pH range for luxuriant growth of blue green algae is 6.5 to 8.5.

Use of chemical fertilizers and pesticides has become an integral part of the present day agriculture. In the presence of fertilizers nitrogen blue green algae are expected to "shut-off" the process of nitrogen fixation. This effect is more pronounced in presence of NH_4^+ than NO_3^- nitrogen. However, upto 40 ppm ammonium nitrogen, no significant reduction in nitrogen fixation by blue green algae occurs.

The blue green algae have been found to accumulate pesticides within their cells, in concentrations several folds higher than that of surroundings. At the recommended field application doses, most of the pesticides do not have any adverse affects on the activity of algae.

Biotic stresses

Varieties of microorganisms inhabit the soil. In an undisturbed soil ecosystem, there always exists equilibrium. A disturbance in this is likely to be met with resistance. The capacity of intruder to withstand, overcome and adjust to the new environment qualifies the organisms to be used as inoculums. Fungi like *Alternaria* and *Cephalosporium* have synergistic effect on algae. Antibiotics producing organisms are expected to have a regulatory effect on algae. Protozoa, mosquito, larvae and snails are common grazers of algae in rice fields.

Blue green algae

Algal Production Technology

The success of any technology usually depends upon its techno-economic feasibility. The algal production technology developed and reported by different Algologists is very simple in operation and easy in adaptability by Indian farmers. The technology has got potential to provide an additional income from the sale of algal biofertilizer. In general, there are four methods of algal production that have been reported, viz. (a) trough or tank method, (b) pit method, (c) field method and (d) nursery cum algal production method. The former two methods are essentially for individual farmers and latter two are for bulk production on a commercial scale.

a. **Trough method:**
   i. Prepare shallow trays (2 m × 1 m × 23 cm) of galvanized iron sheet or permanent tank. The size of the tank can be increased if more material is to be produced.
   ii. Spread 4 to 5 kg of river soil and mix well with 100 g of superphosphate and 2 g sodium molybdate.
   iii. Pour 5 to 15 cm of water in the trays. This will depend upon local conditions i.e. rate of evaporation. Mix the ingredients properly.
   iv. In order to avoid the nuisance of mosquitoes and insects add 10 to 15 g Furadon granules or Malathion, or any other suitable granules.
   v. The mixture of soil and water will settle within 8–10 hours. At this time, add 200 to 250 g mother culture of blue green algae to the surface of water. Then don't disturb water.
   vi. The reaction of the soil should be neutral. If the soil is acidic then add $CaCO_3$ in order to bring the pH of the soil to neutral.
   vii. If sunlight and temperature are normal then within 10–15 days the growth of the blue green algae will look hard flakes on the surface of the water/ soil. Similarly, water level will be reduced due to evaporation.

viii. This way water in the tray/pit is allowed to evaporate and the growth of the algae flakes is allowed to dry.

ix. If soil is dried the algal growth is separated from soil. These pieces of algal growth are collected and stored in plastic bags. In this way from one m² tray or/pit about half-tonnes blue-green algal growth is obtained.

x. Again add water to trays and stair the soil well. Then allow the algae to grow in this way. This time it is not necessary to add mother culture of algae or superphosphate. In this manner one can harvest growth of algae 2–3 times. After this, effect of superphosphate and soil is reduced.

b. **Pit method:** This method of production of blue green algae does not differ from the one described above i.e. trough method. Instead of troughs or tanks pits are dug in the ground and layered with thick polythene sheet to hold the water or one-half cement plastered tanks. Other procedure is the same as in the trough method. This method is easy and less expensive to operate by small farmers.

c. **Field scale method:** The field scale production of blue green algae is really a scaled-up operation of trough method to produce the material on a commercial scale. This type of method of algal production is more common amongst farmers of south India.

i. Demarcate the area in the field for algal production: The suggested area is 40 m². No special preparation is necessary although algal production is envisaged immediately after crop harvest, the stubble is to be removed and if the soil is loamy it should be well puddle to facilitate water-logging conditions.

ii. Prepare a bund with earth so as to store the water.

iii. Flood the area with water to a depth of 2.5 cm. In trough or pit methods flooding is done only in the beginning, while in field scale method flooding is repeatedly needed to keep the water standing.

iv. Then apply superphosphate 12 kg/40 m².

v. To control the insect-pests attach, apply Carbofuran (3% granules) or Furadon 250 g/40 m².

vi. If the field has received previously algal application for at least two consecutive cropping seasons no fresh algal application is required. Otherwise apply the composite algal culture of 5 kg/40 m².

vii. In clayey soils, good growth of algae takes place in about two weeks in clear, sunny weather, while in loamy soils it takes three to four weeks.

viii. Once the algae have grown and formed floating mats they are allowed to dry in the sun in the field and the dried algal flake are then collected in sunny bags for further use.

ix. One can continually harvest algal growth from the same area by reflooding the plot and applying superphosphate and pesticides. In such situations an addition of algal inoculums for subsequent production is not necessary.

       x. During summer months (April-June), the average yield of algae per harvest ranges from 16–30 kg/40 m².

  d. Nursery cum algal production: Farmers can produce algae along with seedlings in their nurseries. If 320 m² of land are alloted to prepare a nursery, an additional 40 m² alongside can be prepared for algal production as described above. By the time rice seedlings are ready for transplantation about 15–20 kg of algal material will be available. This much quantity of algal mass will be sufficient to inoculate one-and-half hectares of area. If every farmer produces the algal material required to inoculate his own land then he will reduce the cost of algal inoculums required to be purchased. So also one can cut the cost of chemical fertilizers to be applied as recommended.

Recommendation of algal biomass for field application:

     i. If mineral nitrogen fertilizers are not used, apply blue green algae biofertilizer in order to gain the benefits of 30–40 kg Nitrogen/ha.

    ii. Broadcast the dry algal material over the standing water in the rice field at a rate of 10–15 kg/ha one week after transplanting the seedlings.

  iii. Addition of excess algal material is not harmful and will accelerate the multiplication and establishment in the field.

  iv. The sun dried algal material can be stored for a long time in a dry state without any loss in viability.

    v. Do not store the algal material in direct contact with chemical fertilizers or other chemicals.

  vi. Apply algae for atleast three consecutive seasons so that there will be sufficient algal inoculums found in the field.

 vii. Recommended pest control measures and other management practices don't interfere with the establishment and activity of algae in the field.

Blue green algae (Algalization and crop yield)

The significance of algal biofertilizer lies in the fact that unlike the chemical fertilizers, these are not directly utilized by the crop. Only the products of their activity are used. During the crop growth cycle, the algae grow, multiply, fix atmospheric nitrogen and make it available to the crop by way of excretion and autolysis. During unfavorable season, they form perennating bodies which germinate with the onset of congenial conditions. Thus, there is a possibility to build up populations of these algae in the soil, through superimposed inoculations for 3–4 consecutive seasons. Algalization of rice crops has been found to supplement nitrogenous fertilizers to the extent of 30–40 kg N/ha/season.

Successful establishment of desired algae in the rice fields has been found to form a source of slow release of nitrogen for the crop plants. They have also been found to protect a part of the applied fertilizer nitrogen from being lost. Studies using N^{15} have been shown that the nitrogen fixed by the blue green algae is actually taken up by the crop plants.

Algalization in problematic soils

Saline-alkali soils are generally unsuitable for raising crops. Blue green algae have been shown to help in reclamation of such soils. This is because of the preferential absorption or adsorption of sodium by them. The growth of these blue green algae in saline–alkaline habitats reduces salinity by 25–30%, pH, electrical conductivity and exchangeable sodium. It also increases aggregation, hydraulic conductivity, soil nitrogen and permeability.

However, we still don't know the mechanism by which the blue green algae scavenges sodium (Na). Attempts are to be made to investigate as to what happens to this absorbed/adsorbed sodium. It is also essential to develop an adaptable technology which can be used to grow and multiply the salt tolerant algal strains in such areas. Acidic soils pose another problem in getting good results from algalization. Majority of blue green algae have a wide pH range of 6.5 to 8.5. However, some algal species are delicate. Quite a few of them have been found to be true acidic forms showing optimum growth only when the pH is below 5.0. On the other hand, there are forms, which prefer only alkaline pH. Thus, it is possible to isolate pH specific algal forms from the natural algal flora which can be used in acidic soils without any soil amendments.

3.2 CONSTRAINTS OF BIOFERTILIZERS

The major limiting factors include:

i. Narrow genetic base of mother cultures and lack of efficient and virulent strains suitable to various agro-environments.

ii. Unsatisfactory carrier material with uniform and consistent good quality comparable to imported peat material.

iii. Contamination in broth mixing and packing stages, not using completely closed system of production.

iv. Unsatisfactory packing material which reduces shelf life.

v. Unsatisfactory storing conditions, particularly during the distribution period.

vi. Exposure to high temperatures and sunlight destroy the microbial culture.

vii. Biofertilizer should be preferably be kept in cold storage conditions. Lack of quality controls and certification procedures.

viii. At field level: The efficiency when applied to soils is limited by several factors. Some important factros influencing efficiency of biofertilizers in field in situ are drought and high summer temperature, water logging, unfavourable soil pH, antagonism from other organisms and nutrient deficiency. There is an acute awareness gap among the farmers on the subject.

3.3 BIOGAS PRODUCTION

Biogas typically refers to a gas produced by the biological breakdown of organic matter in the absence of oxygen. Biogas originates from biogenic material and is a type of biofuel. One type of biogas is produced by anaerobic digestion or fermentation of biodegradable materials such as biomass, manure or sewage, municipal waste, green waste and energy crops. This type of biogas comprises primarily methane and carbon dioxide. The other principal type of biogas is wood gas which is created by gasification of wood or other biomass. This type of biogas is comprised primarily of nitrogen, hydrogen, and carbon monoxide, with trace amounts of methane. The gases methane, hydrogen and carbon monoxide can be combusted or oxidized with oxygen. Air contains 21% oxygen. This energy release allows biogas to be used as a fuel. Biogas can be used as a low-cost fuel in any country for any heating purpose, such as cooking. It can also be used in modern waste management facilities where it can be used to run any type of heat engine, to generate either mechanical or electrical power. Biogas can be compressed, much like natural gas, and used to power motor vehicles and in the UK, for example, is estimated to have the potential to replace around 17% of vehicle fuel. Biogas is a renewable fuel, so it qualifies for renewable energy subsidies in some parts of the world.

Biogas is practically produced as Land Fill Gas (LFG) or digester gas. A biogas plant is the name often given to an anaerobic digester that treats farm wastes or energy crops. Biogas can be produced utilizing anaerobic digesters. These plants can be fed with energy crops such as maize silage or biodegradable wastes including sewage, sludge and food waste.

Landfill gas is produced by wet organic waste decomposing under anaerobic conditions in a landfill. The waste is covered and compressed mechanically and by the weight of the material that is deposited from above. This material prevents oxygen from accessing the waste and anaerobic microbes thrive. This gas builds up and is slowly released into the atmosphere if the landfill site has not been engineered to capture the gas. Landfill gas is hazardous for three key reasons. Landfill gas becomes explosive when it escapes from the landfill and mixes with oxygen. The lower explosive limit is 5% methane and the upper explosive limit is 15% methane. The methane contained within biogas is 20 times more potent as a greenhouse gas than carbon dioxide. Therefore uncontained landfill gas which escapes into the atmosphere may significantly contribute to the effects of global warming. In addition to this volatile organic compounds (VOCs) contained within landfill gas contribute to the formation of photo-chemical smog.

The composition of biogas varies depending upon the origin of the anaerobic digestion process (Table 3.1). Landfill gas typically has methane concentrations around 50%. Advanced waste treatment technologies can produce biogas with 55–75% CH_4 or higher using *in situ* purification techniques biogas also contains water vapor, with the fractional water vapor volume of biogas temperature correction content and thermal expansion can be easily done via algorithm.

Table 3.1: Composition of biogas

Compound	Concentration (%)
Methane(CH_4)	50–75
Carbon dioxide(CO_2)	25–50
Nitrogen(N_2)	0–10
Hydrogen(H_2)	0–1
Hydrogen sulfide(H_2S)	0–3
Oxygen(O_2)	0–2

Applications

Biogas can be utilized for electricity production on sewage works, in a CHP gas engine, where the waste heat from the engine is conveniently used to heat the digester; cooking, space heating, water heating and process heating. If compressed, it can replace compressed natural gas for use in vehicles, where it can fuel an internal combustion engine or fuel cells and is a much more effective displacer of carbon dioxide than the normal use in on-site CHP plants.

Scope and potential quantities

In India biogas produced from the anaerobic digestion of manure in small-scale digestion facilities is called *Gober gas* it is estimated that such facilities exist in over 2 million households. The digester is an airtight circular pit made of concrete with a pipe connection. The manure is directed to the pit, usually directly from the cattle shed. The pit is then filled with a required quantity of waste water. The gas pipe is connected to the kitchen fire place through control valves. The combustion of this biogas has very little odour or smoke. Owing to simplicity in implementation and use of cheap raw materials in villages, it is one of the most environmentally sound energy sources for rural needs. Some designs use vermiculture to further enhance the slurry produced by the biogas plant for use as compost.

Deenabandhu Model

This is a new model of biogas unit popular in India. The word 'Deenabandhu' means "helpful for the poor". The unit usually has a capacity of 2 to 3 cubic metres. It is constructed using bricks or by a ferrocement mixture. The unit is subsidised by the Ministry of Non-Conventional Energy Sources of the Government of India. A turn key agent is also provided to the approved mason for maintenance of the unit around for three years. The total cost of construction of a 2 cubic meter unit comes to ₹ 18,000 for the brick model and ₹ 14,000 for the Ferrocement model.

3.4   BIODEGRADATION

Bacteria and fungi, including yeasts and molds, are the microorganisms responsible for biodegradation. Environmental managers want to use biodegradation when it is needed and prevent it when preservation is important. Chemicals are live creosote or copper compounds commonly used to treat wood in buildings and other structures to prevent biodegradation. Compounds that inhibit biodegradation are often added to automobile anti-freeze solutions, aircraft deicer formulations, and other products to preserve the original qualities of the product. These products and chemicals can enter the environment and become contaminants. The inhibitors have a negative effect when the product becomes a waste and is to be biodegraded. For example, biodegradation of aircraft deicer formulations in airport run-off is often inhibited because of the benzotriazoles that are present to preserve the formulation.

Biodegradation is the chemical breakdown of materials by a physiological environment. The term is often used in relation to ecology, waste management and environmental remediation. Organic material can be degraded aerobically with oxygen, or anaerobically without oxygen. A term related to biodegradation is biomineralisation, in which organic matter is converted into minerals. Biosurfactant, an extracellular surfactant secreted by microorganisms enhances the biodegradation process. Biodegradable matter is generally organic material such as plant and animal matter and other substances originating from living organisms or artificial materials that are similar enough to plant and animal matter to be put to use by microorganisms. Some microorganisms have the astonishing, naturally occurring, microbial catabolic diversity to degrade, transform or accumulate a huge range of compounds including hydrocarbons (e.g. oil), polychlorinated biphenyls (PCBs), polyaromatic hydrocarbons (PAHs), pharmaceutical substances, radio nuclides and metals. Major methodological breakthroughs in microbial biodegradation have enabled detailed genomic, metagenomic, proteomic, bioinformatic and other high-throughput analyses of environmentally relevant microorganisms providing unprecedented insights into key biodegradative pathways and the ability of microorganisms to adapt to changing environmental conditions.

Pesticides

4.1 HISTORY

Before 2500 BC, humans have utilized agricultural chemical to protect their crops. The first known pesticide was elemental sulfur dusting used in Sumer about 4,500 years ago. By the 15th century, toxic chemicals such as arsenic, mercury and lead were being applied to crops to kill pests. In the 17th century, nicotine sulfate was extracted from tobacco leaves for use as an insecticide. In the 19th century, the two more natural pesticides introduced, pyrethrum which is derived from chrysanthemums, and rotenone which is derived from the roots of tropical vegetables.

In 1939, Paul Müller discovered DDT; which was a very effective insecticide. It quickly became the most widely used pesticide in the world. In the 1940s manufacturers began to produce large amounts of synthetic pesticides and their use became widespread. Some sources consider the 1940s and 1950s to have been the start of the "pesticide era." Pesticide use has increased 50-fold since 1950 and 2.3 million tonnes of industrial pesticides are now used each year. Seventy-five per cent of all pesticides in the world are used in developed countries, but use in developing countries is increasing. In the 1960s, it was discovered that DDT was preventing many fish-eating birds from reproducing, which was a serious threat to biodiversity. Rachel Carson wrote the best-selling book *Silent Spring* about biological magnification. The agricultural use of DDT is now banned under the Stockholm Convention on Persistent Organic Pollutants, but it is still used in some developing nations to prevent malaria and other tropical diseases by spraying on interior walls to kill or repel mosquitoes.

Instead of 50 years of pesticide use, most pesticides have never been systematically reviewed for their full range of long-term health effects on humans, such as potential damage to nervous, endocrine or immune systems.

4.1.1 Introduction

Pest of Crops

Pest organisms causes economic loss in crop production. Pest has been defined as any organism detrimental to man or his property in causing damage significant of economic importance. Checking these organisms by various ways are grouped under the principles of plant protection. The pests are classified as follows:

I. Plant Kingdom Pests	II. Animal Kingdom Pests	III. Viruses
1. Bacteria	1. Nematodes	
	(Ph. Nematohelminthes Cl. Nematoda)	
2. Fungi	2. Mollusca (Ph.)	
	(Cl. Gastropoda) e.g. snail, slugs	
3. Algae	3. Crustacea (Cl) e.g. crabs	
4. Arborell	4. Archnida (Cl) e.g. mites	Arthropoda (Phylum)
5. Weeds	5. Hexapoda (Cl) e.g. insects, bugs beetles	
	6. Aves (Cl) e.g. birds	
	7. Mammalia (Cl) e.g. mice, rabbit	Chordata (Phylum)

4.1.2 Principles of Plant Protection

Pest control may be defined as any method or procedure employed to reduce the pest population and prevent damages caused by them. There are certain methods or techniques by which losses sustain by the cultivator due to the pests, which can be minimised.

1. **Mechanical Control:** These methods aim in reducing the population of pests particularly insects by manual devices. e.g. a specially designed hopper doser is employed to collect grasshoppers and *Pyrilla* in some countries.

2. **Cultural Control:** It is concerned with the use of farming or cultural practices associated with the crop production to make environment less favourable for the survival, growth and reproduction of pest species, e.g. crop rotation, post harvest ploughing etc.

3. **Physical Control:** Control of pests through manipulation of physical environment or employment of physical sources, e.g.

   i. *Light energy (Light trap):* It requires 100 watt lamp and for collection of insects, a funnel is in a bottle containing kerosene-water mixture or calcium cyanide solution.

   ii. *Electromagnetic energy:* X-ray and γ-ray are used for male sterility of insects.

   iii. *Sound energy :* A source of ultrasound are used for :

       a. cytoplasm precipitation. and
       b. nucleo membrane breakage of insects

4. **Chemical Control:** Pests are controlled by (i) plant products/other natural products (ii) synthetic inorganic compounds and (iii) synthetic organic compounds. These chemicals are known as pesticides.

   The chemical protection of plants is based on the use of various organic and inorganic compounds toxic to harmful organisms. With the developing chemical technology and progressive use of greater quantity of pesticides, various pesticides belonging to diverse chemical groups with varying structures are now available for pest control. The main requirements of satisfactory application of pesticides are:

    a. Inherent toxicity and easy availability of active constituent for pest control;

    b. Low phytotoxicity;

    c. Low toxicity to man and animals;

    d. Stability in storage as concentrate; and

    e. Stability when diluted to prepare active spray strength.

5. **Use of Resistant Varieties and Transgenic Varieties:** Genetical improvement of host plant against the different pests through breeding (resistant varieties) and through incorporation of genes (transgenic varieties) from different living organisms (microorganisms, plants and animals).

6. **Biological Control:** Biological control has been broadly defined as the encouragement of beneficial organisms already existing in a locality or of the introduction of suitable new specie(s) of exotic parasitic organism(s), which are parasites on harmful insects in a locality where the pest is thriving with a view to control the pest, e.g. insect-insect, insect-microorganism, microorganism-microorganism, plant-plant.

    e.g. *Bacillus thuringiensis, Neoaplectena glasseri* (parasitic nematode against Japanese bettle)

7. **Legal Control/Legislative Measures:**

    i. Quarantine — International / Domestic

    Quarantine measures are introduced by the relevant authorities of a country to prevent (biosecurity) the admission into it and spreading of the most dangerous plant diseases, pests and weeds.

    ii. Pest controlling laws.

    iii. Certification of planting materials.

8. **Integrated Pest Management (IPM):** Integrated pest management signifies the combination of all pertinent methods– chemical, cultural, biological, use of resistant varieties, etc.

Pesticide

Pesticides means any substance intended for preventing, destroying or controlling any pest including unwanted species of plants or animals during storage, transport, distribution and processing of food, agricultural commodities or animal feed or which may be administered to the animal for the control of ectoparasites.

Use of pesticides in India began in 1948, just after independence, when DDT was imported for malaria control and BHC for locust control. The first plant, ICI to produce BHC was established in 1952 in the private sector at Rishra, near Kolkata.

In 1954, Hindustan Insecticides Ltd., first Govt. of India enterprise was set up at Delhi to manufacture DDT for malaria control programme. Since then, the production of pesticides has increased tremendously. At present 241 pesticides are registered for use in India; 61.0% are in the form of insecticides, 16.0% are herbicides, 18.0% fungicides and 5.0% other pesticides. The per hectare consumption of pesticides is estimated at 0.480 kg.

4.1.3 Classification of Pesticides

Depending on the purpose for which they are used, pesticides are divided into the following basic groups:

According to use

I. **Direct Action Agrochemicals**
   1. Bactericides : Chemicals used to control the bacterial diseases
   2. Fungicides : Chemicals used to control the plant diseases caused by various fungi
   3. Antiseptics : For the protection of non-metallic materials (wood, cane, bamboo etc.) from damage by microorganisms
   4. Algicides : For the destruction of algae and other aquatic vegetation
   5. Herbicides : For control of weeds (herbaceous weeds)
   6. Arboricides : Destruction of undesirable arborell and bushy vegetation
   7. Nematicides : For the control of nematodes
   8. Limacides or Molluskicides or Molluscides : For the control of various mollusks, including gastropods
   9. Acaricides : For the control of mites or ticks
   10. Insecticides : Chemicals used for control of insects
   11. Zoocides or Rodenticides : For the control of rodents/mice

II. **Indirect Action Agrochemicals**
   1. Attractants : chemical which attracts some harmful pests, e.g. food lure and sex lure (pheromone).
   2. Repellents : which repel some harmful pests, e.g. Indalone, Rutger 612, MGK 326.
   3. Chemosterilants : chemical which use to sterilize the harmful pest reproductive organ, e.g. Tepa, Apholate.
   4. Antifeedants : which prevent the feeding of a pest on a treated material without necessary killing the pest. The insect remains on the treated material on starvation, e.g. Clerodin A.
   5. Synergent : which activate on the action of pesticide chemical, e.g. Piperonyl butoxide in pyrethroid insecticides.

Chemicals used for stimulating or retarding the growth of plants (growth regulators), for removal of leaves (defoliants), for desiccating plants (desiccants) are also included among the pesticides. However, out of these, insecticides, fungicides and herbicides in that order are most widely used.

According to the nature of their penetration into the target organism:

Insecticide

1. *Contact insecticides,* which kill insects by means of intimate and direct contacts with any part of the body, e.g. naturally occurring compounds like nicotine, pyrethrum and rotenone; lindane, DDT, parathion.

2. *Stomach insecticides,* which penetrate into the insect through the organs of its alimentary system and kill it as a result of the poison entering the gut (i.e. alimentary system) e.g. lead arsenate, calcium arsenate, methoxychlor etc.

3. *Systematic insecticide,* which are capable of moving through the vascular system of plants and poisoning insects that feed on the plants. Systemic poisons are those which are applied to one part of the crop like root or the leaf and are translocated to other parts of the plant in the fluid systems for tendering the whole plant toxic to insect. Most of the systemic poisons are stomach poisons in that the attacking insect must either chew the tissue or suck the juice of the plant before it is killed e.g. phosphoric or thiophosphoric acids esters.

4. *Fumigants,* which penetrate into the insect through its respiratory organs. e.g. liquid nicotine, naphthalene, carbon disulphide, methylbromide. Majority of pesticides can penetrate the insect organism simultaneously by different routes. Based on their main route of penetration into the insect, they are assigned to one or other subgroup. For example, though *lindane* shows contact, stomach and fumigant action, still it is assigned to the contact insecticides group.

Fungicides

1. *Seed disinfectants:* The application of fungicides to seeds before planting is known as seed disinfection and the chemical/fungicide used for this purpose is seed disinfectant. The purposes for seed disfection are (a) to control diseases caused by seed borne infection and (b) to protect germinating seeds or seedlings from the attack of soil-borne pathogens. Treatment of seeds by chemicals may be effected by (i) in liquid (ii) dry seed treatment, or (c) slurry treatment; e.g. thiram, captan, chloranil, benomyl etc.

2. Fungicides used for control the diseases of growing plants:
    i. preparations with a prophylactic effect, that are used to protect plants from various infections, e.g. agalol, captan.
    ii. preparation with an eradicative effect (curatives), that are used to cure the disease-affected plants, e.g. blitox, bavistin etc.

3. Fungicide for disinfectants for non-metallic materials and bactericides
    i. *Contact fungicide:* Which kill the fungi by means of direct contact, e.g. blitox, captan.
    ii. *Systematic fungicide:* It moves through the vascular system of plants e.g. terrazole, benlate, clolroneb, 1-4-oxathins.

Herbicide

Classification with respect to their action on plants:
1. Non-selective herbicides, acting on all species of plants e.g. Butachlor, Paraquat, PCP.
2. Selective herbicides, which attack/kill only certain species of plants and are safe for others e.g. 2,4-D, I.P.C, CIPC dalapon.

This division is conditional, since the majority of the compounds depending on the concentrations used and the rate of application per unit area treated, may be either non-selective or selective herbicides.

Classification on the basis of the manner of absorption:
1. Soil herbicide: A herbicidal agent taken up by the plant via the root is termed a soil herbicide.
2. Foliage herbicide: It enters via the green, aerial plant parts.
3. Contact herbicides: It include compounds injurious to plant foliage and stems that come in direct contact with them. When such compounds contact the foliage, the normal life processes of the plant are disturbed and it dies.
    It is necessary, however, to note that such herbicides injure only those parts of the plant with which they come in contact, and in some cases sprouting of new shoots and further development of the injured plant are observed.
4. Systemic herbicides: This includes compounds that are capable of moving through the vascular system of plants. When such herbicides come in contact with the foliage and roots of a plant, they are quickly distributed through the whole plant causing its death.
    The use of systemic herbicides is especially valuable in controlling weeds with strong root systems and perennial weeds.
5. Herbicides acting on the root system of plants or on germinating seeds: It consists of herbicides that are introduced into the soil to destroy seeds, germinating seeds and the roots of seeds.

Apart from the quantity of herbicide applied, the timing of the application is also important for an optimal control of weeds. Three timings are differentiated according to *the state of development of the crop plants* when the herbicide is applied.
1. Pre-sowing;
2. Pre-emergence;
3. Post-emergence.

The type of herbicide used is selected according to the nature and state of development of the target weed. Soil applied herbicides are used for weeds that not yet emerged; foliar or soil applied herbicides are used for post-emergence.

Criteria of an ideal pesticide

1. Chemical must be non-phytotoxic (desirable crop).
2. Inherent toxicity and easy availability of active constituent for pest control.
3. Quick toxic action.
4. Stability on treated surface (persistence) for a reasonable period.
5. Toxic to as many stages of target organisms.
6. Harmless to higher animals, including human being.
7. Harmless to beneficial flora and fauna.
8. Compatible with the group insecticides, fungicides and herbicides.
9. Relatively non-accumulation in soil and edible plant product.
10. Seasonal stability under conditions of storage and transport.
11. Non-erosive action on the metal and rubber parts of the appliances.

4.1.4 Pesticide Formulations

Formulation is an art and science of wrapping up the active chemical/toxicant into suitable forms so as to make it more effective.

Advantages of formulation

1. Formulations dilute the active ingredient (a.i.).
2. It provide the doses and uniform coverage of crop field.
3. Pesticide formulation can be applied according to situation demand.
4. Formulations are safe, economic and efficient.
5. It minimizes the environmental hazards.

General classification of formulation

Dry/Solid formulations :
1. Dusts
2. Granules
3. Wettable powders
4. Seed disinfectants

Liquid formulations :
1. Emulsion concentrates
2. Solution of pesticides in water and organic solvents
3. Aerosol

Criteria for choice of pesticide formulation

1. Purpose for which we apply the pesticide.
2. Type of machinery materials for application of respective formulation (duster, sprayer etc.).

3. Pest itself govern the choice (soil inhabiting insect, flying insect, crawling insect etc.).
4. Physico-chemical properties of pesticide (water solubility, ionizibility etc.).
5. Local weather condition (e.g. high velocity of wind, rainy weather etc.).
6. Availability of applied equipment.
7. Economy of the pesticide formulation.
8. Whether the pest should control or preventive measure.

Dusts (Powders)

Pesticidal dusts consist of a mechanical mixture of the active ingredient with or without an inert diluent pulverized to a particle size of 3 to 30.

Classification of dusts

i. *Undiluted toxic agent* : insecticides, which may be applied as dusts without any diluent, e.g. Calcium arsenates, sodium fluoride, ground pyrethrum flowers etc.

ii. *Toxic agent with an active diluent* : Some insecticides like rotenone can be mixed with other active pesticides like sulphur (fungicide) and then applied.

iii. *Toxic agent with an inert diluent* : The powdered material of the pesticide is diluted with relatively inert diluents (carriers) like tale in order to cover more area or to reduce the phytotoxicity or to improve the chemical or physical properties.

Type of carriers

1. Mineral: i. Chemically active/adsorptive materials
   a. Carbonate : Dolomite
   b. Phosphate : Appatite
   c. Oxide : Ca lime Mg lime Silicon oxide (Pyrollite)
   ii. Relatively inert materials : Talc (Montmorillonite, Kaolinite, Illite, Pyrophylite)

2. Biological source: i. Rice hull
   ii. Ground grains
   iii. Corn-cob
   iv. Wallnut shell

Granulated Formulations

Two types must be differentiated in products of Granular (G) form:

A. Products made by impregnation with liquid pesticides or solutions of them (soaking or coating) of granular carriers (perlite or vermiculite) [a.i. 20% max technically feasible]

B. Products made by granulation of powdery mixtures of active ingredient and formulation aids [a.i. same order as those in dispersible powder] simultaneously.

Advantages

i. Granulated formulations are widely used for the control of soil inhabiting pests and also for making plants poisonous to the sucking pests.

ii. Granular applications are becoming popular as they are more convenient and leave a smaller residue on the plants.

The most widely used granular formulations are of 0.2 to 1 mm size.

Low strength granule   -   for plants (e.g. 3G Furadan)

High strength granule   -   weeds in water reservoirs

Wettable Powders

Powdered formulations that on dilution with water yield rather stable suspensions are called Wettable Powders (W.P.).

Advantages

i. 90% of WP adheres to plant leaf (whereas 10% in case of dust).

ii. Pesticide penetrate in fruit and other parts in case of EC/liquid formulation but lower percentage of penetration in case of W.P. W.P. adhere well to the surfaces and do not penetrate and can be washed out if required.

iii. Low drifting in case of W.P. in comparison to dust formulation.

Important conditions for the wettable powders to be effective are:

i. Rapid formation of a suspension and slow settling out of solid particles.

ii. Good wettability of sprayed objects (e.g. leaf, fruit etc.) and easy spreading over their surface.

iii. Retention on sprayed surfaces for a more or less prolonged time.

iv. It should be stable in storage and should not cake.

Emulsive Concentrates

Emulsive concentrates (E.C.) are that formulation which upon dilution with water give stable emulsions suitable for spraying plants and surfaces.

> Emulsion: fine dispersion of one liquid in another

E.C. =	A.I.	+	Carrier (solvent)	+	Emulsifier
	Pesticide (active ingredient)		Example: Aromax, Methyl isobutyl ketone (MIBK), Xylene, kerosene		Example: Na-sterate, Ca-sulphonate, Ether polyethylene glycol, Ether polypropylene glycol, LOVO (emulsifier for air spraying: to decrease the evaporation)

Solutions of Pesticides in Water and Organic Solvents

Water: Only compounds that are rather soluble in water can be used in the form of aqueous solutions.

e.g.   herbicides (salts of organic acids with different bases)
Organophosphate insecticides (water soluble)
Fungicides
Seed disinfection with aqueous solutions of organic Hg compounds

Solvents: Various solutions of pesticides are also used to control some plant domestic pests by mixing in organic solvents (xylene, kerosene, cyclohexanone, methyl ethyl ketone etc.)

e.g. Baygon

Aerosols

One of the new forms in which pesticides are used in public health and agriculture is the aerosol. Aerosols obtained by atomizing solution of insecticides in volatile solvents (petroleum products) usually are recommended for control of flies and other flying insects in enclosed premies. Such solutions are placed in metal aerosol cylinders equipped with an atomizing device. With the aid of CO_2 or a low-boiling solvent (freon, methyl chloride, etc.) pressure is created in the cylinder that facilitates good atomization of the preparation. After the solution has been sprayed into the air and the solvent has evaporated, the pesticide remains in the atmosphere in a finely dispersed condition.

Fumigants

Pesticide fumigants must be sufficiently volatile to produce a toxic concentration of vapour in closed space.

Pesticides in gaseous form are known as fumigants and are used in storage house, buildings, ship and air cargo and even in soil where the gas can be confined.

e.g. Crop fumigation (Citrus trees) by HCN.

Soil fumigation by celphos or phosphine or hydrogen phosphide gas is released from tablets containing aluminium phosphide or zinc phosphide in the presence of moisture.

Adjuvants or Auxiliary Spray Materials in Pesticide Formulation

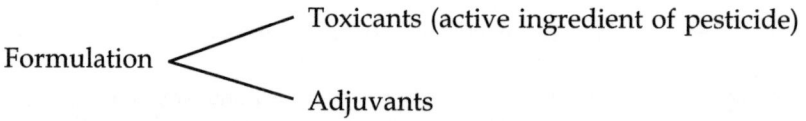

Formulation
- Toxicants (active ingredient of pesticide)
- Adjuvants

Adjuvants are accessory or supplementary agents or substances added to the plant protecting chemicals in order to increase the efficiency of the toxicants.

1. Wetting and spreading agents
2. Emulsifying agents (emulsifiers) and detergents

3. Dispersing agents or deflocculating agents
4. Adhesives or stickers
5. Penetrante
6. Humicant
7. Deodorant
8. Stabilising agent
9. Synergists or activators
10. Propellant
11. Correctners/Correcters

1. **Wetting and spreading agents:** Spreaders are to prevent the spray solution to form large droplets and their roll down the leaves so that the material gets evenly spread out. A spreader has to do wetting before it can spread and wetting-spreading are closely related.
   e.g. long chain alcohols, soap, gelatin, sulphite lye (available as a by-product of paper industry).

2. **Emulsifying agents and detergents:** Materials which stabilize the emulsion of two liquids which are not miscible and tend to soluble in each other are emulsifying agents. There are a number of sprays in which the active ingredient is dissolved in an organic solvent, but later this solvent had to be dispersed in water for spraying. The emulsifying agents maintain the stability of the concentrate within limits.
   Detergents are emulsifiers which have got the additional property of wetting also.
   e.g. sodium stearate, calcium sulphonate, LOVO.

3. **Dispersing agents/deflocculating agents:** Materials used to keep the particles separate (e.g. W.P.) and prevent their aggregation into lumps are termed as deflocculating agents. e.g. Sodium carboxymethyl cellulose, methyl cellulose etc.

4. **Adhesives or stickers:** Substances which are adhesive in nature and improve the retentivity of the spray deposit are termed as stickers.
   e.g. Synthetic resins, gelatin, polyvinyl acetate.

5. **Penetrants:** The substances which enhance the penetration of the insecticide into the target insect, e.g. petroleum oil enable to insecticide to penetrate the target insect with waxy cutile (Coleoptora insect, locust etc.)

6. **Humictant:** The substance that are added to the spray to delay evaporation of water, in dry area, e.g. glycerol.

7. **Deodorant:** Some insecticides are offensive in smell, such as pyrethrin, thiocyanate; the unpleasant odour is musked by methyl pine oil, cider wood oil, at various concentration (0.1 to 1% concentration).

8. **Stabilising agent:** Some pesticides are degraded very fast and these can be comparatively controlled by using stabilising agent.

e.g. Toxaphane $\rightarrow$ Dehydro-carbonate (de chlorination checked)

Aldrin $\rightarrow$ Epichlorohydrine

Pyrethrin $\rightarrow$ Antioxidants Isopropyl cresol in loose powder

9. **Synergists or activators:** Synergism is said to occur when two materials give greater physiological action when applied together than when applied separately. For example, compound A gives 20% mortality and compound B gives 30% mortality, when applied separately to a species of insect, but when mixed and applied together the combination gives 90% mortality or increase of 40% over result to be expected from the individual one, e.g. Piperonyl butoxide in pyrethroids (Sesame oil).

10. **Propellant:** An inert compressed fluid in which the active contents of an aerosol are dispersed; e.g. hydrocarbon, flurocarbons or dimethyl ether.

11. **Correctners:** Which reduce the phytotoxicity of the pesticide chemicals.

   e.g. $CuSO_4$ is phytotoxic (in Bordeaux mixture) by using lime, phytotoxicity can be reduced. In lime sulphur, $FeSO_4$ is added which acts as correctner.

4.1.5 Toxicology of Pesticides

Toxicology (*toxicum* – poison, *logia* – speech, word) is a science dealing with poisons and their action on organisms.

Poisons are substances which when they enter an organism in different ways (through the respiratory tract, integument, alimentary tract) in insignificant amounts are capable of causing malfunctions of its vital activity which in definite conditions results in an unhealthy state, i.e. produce a toxic effect.

Toxicity: It is the property of a pesticide, when used in small amounts, to upset the normal vital activity of an organism and cause it to be poisoned, to perish. There are two types of toxicity e.g.

Acute poisoning and Chronic poisoning.

Acute poisoning: Acute poisoning of an organism by a pesticide occurs when the pesticide acts at once. It manifests itself in upsetting of the vital activity of the organism with a possible lethal outcome. It is attended by rapid development of the ailment, e.g.

Pesticide	Vital activity
Malathion, Quinalphos	Cholinesterase inhibition
Decamethrin, Fenvalerate	'Knock-down effect' due to rapid cholinesterase inhibition
Celphos	Oxidation-reduction processes inhibition etc.

Chronic poisoning: Chronic poisoning of an organism is the result of the repeated action of relatively small amounts of a pesticide and manifests itself in slowly developing malfunctioning of normal vital activity, e.g.

Warfarin: Anticongulation

Dose: A measure of the toxicity of pesticides for various organisms is the dose on the amount of a pesticide causing a definite effect.

The degree of toxicity of a substance is characterized by the following terminologies:

i. **Threshold dose:** The threshold dose is the smallest amount of a substance causing changes in an organism that are determined by the most sensitive biochemical and physiological tests in the absence of external indications of poisoning of an organism/animal.

ii. **Toxic sublethal dose:** It is the dose causing visible manifestations of poisoning of an organism without a lethal outcome.

iii. **Toxic lethal dose:** A toxic lethal dose causes poisoning of an organism terminating in its perishing.

Dose(s) of pesticide is expressed in units of mass of the pesticide per unit of area, volume or mass of the object being treated.

Active ingredient (a.i): a.i is the element, group or groups of the chemical compound which are responsible for insecticidal or fungicidal action of the formulation.

The toxicity indices of pesticide are designated by the following symbols:

LD   (Lethal Dose)

LC   (Lethal Concentration) and

ED   (Effective Dose)

If the effect of the action of a pesticide is evaluated according to the number of perished objects the indices LD and LC are used.

If the effect of the action of a pesticide is evaluated according to the degree of violation of separate vital activity processes (the accumulation of dry matter, inhibition of growth, the onset of separate reactions and so on) ED is the quantitative index.

LD_{50}: The amount of poison which will kill one-half of a group of experimental animals is called as Median Lethal Dose or LD_{50}.

The toxicity of pesticides varies and depends on their amount, the ways of entrance, the duration of action, the state of the organism, the environment, etc.

Toxicity according to ways of entrance:

i. **Oral toxicity:** Toxicity or toxic chemicals when ingested into the stomaches of test animals (e.g. rats) through mouth.

ii. **Dermal toxicity:** Toxicity or toxic chemicals in entering through the skin.

Classification of toxic chemicals

Based on toxicity tests, Bailey and Surft (1968) have classified the chemicals into six broad categories as stated in Table 4.1.

Table 4.1: Classification of chemicals based on toxicity

Toxicity Rating	Oral–rats LD$_{50}$ (mg/kg)	LD$_{50}$ (mg/kg) by single dose dermal rabbits	Possible lethal dose (man)
Extremely toxic	1 or less	20 or less	A taste to a grain
Highly toxic	1–50	21–200	A pinch to one tea-spoonful
Moderately toxic	51–500	201–1000	1 tea spoonful to 1 table spoonful
Slightly toxic	501–5000	1001–2000	28–560 g
Practically non-toxic	5001–15000	2001–20,000	560–1120 g
Relatively harmless	> 15,000	> 20,000	> 1120 g

In the Insecticides Act of Government of India (1968), the chemicals have been put into four categories detailed in Table 4.2.

Table 4.2: Classification of pesticides based on insecticide act

Classification of the insecticide/pesticide	Medium lethal dose by the oral route (acute toxicity) LD$_{50}$ mg/kg of the body weight of test animals	Medium lethal dose by the dermal route (dermal toxicity) LD$_{50}$ mg/kg of the body weight of animals	Single word in upper triangle	Colour of the identification band on the label
Extremely toxic	1–50	1–200	Poison	Bright red
Highly toxic	51–500	201–2000	Poison	Bright yellow
Moderately toxic	501–5000	2001–20,000	Danger	Bright blue
Slightly toxic	More than 5000	More than 20,000	Caution	Bright green

4.1.6 Steps for Minimization of Pesticide Toxicity

1. Antidote

A substance given to a patient to counteract the effect produced by the ingestion of a poisonous or toxic chemical is known as antidote.

Example:

Pesticide	Antidote
Group-I	
OP compounds (e.g. methyl parathion, phosphamidon, dursban, metasystox etc.)	Atropine sulphate is used. Injection should be repeated as symptoms recur.
Group-II	
Carbamate (Aldicarb, Carbfuran, Carbaryl etc.)	Atropine sulphate
Group-III	
O-Cl (Dieldrin, aldrin, endosulfan, BHC, DDT, toxaphase)	Calcium gluconate given intravenously

Contd.

Contd.

Group-IV	
Inorg. Arsenicarb (Sodium arsenite)	BAL (dimercaprol) is specific for arsenic poisons (intramuscular injection)
Group-V	
Cyanides–HCN or cyanogas	Sodium nitrite/sodium thiosulphate given intravenously
Group-VI	
Anticoagulants – Warfarin, Pival, Indalone, Diphacin	Vitamin K by month intravenously or intramuscularly. Vitamin C is a useful adjunct.

Universal antidote preparation

A mixture containing 80 g of activated charcoal, 4 g of tannic acid and 4 g of magnesium oxide in warm water will adsorb and neutralize the poison. Charred papad can act as a substitute for activated charcoal and strong tea decoction for tannic acid.

2. Insecticide Act

Insecticide Act, 1968

Govt. of India, No. 46 of 1968

and

The Insecticides (Amendment) Act, 1977

Govt. of India, No. 24 of 1977

and

The Insecticide Rules, 1971 and its amendment in 1977,

Govt. of India

An act to regulate the import, manufacture, sale, transport, distribution and use of insecticides with a view to prevent risk to human beings or animals and matters connected therewith. The enforcement of this Act is the joint responsibility of the Central and State Government.

Central Insecticides Board (CIB) is constituted to advise the Central Govt. and State Govts. on all technical matters arising out of the administration of this Act and to carry out other functions assigned to the Board by or under the Act.

A **Registration Committee (RC)** has been constituted to register insecticides, scrutinizing formulae, verifying claims of efficacy and safety to human beings and animals, specify the precaution against poisoning and any other function.

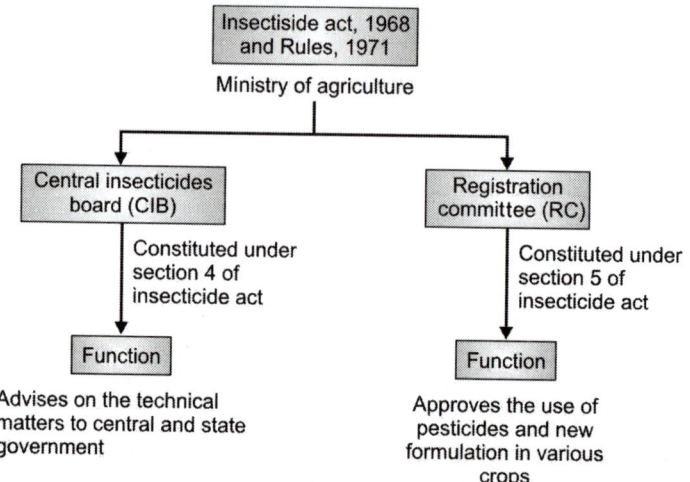

4.2 NATURALLY OCCURRING INSECTICIDES OR BOTANICAL INSECTICIDES

Nicotine: Alkaloids-alkali like compounds, found in plant kingdom [all organic bases are nitrogenous compounds possessing one pair of electron]

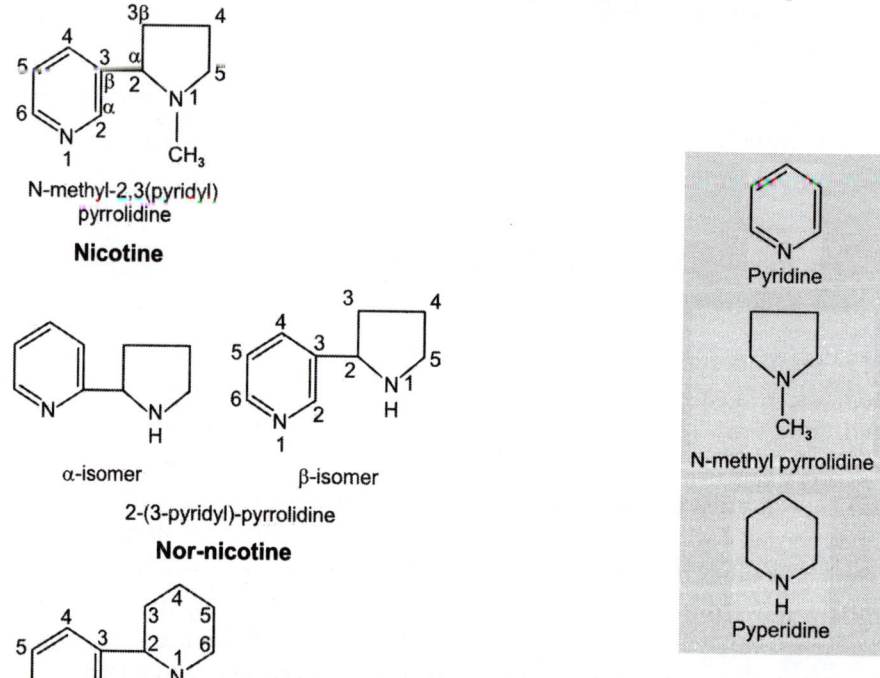

Source : Nicotine   : *Nicotiana tabacum*
                                      Nicotiana rustica

         Nor-nicotine : *Nicotiana sylvestris*
                                        Duboisia hopwoodii

         Anabasine   : *Anabasis aphylla*
                                        Nicotiana glauca

Mode of action : Nicotine has a comparatively high vapour pressure (volatility mgHg 0.0425 at 25 °C) mainly acts in vapour phase. Nicotine vapour penetrates through the cuticle and gut wall of the insects or through the spiracles in the tracheal system and paralyses the nervous system by blocking the motor nerves in the ventral nerve code. It is particularly effective against most soft-bodied insects particularly aphids.

Extraction of nicotine from plant

The mixture of alkali (generally Ca(OH)$_2$) and plant tissue is subjected to alternative pressure and vacuum which ruptures the cells of the tobacco tissues and permits the complete extraction of the alkaloid. It is sold in the market in the form of the 40% solution of sulphate i.e. nicotine sulphate.

Rotenoid

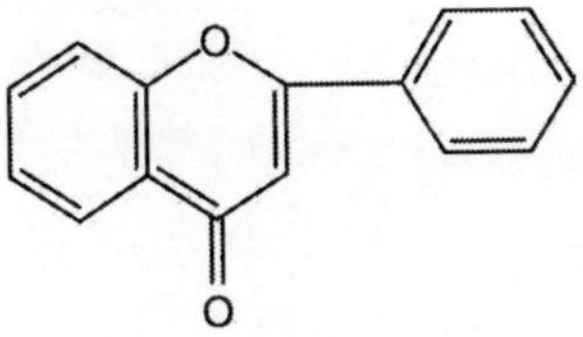

Flavanone 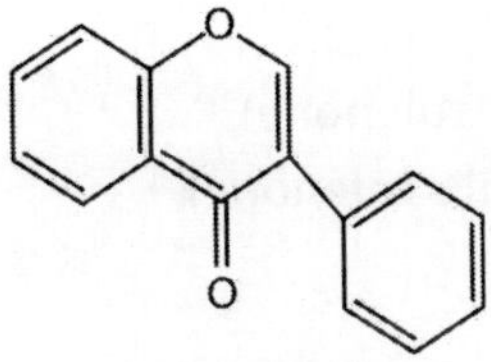   Isoflavanone   Isoflanone

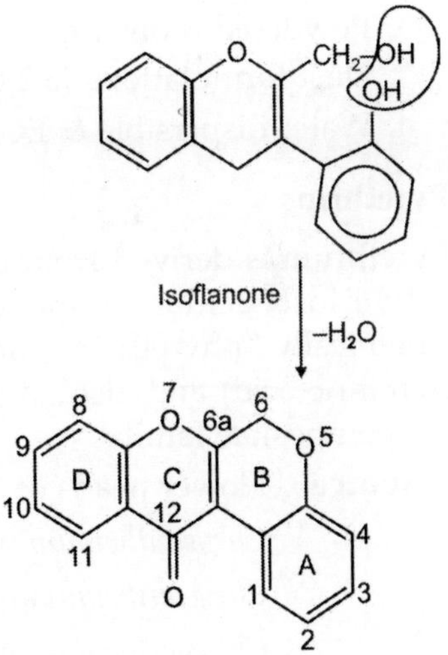

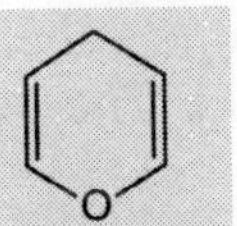

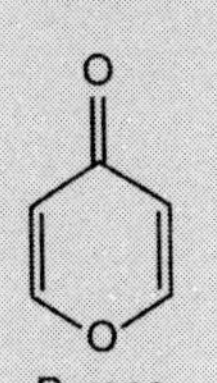

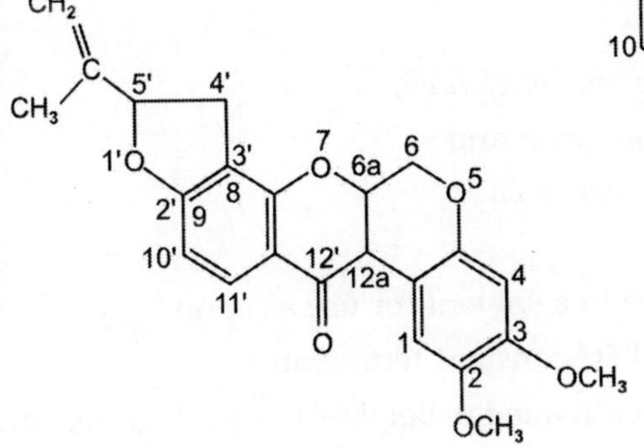

6a,12a,4′, 5′-Tetrahydro-2,3-dimethoxy-5′-isoprophenyl-furano(3′, 2′, 8, 9)-6H-rotoxen-12-one

Source: Commercial purposes : *Derris elliptica*
(Leguminous plants) : *D. malaccensis* } root
Other : *Tephrosia* spp.
Lonchocarpus spp.

Derris sp. and *Lonchocarpus* sp. are toxic to fish (i.e. Pisicidal effect)

Mode of Action: The exact mode of action of rotenoids is not yet known; but the respiratory system and heart beat of insects are depressed and slowly paralysed resulting in death. Rotenoid is believed to inhibit oxygen utilization of insect by the body cells. Poisoned insects exhibit a steady decline in oxygen consumption followed by paralysis and death.

Properties:

i. Rotenoids are highly toxic to fish, but they are virtually non-toxic to warm blooded animals.
ii. It is active against a wide range of insects and leaves no toxic residue.
iii. Rotenone is sparingly volatile.

Formulation:

i. Powdered roots are normally used.
Dust formulations (0.2-0.5% rotenone)
ii. Water dispersible & EC (1–6% rotenone).

Pyrethrins

Pyrethrum is derived from flowers of *Chrysanthemum* sp. The name given to the active insecticidal components of the dried flowers is known as pyrethrins. Chemically "phyrethrins" are organic esters of carboxylic acid (chrysanthemic/pyrethric acid) and alcohol (pyrethrolone, cineralone and jasmoline). The plants are compositae family

Source: Flower heads of
Chrysanthemum cinerariefolium,
Chrysanthemum roseum and
Chrysanthemum marshalli

Use: Dusts

Extractives are suspended in a solvent for use as spray.

Flower head dried in 54.4 °C constant temperature.

Formerly from Japan, now, cultivated in Belgian, Congo, Uganda, India, Yugoslavia and the USA.

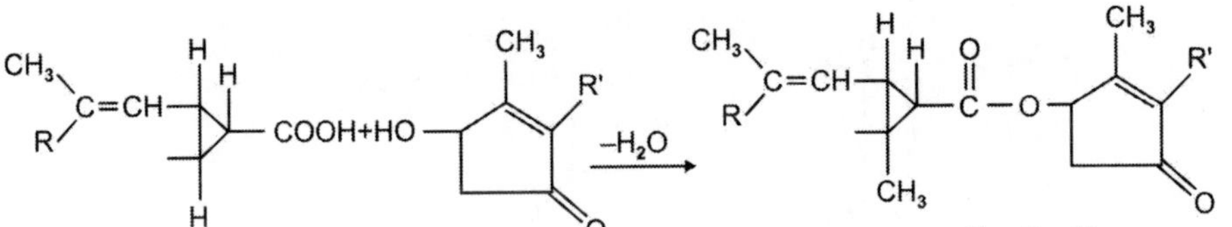

Acid moiety   Alcohol moiety   Pyrethroid
(Pyrethroid are esters compounds)

Structure of Pyrethrin and Cinerin and Jasmolin

Pyrethrin

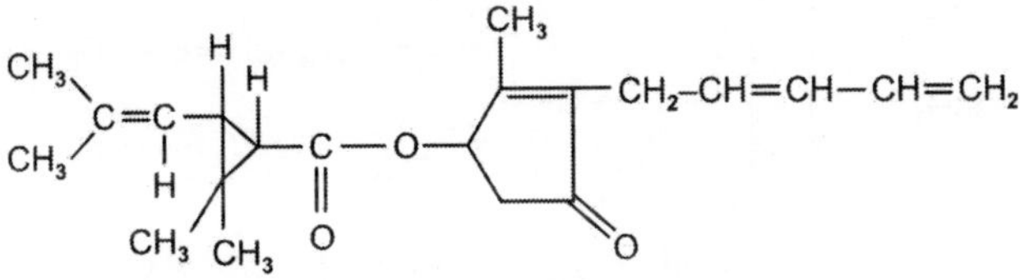

Chrysanthemic acid   Pyrethrelone
(acid part)   (alcoholic part)

Pyrethrin – I

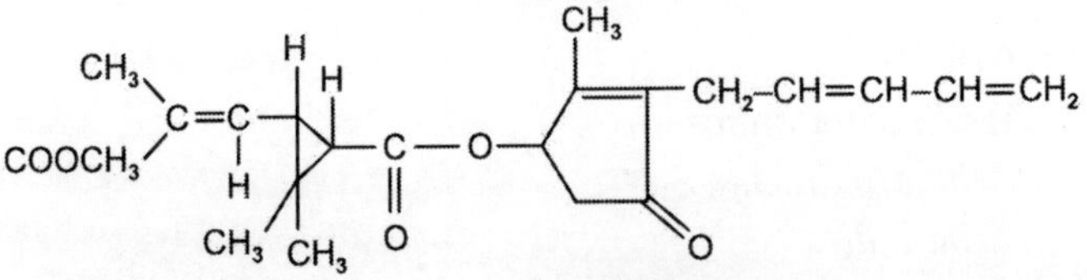

Chrysanthemic acid   Pyrethrelone
(acid part)   (alcoholic part)

Pyrethrin – II

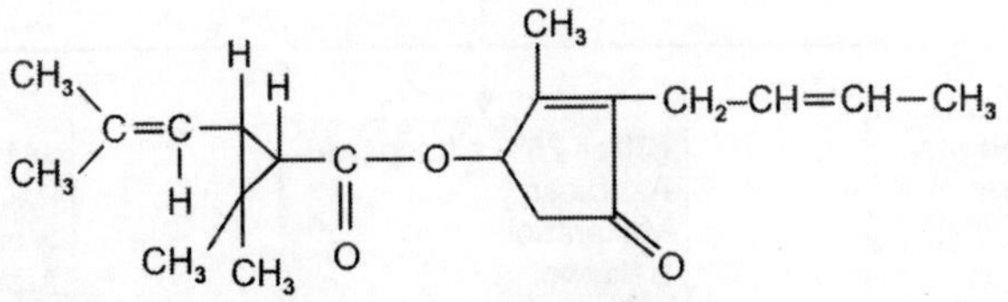

Chrysanthemic acid   Cineralone
(acid part)   (alcoholic part)

Cinerin – I

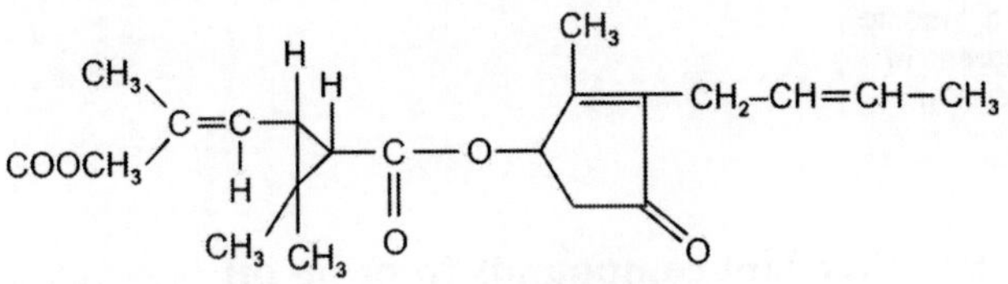

Chrysanthemic acid   Cineralone
(acid part)   (alcoholic part)

Cinerin – II

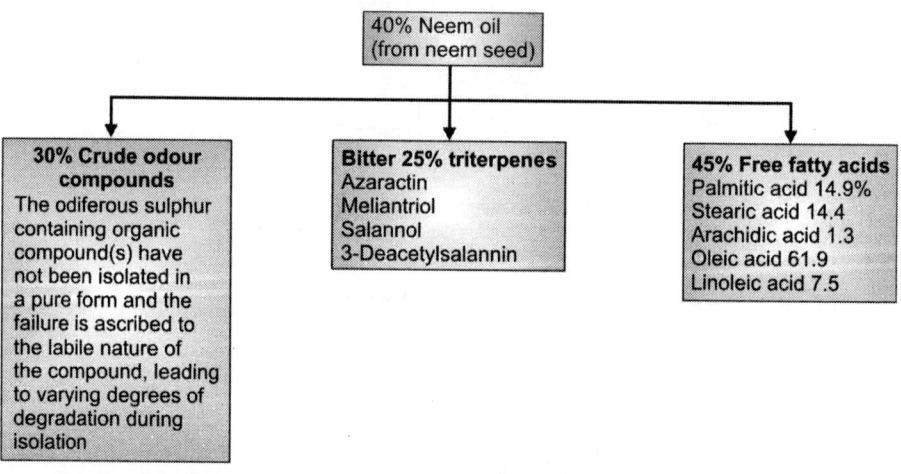

Chrysanthemic acid
(acid part)

Jasmoline
(alcoholic part)

Jasmolin – I

Chrysanthemic acid
(acid part)

Jasmoline
(alcoholic part)

Jasmolin – II

Neem oil

Botanical description

Neem spp.   *Azadirachta indica*
              Melia azadirachta
              Melia indica

Neem oil kernels (crushing of seed or fried fruits)

40% Neem oil
(from neem seed)

30% Crude odour compounds	Bitter 25% triterpenes	45% Free fatty acids
The odiferous sulphur containing organic compound(s) have not been isolated in a pure form and the failure is ascribed to the labile nature of the compound, leading to varying degrees of degradation during isolation	Azaractin Meliantriol Salannol 3-Deacetylsalannin	Palmitic acid 14.9% Stearic acid 14.4 Arachidic acid 1.3 Oleic acid 61.9 Linoleic acid 7.5

Insect repellent/Antifeedant compounds in neem oil

The bitter principles present in various tree plants were believed to be responsible for beneficial effects. Several compounds have been isolated and characterized.

The main feature is that they belong to a class of triterpenes with 26 carbons.

Azadirachtin, the most important triterpenes, insect repellent or antifeedant, reducing the feed consumption of at least 40 species. It appears to be safe to beneficial insects, fish, animals and most crop plant. It is a systemic pesticide.

Meliantriol is a locust antifeedant in extremely low concentration. *Salannol* and *3-deacetylsalannin* are two antifeedants recently isolated from neem. *Nimbin* was first compound isolated in a pure form from alcohol extract of neem oil.

Formulation:

1. Repelin and Wellgro (I.T.C. Ltd.)
   Control of cut worms and boll worm (*Heliothis armigera*) of tobacco and cotton
2. Nimbosol and Biosol (AV Thomos and Co.) Control of white flies and lepidopterian pests
   Azadirachtin-rich formulation: Neemark granule : recommended for cotton, paddy, tobacco, groundnut, sugarcane, chilli, brinjal vegetables, legumes and food grains.

4.3 SYNTHETIC INSECTICIDES

4.3.1 Organochlorinated Hydrocarbons

Organochlorine group of insecticides includes substances varying in their chemical structure. But the common nature of some of their properties (high insecticidal activity, chemical and biological persistence) makes it possible to combine them into one group. All organochlorine insecticides are poorly soluble in water and well soluble in organic solvents, including fats. Many of them are quite volatile. The representatives of this group are mainly contact insecticides with prolonged residual effects and a broad spectrum of action. Organochlorine insecticides upon entering an insect's organism act on its nervous system, violating, as is assumed, the lipid equilibrium of the nerve cell membranes, and preventing the transmission of nerve impulses. Insects system, attended by tremors and paralysis.

DDT and its analogous

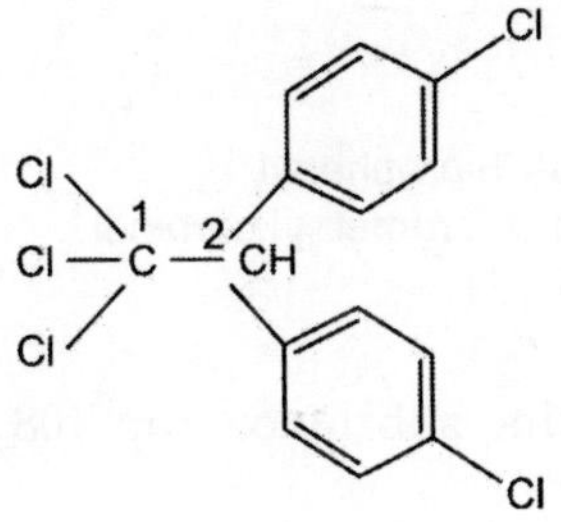

DDT
Dichloro diphenyl trichloroethane
D   D   T
1,1,1 Trichloro-2,2-*bis*(*p*-chlorophenyl) ethane, pp′-DDT

DDT was discovered in 1939 by Paul Muller and patented by the Swiss Firm of J.R. Geigy A.G. for insecticidal purpose in 1942. Because of environmental pollution and toxic hazards to human health some countries such as Sweden, Great Britain, Canada and the USA have banned the use of DDT. The World Health Organization, however, is in disfavour of the total ban on DDT, as no satisfactory substitute is yet known particularly for the control of insect vectors of human diseases in the tropics.

The technical product is a mixture of compounds and may contain upto 30% *op'* isomer. The universally accepted and WHO approved specification calls for at least 70% *pp'* isomer, which has more potency as an insecticide.

It was marketed in 1942 under the name Gesarol in the crop protection field and under the name Neocide in the field of human hygiene.

Preparation/Synthesis

1. Condensation of chlorobenzene with chloral:

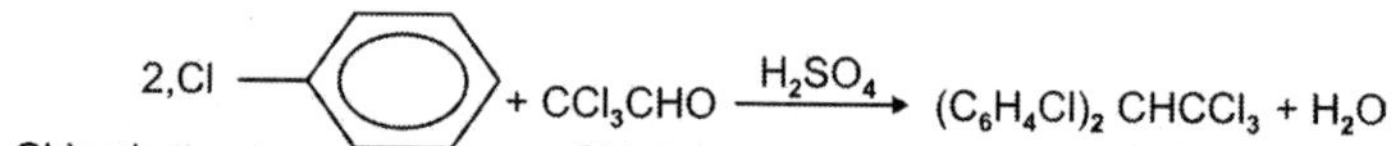

$$2,Cl - \text{(Chlorobenzene)} + CCl_3CHO \text{ (Chloral)} \xrightarrow{H_2SO_4} (C_6H_4Cl)_2 CHCCl_3 \text{ (DDT)} + H_2O$$

This reaction takes place in the presence of condensing agent such as conc. H_2SO_4, oleum, chlorosulfonic acid, HF, anhydrous NH_4Cl and in industry conc. H_2SO_4 or weak oleum is used at a temperature not higher than 20 °C.

2. An interesting method for the synthesis of DDT is the reaction of chlorobenzene with p-chlorophenyl trichloromethyl carbinol, i.e. $ClC_6H_4CH(OH)CCl_3$:

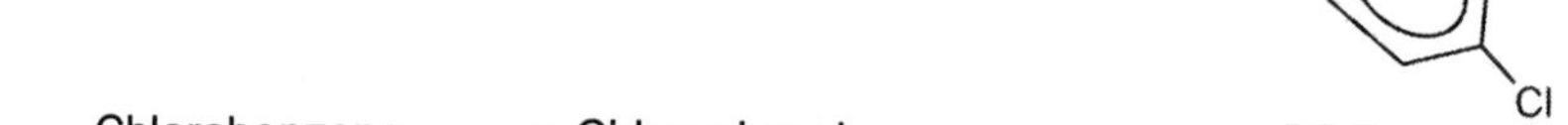

Chlorobenzene   p-Chlorophenyl trichloromethyl carbinol   DDT

Physical properties:

i. DDT is a white crystalline substance, mp 108.5°–109 °C, solubility in water about 0.001 mg/litre.

ii. The best solvents for DDT are ketones, esters of the lower fatty acids, aromatic hydrocarbons, and halogen derivatives of hydrocarbons of the aliphatic and aromatic series.

iii. Technical grade DDT contains 75–76% pp' isomer.

Chemical properties:

1. The pure, pp'-isomer of DDT is thermally stable. Its decomposition starts about 195 °C and proceeds according to the equation:

$$(C_6H_4Cl)_2CHCCl_3 \xrightarrow{195°C} (C_6H_4Cl)_2C=CCl_2 + HCl$$

1,1 – dichloro – 2, 2 – bis –
p – chlorophenylethylene (DDE)

2. Under the influence of sunlight in alcohol, DDT decomposes in the following way:

$$2(C_6H_4Cl)_2CHCCl_3 + 2C_2H_5OH \rightarrow$$
$$2CH_3CHO + (C_6H_4Cl)_2CHCCl = CClCH(C_6H_4Cl)_2 + 4HCl$$

In the presence of the oxygen of the air, the process goes further and pp'-dichlorobenzophenone is obtained:

$$(C_6H_4Cl)_2CHCCl = CClCH(C_6H_4Cl)_2 \rightarrow [(C_6H_4Cl)_2C=C=C=C(C_6H_4Cl)_2]$$
$$\downarrow$$
$$2, C_6H_4Cl-C-C_6H_4Cl + 2CO_2$$
$$\underset{O}{\overset{||}{}}$$

p, p'–dichlorobenzophenone

3. Pure DDT at room temperature does not affect most metals, but technical preparations, especially those containing water and salt solutions cause more or less corrosion. Probably this is associated with the evolution of HCl as a result of hydrolysis of DDT by water:

$$(C_6H_4Cl)_2-CHCCl_3 + 2H_2O \rightarrow (C_6H_4Cl)_2-CH-COOH + 3HCl$$

DDA
Dichloro-diphenyl acetic acid (biologically inactive)

Toxicity

i. DDT may be used as a broad spectrum insecticide, as its effect on a large number of species of insects.

ii. DDT is both stomach as well as contact insecticide. It has been mainly used against biting and chewing insect pests, domestic insects and mosquitoes.

iii. DDT is toxic to warm-blooded animals in the sense that it is not degraded in the body and may persist in the body fat.

Formulation: Dust 1–10% a.i. 5% usual, W.P. 20–50% (usual 50%), aerosol EC

Analogs of DDT

DDD or TDE

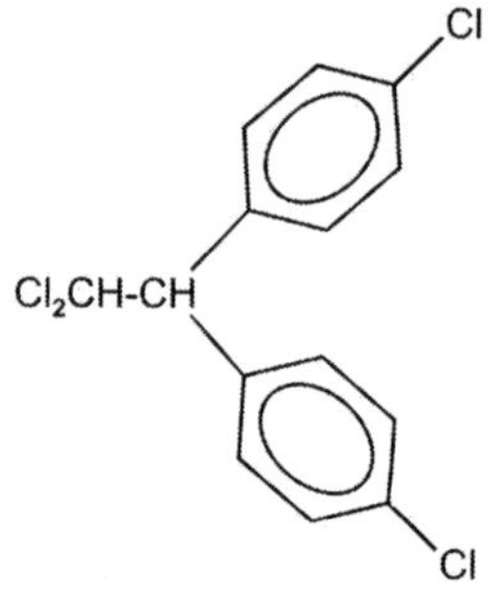
Cl
Cl2CH-CH
Cl

TDE (tetrachloro diphenyl ethane)
1,1-dichloro-2,2-*bis*(*p*-chlorophenyl)ethane
DDD(Dichloro diphenyl dichloroethane)

Synthesis:

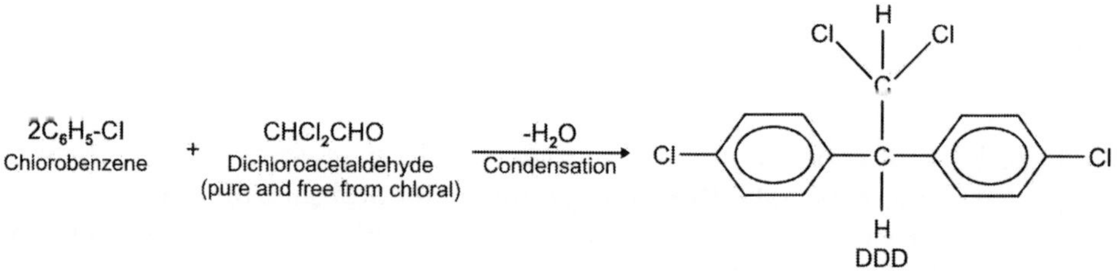
2C6H5-Cl
Chlorobenzene
+
CHCl2CHO
Dichloroacetaldehyde
(pure and free from chloral)
-H2O
Condensation
H
Cl
Cl
C
Cl
C
Cl
H
DDD

Properties:

It consists of white crystals, mp. 112 °C. The technical grade preparation has a setting point of about 86 °C.

Toxicity: Low mammalian toxicity and low level of accumulation in the fatty tissues and milk of mammals.

Methoxychlor

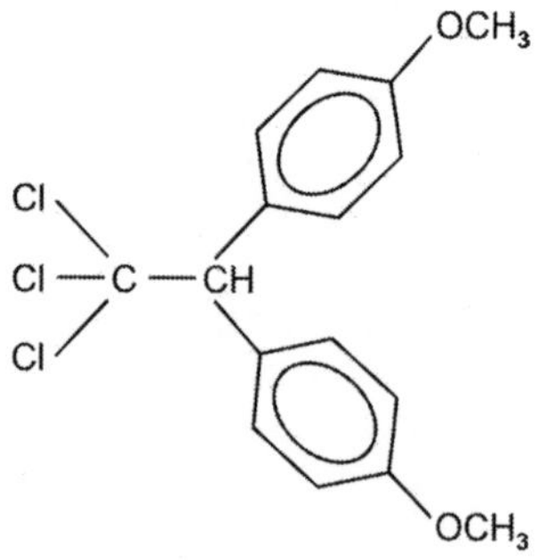
OCH3
Cl
Cl —C —CH
Cl
OCH3

1,1,1-trichloro-2,2-*bis*(*p*, *p'*-methoxy phenyl) ethane

Synthesis:

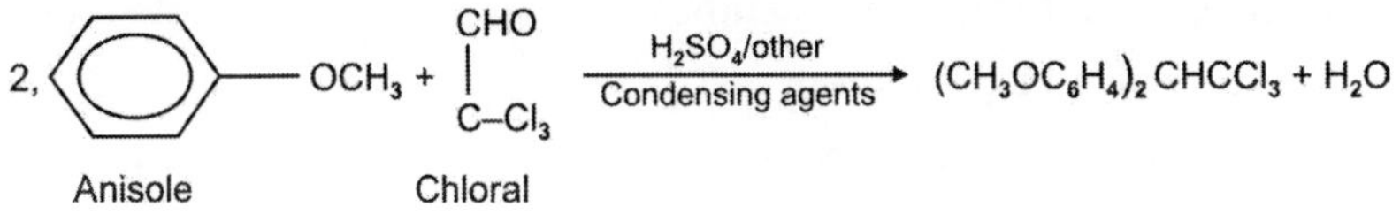

$$2, \text{Anisole} - OCH_3 + \underset{\text{Chloral}}{\overset{CHO}{\underset{C-Cl_3}{|}}} \xrightarrow[\text{Condensing agents}]{H_2SO_4/other} (CH_3OC_6H_4)_2 CHCCl_3 + H_2O$$

Anisole   Chloral

Properties:

i. Technical grade product contains 88% of the *pp'*-isomer and small amount of *op'*-isomer.

ii. White crystalline substance, mp. 89 °C.

iii. Methoxychlor is similar to DDT in its chemical properties.

Kelthane/Dicofol

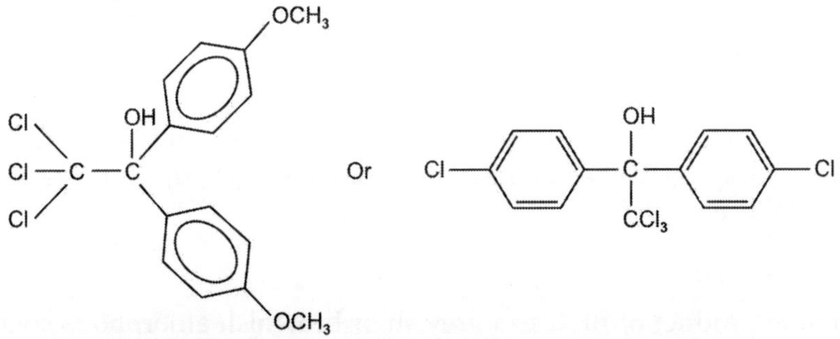

Or

2,2-*bis*(*p*-chlorophenyl)-2 hydroxy-1,1,1-trichloroethane

Used as acaricide.

Physical properties

i. It is insoluble in water but soluble in petroleum, ether, toluene, ethanol.

BHC

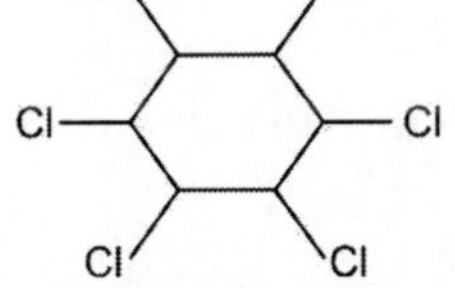

1,2,3,4,5,6-hexachlorocyclohexane

BHC was first synthesised by Michael Faraday in 1825 and its structure was determined in 1836. In 1936, Bender discovered the insecticidal properties of BHC, and took out a patent. The important discovery that, among the various isomers formed, the γ-isomer of BHC is the carrier of insecticidal properties is linked with the name of Thomas (1945). According to Mullins (1955) the molecule of γ BHC (size and shape) is smaller than those of the other sterioisomers and so can penetrate more easily.

Other names: BHC (Benzene hexachloride)

HCH (Hexachloro cyclohexane)

γ-BHC/γ-HCH (Lindane)

Gammexane (γ-cyclohexane)

BHC Stereoisomers : The molecule of 1,2,3,4,5,6-hexachlorocyclohexane may exist in 16 possible sterio-isomeric forms. The BHC molecule has to be thought of as 3-dimensional structure. All the six carbon atoms do not lie in one plane. Three of them lie in one plane while the other three lie in another plane.

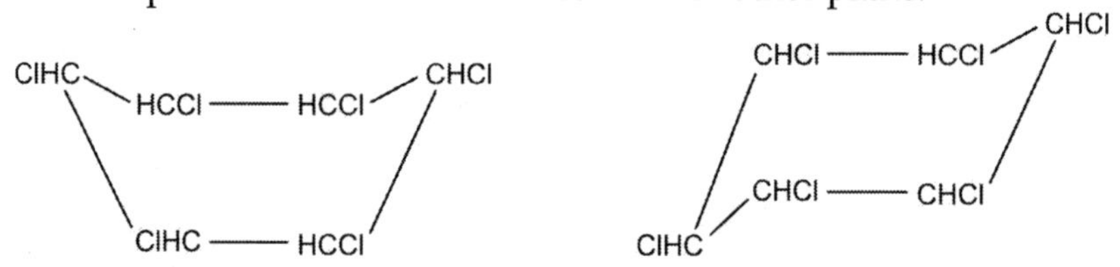

Cis (boat form)   *Trans* (chair form)

According to the position of bonds between carbon and chlorine atom 8 isomers are known and these have been named as α, β, γ, δ (ξ, ζ, η, θ). Of these γ isomer is highly toxic to insect.

Physical properties:

1. The crude product of BHC is a greyish or brownish amorphous solid with a musty odour, melting at 65 °C. It consists of 10 to 18% of the active γ-isomer.
2. BHC is considerably more volatile than DDT which accounts for the shorter residual action of BHC.
3. The γ-isomer is 500 to 1000 times active than the δ-isomer.
4. Lindane (at least 99% pure γ-isomer) is almost odourless.

Synthesis of BHC :

i. Chlorination of cyclohexane

$$\underset{\text{Cyclohexane}}{C_6H_{12}} + 6Cl_2 \rightarrow C_6H_6Cl_6 + 6HCl$$

ii. Chlorination of cyclohexene

$$\underset{\text{Cyclohexene}}{C_6H_{10}} + 5Cl_2 \rightarrow C_6H_6Cl_6 + 4HCl$$

iii. Photochemical chlorination of benzene

Benzene when react with Cl_2 in presence of sunlight form hexachloro cyclohexane. In industry, chlorination is carried out under UV irradiation and in the presence of excess of benzene or chlorinated organic solvents, usually methylene chloride and in the presence of different initiators like organic peroxides, unsaturated compounds like ethylene terpenes.

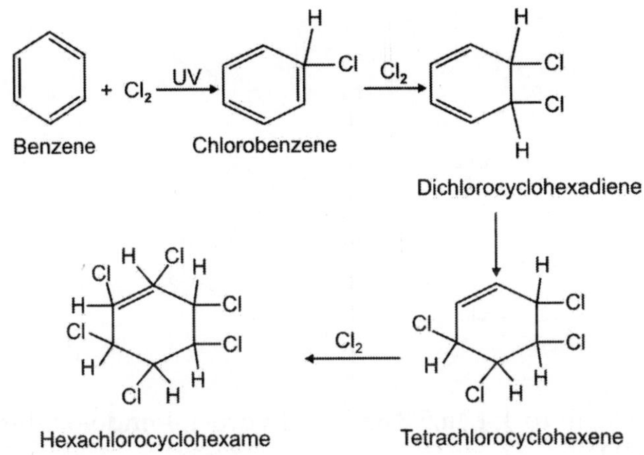

Benzene   Chlorobenzene   Dichlorocyclohexadiene

Hexachlorocyclohexame   Tetrachlorocyclohexene

Chemical properties:

The isomers of BHC are stable to light, heat, air, CO_2 and strong acids. In the presence of alkalies the α, β, γ, δ and ξ isomers are readily dehydrochlorinated, to form trichlorobenzene. The dehydrochlorination of BHC is accelerated by water, light and bases (lime, NH_3 and organic amines) and also at elevated temperature of 250° to 350°C.

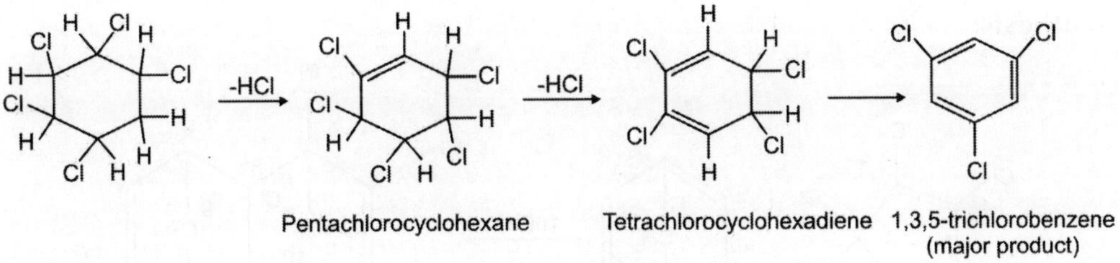

Pentachlorocyclohexane   Tetrachlorocyclohexadiene   1,3,5-trichlorobenzene (major product)

$\left.\begin{array}{l} 1,2,4 \\ 1,3,5 \\ 1,2,3 \end{array}\right\}$ Trichloro benzene (75–90%) (minor product)

Formulations:

Dust formulations (0.2 to 0.65% γ-BHC) 5% and 10%

    EC formulations (12–20% γ-BHC)

    Pellets (for smoke generators)

    Seed dressings (20–40% γ-BHC)

Polychlorocyclodienes or Cyclodiene Insecticides

With hexachlorocyclopentadiene as the starting point, a series of hydrocarbons are prepared by Diels-Alder reaction, a well known process in organic chemistry. Of them the following have been utilized as insecticides for commercial purposes:

Aldrin

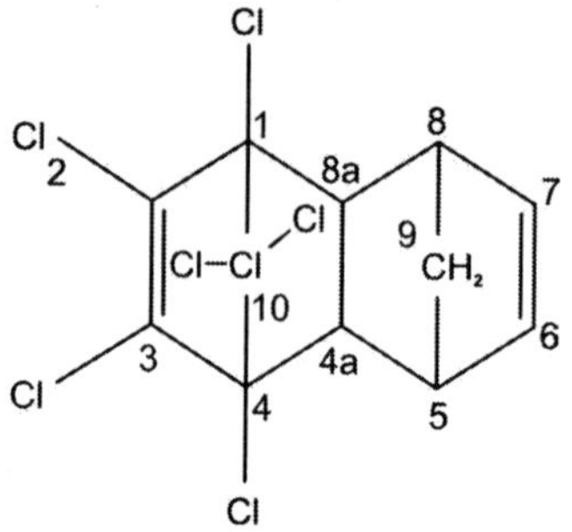

1,2,3,4,10,10-Hexachloro-1,4,4a,5,8,8a-hexahydro-1,4-endo-5,8-hexo-dimethano naphthalene, HHDN.

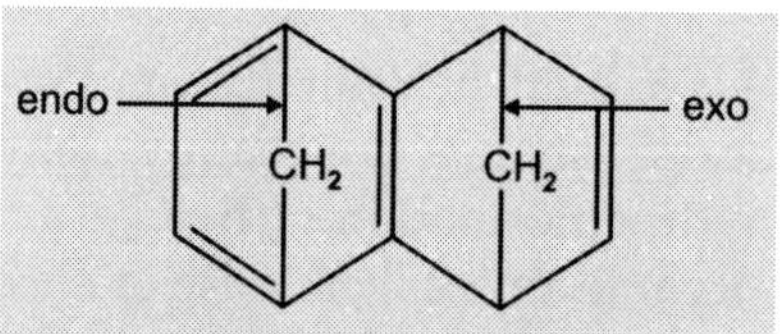

Dimethane napthalene

Synthesis:

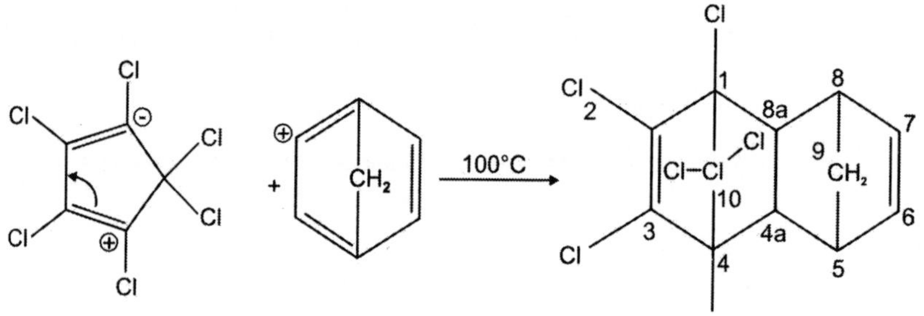

| Hexachlorocyclopentadiene (Diene) | Bicycloheptadiene (Dienophile) (Diel-Alder's reaction) | Aldrin |

Properties:

1. Solid product, mp 104 °C.
2. Stereoisomer is known as – isodrin and this can be differentiated from Aldrin by the fact that it has endo-endo configuration.
3. Aldrin is thermally stable, no noticeable decomposition on prolong exposure to a temperature 240 °C.
4. The double bond in the chlorinated ring is unreactive, but the double bond in the unhalogenated ring is extremely reactive and undergo number of

reaction, e.g. Br, Cl add easily to the double bond and oxidizing agent like KMnO$_4$, K$_2$Cr$_2$O$_7$ easily attract the reactive double bond.

5. Peroxides, peracetic acid and other organic acids convert aldrin to dieldrin in soil, plants, insects and vertebrates.

Formulation:

Dust formulation (1.5–2% aldrin)

EC (20%)

Seed dressing (30% aldrin)

Toxicity:

i. against insect is very high

ii. long-term effect of its persist

Dieldrin

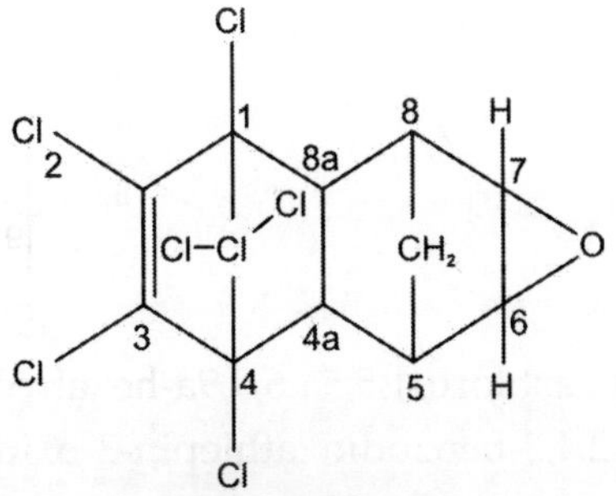

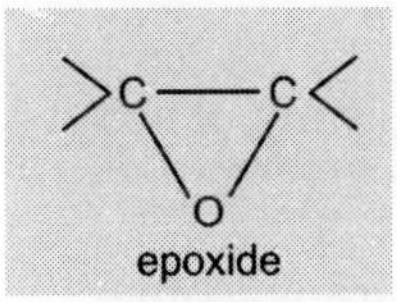

epoxide

1,2,3,4,10,10-Hexachloro-6,7-epoxy-1,4,4a,5,6,7,8,8a- epoxide octahydro-1,4-endo-5,8-exo-dimethanonaphthalene, HEOD

Synthesis:

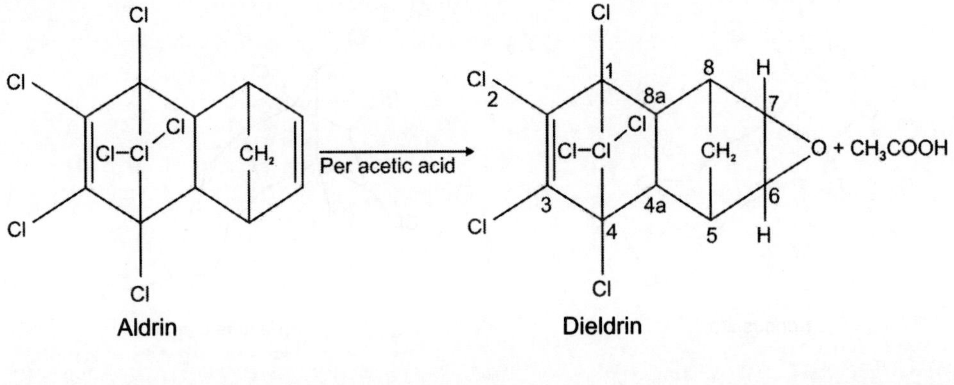

Aldrin   Dieldrin

Properties of Dieldrin:

i. m.p. 176 °C.

ii. Dieldrin is less reactive (biologically) than aldrin.

iii. it has a very wide spectrum of insecticidal activity and has been recommended and used against soil and foliage sprays.

iv. Stereoisomer of dieldrin is endrin (-1,4,5,8-endo-endo). Chemical reactions and biological properties are more or less similar to dieldrin. But the biological properties of endrin is to some extent better than dieldrin.

Endosulfan

Trade name: Thiodan, Endocel

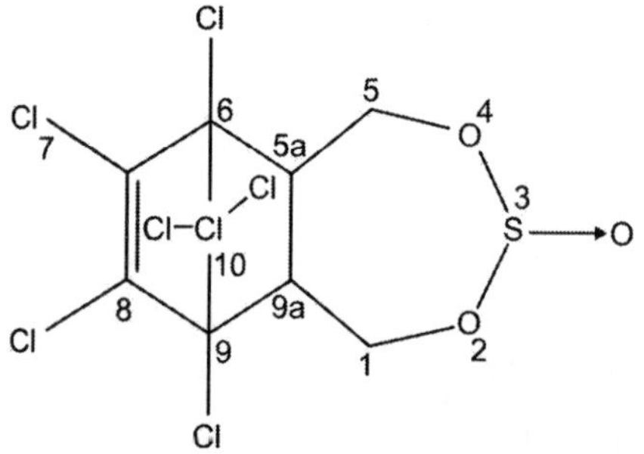

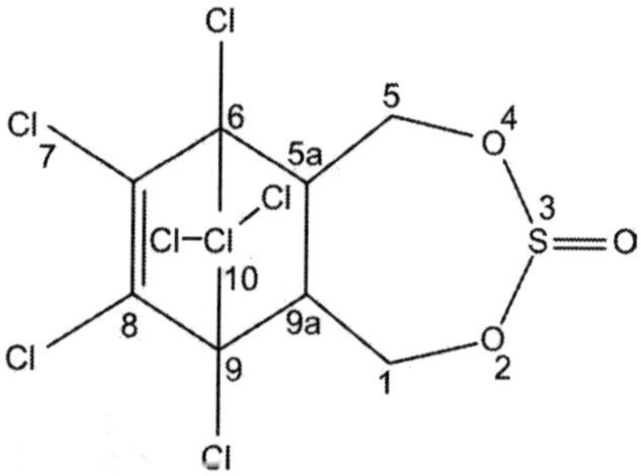

6,7,8,9,10,10-hexachloro-1,5,5a,6,9,9a-hexahydro-6,9methano-2,4,3-benzodioxathiepin-3-oxide

Properties:

i. mp 70–100 °C, tech. grade consisting of about 4 parts of a-cis-isomer (mp 108 °C) and one part of β-isomer (mp 206 °C)

ii. α-cis-isomer $\xrightarrow[\text{at high temp.}]{\text{slowly}}$ β trans-isomer

iii. α,β-isomer $\xrightarrow{\text{Oxidised}}$ endosulfan sulfate
   (a) Air
   (b) Biological systems
   (c) Peroxides/permanganate

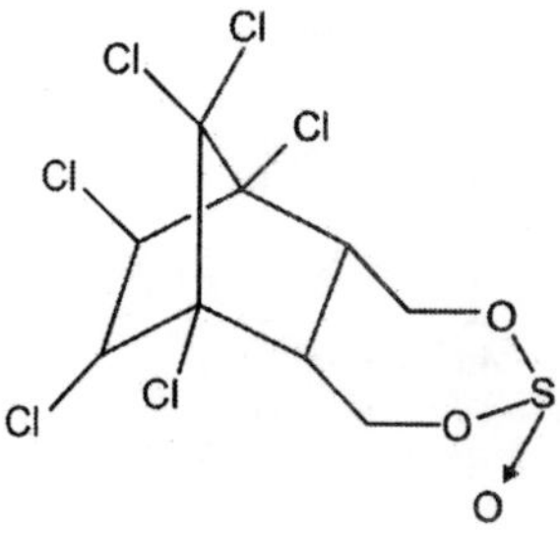

α-endosulfan

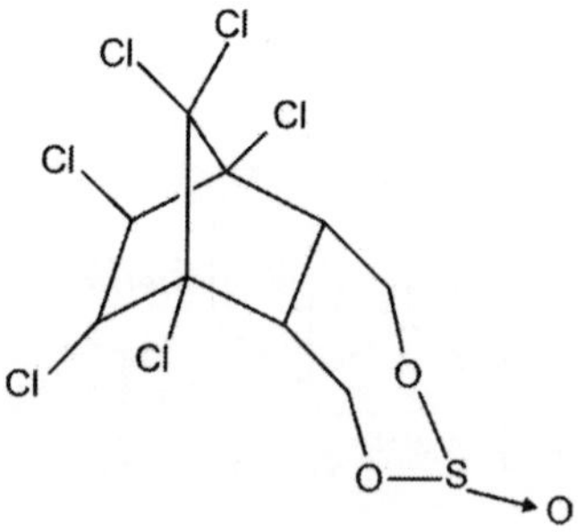

β-endosulfan

Chlorodane

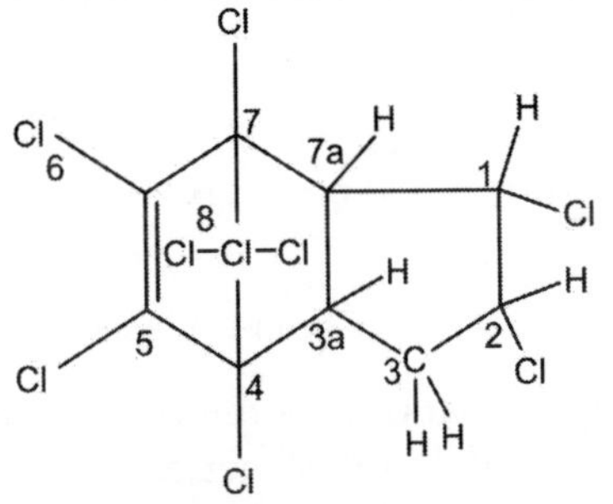

α,β-isomer

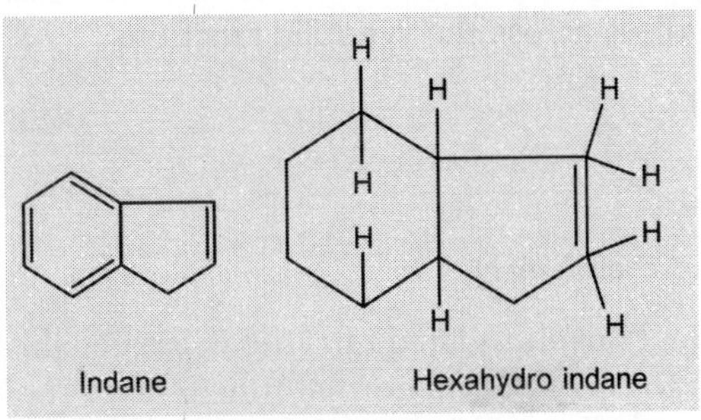

1,2,4,5,6,7,8,8-Octachloro-1,2a,3a,4,7,7a- hexa hydro-4,7,endo methylene indene Dust (5–10%), transform of endosultan is 8 times toxic than cis form WP (40–50%), 40–75% EC

Heptachlor

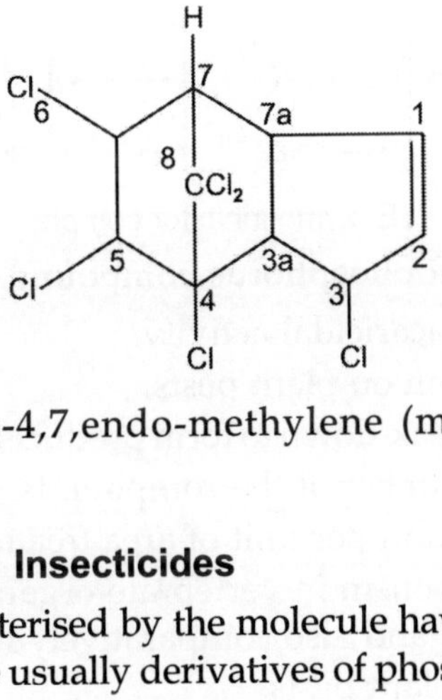

3,4,5,6,7,8,8-heptachloro-4,7,endo-methylene (methano), 3a,4,7, 7a-tetra-hydroindene.

4.3.2 Organophosphorus Insecticides

These insecticides are characterised by the molecule having one or more rarely two atoms of phosphorus and are usually derivatives of phosphates, i.e. phosphoric acid.

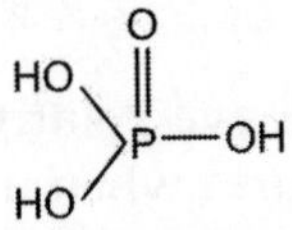

Phosphoric acid

Schrader is the pioneer worker in this new group of insecticide, during World War II. He synthesized nearly 300 OP compounds.

Mode of Action

The biological activity of the OP compounds is due to the capacity of the central P-atom to phosphorylate the active site of the enzyme cholinesterase, an essential constituent of the nervous system, not only of insects, but also the higher animals. Cholinesterase hydrolysis acetylcholine which act as the chemical mediator of nerve impulses across the synaptic junctions.

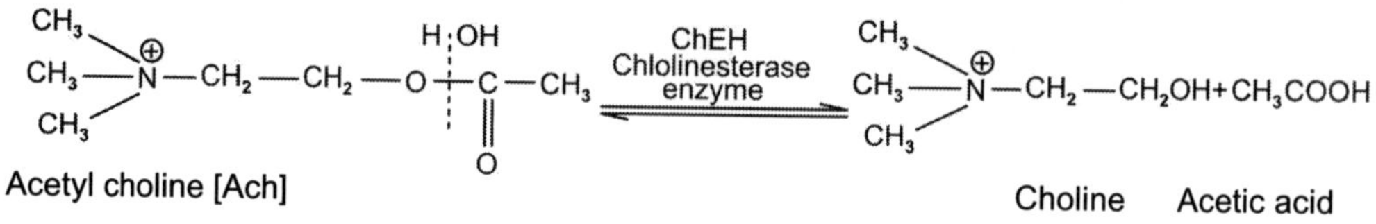

Acetyl choline [Ach]   Choline   Acetic acid

The phosphorylated enzyme is irreversibly inhibited and is therefore no longer able to carry out its normal functions of rapid removal and destruction of neuro-hormone (acetyl choline) from the nervous synapse. This results in accumulation of acetyl choline with consequent disruption of the normal functioning of the nervous system giving rise to typical cholinergic symptoms associated in insects with OP poisoning like hypersensitivity, hyperactivity, tremor, convulsions, paralysis and death.

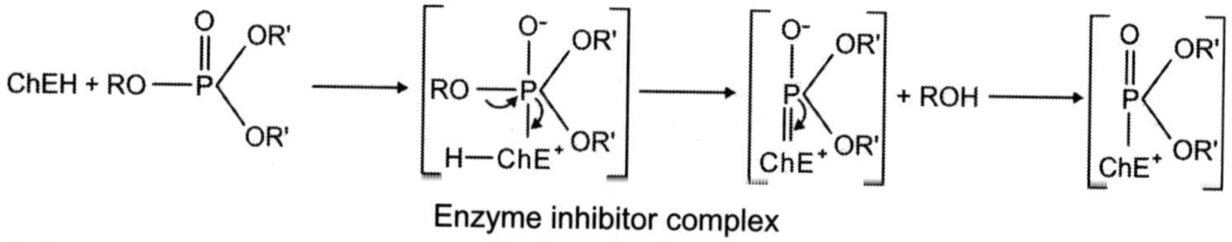

Enzyme inhibitor complex

Advantages of the organophosphorus compounds as pesticides:

1. High insecticidal and acaricidal activity.
2. Wide spectrum of action on plant pests.
3. Low persistence and break-down to form products nontoxic to man and animals.
4. Systemic action of a number of the compounds.
5. Low dosage of compound per unit of area treated.
6. Relatively rapid metabolism in vertebrate organisms and absence of accumulation in their bodies, and also comparatively low chronic toxicity.
7. Rapidity of action on plant pests.

Disadvantages

Organophosphorus compounds have relatively high toxicity to vertebrates, requiring suitable protective measures when using them.

Structure and classification

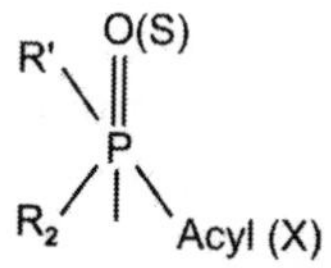

where X is a labile leaving group/groups that can be metabolized *in-vivo* to a labile group.

R^1 and R^2 are short chain alkyl, alkoxy, alkylthio or amide groups.

Most organophosphates are regarded as esters of alcohols with a phosphoric acid or as anhydrides of phosphoric acid with some other acid. Compounds of this category with insecticidal action may be grouped as follows:

1. Derivatives of phosphoric acid, e.g. phosphamidon (Demecron)

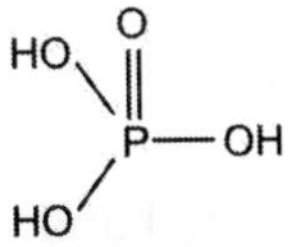

HO\
|| O\
P—OH\
HO/

2. Derivatives of thio phosphoric acid, e.g. parathion

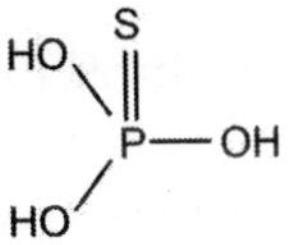

HO\
|| S\
P—OH\
HO/

3. Derivatives of dithiophosphoric acid, e.g. malathion

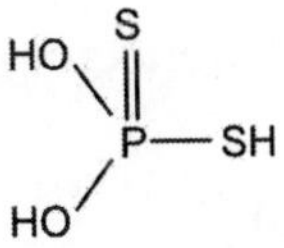

HO\
|| S\
P—SH\
HO/

4. Derivatives of pyrophosphoric acid, e.g. TEPP

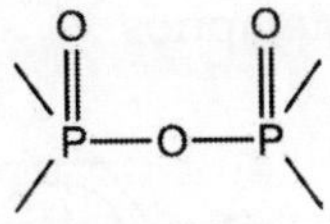

O   O\
|| ||\
P—O—P

5. Derivatives of phosphonic acid, e.g. EPN

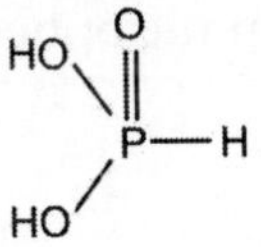

HO\
|| O\
P—H\
HO/

6. Others, e.g. Isopestox

Derivatives of phosphoric acid

Phosphamidon

Trade name: Demecron

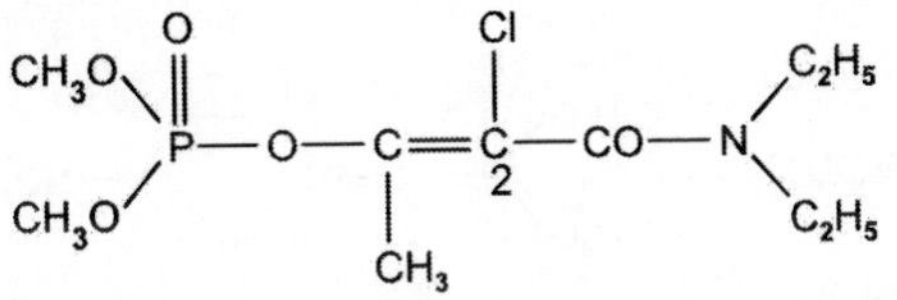

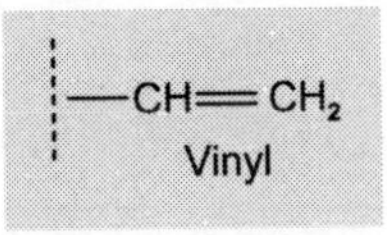

CH₃O\
|| O\
P—O—C=C—CO—N\
CH₃O/ | |Cl   \C₂H₅
       CH₃ 2   /C₂H₅

—CH=CH₂
Vinyl

O,O-dimethyl-O(2-chloro-N,N-diethyl-carbamoyl)-methylvinyl phosphate

Synthesis:

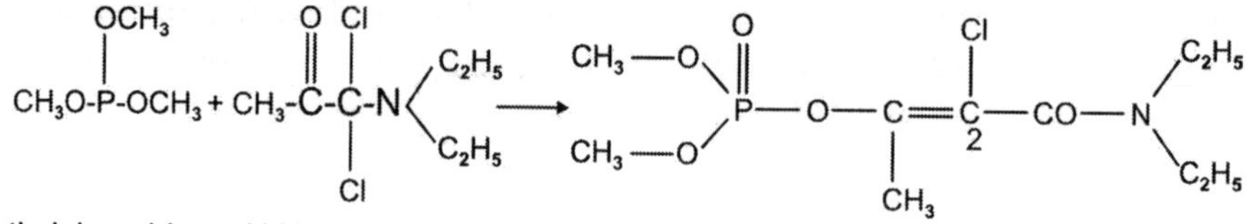

$$CH_3O\text{-}P\text{-}OCH_3 + CH_3\text{-}\overset{O}{\overset{||}{C}}\text{-}\overset{Cl}{\overset{|}{C}}\text{-}N\overset{C_2H_5}{\underset{C_2H_5}{\big<}} \longrightarrow$$

Trimethylphosphite   N,N-diethylacetamide

Phosphamidon

Properties:

i. It is highly soluble in water, alcohol and acetone.

ii. Stable in neutral and weakly acidic aqueous solution but rapidly hydrolysed in alkaline medium.

iii. It is systemic insecticide. It gets absorbed into the plant within one to three hours and is translocated more towards the top.

iv. It is compatible with most pesticides except the alkaline ones like Bordeaux mixture, lime sulphur, nicotine sulphate and copper oxychloride based fungicides.

Other phosphoric acid derivatives : Monocrotophos, Dicrotophos, Chlorfenvinphos, Tetrachlorvinphos

Derivatives of thiophosphoric acid

Methylparathion

Trade name: Folidol, Metacide, Metaphos

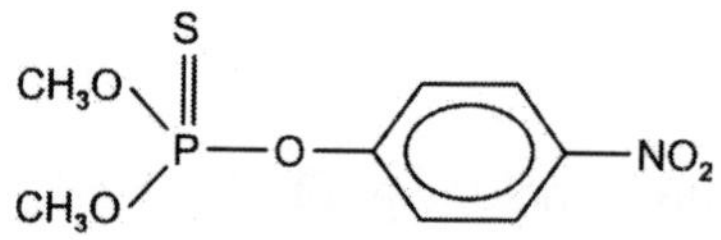

O,O-dimethyl-O-p-nitrophenyl thiophosphate

Parathion

Trade name: Thiophos

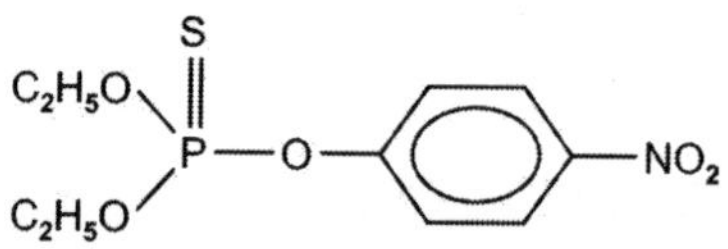

O,O-diethyl-O-p-nitrophenyl thiophosphate

Synthesis:

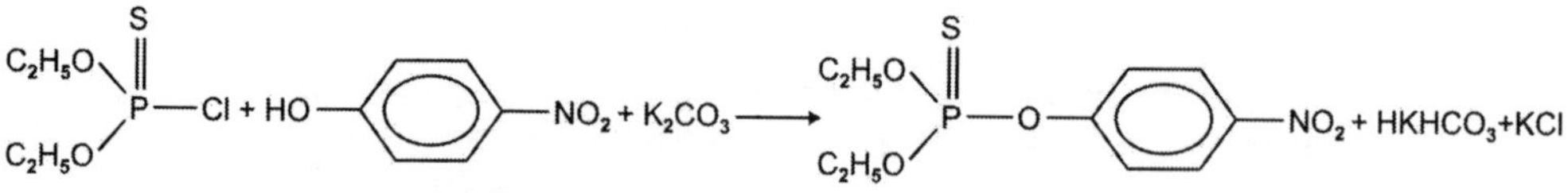

p-nitritrophenol

Diethylchlorothiophosphate

Parathion

Properties of parathion:

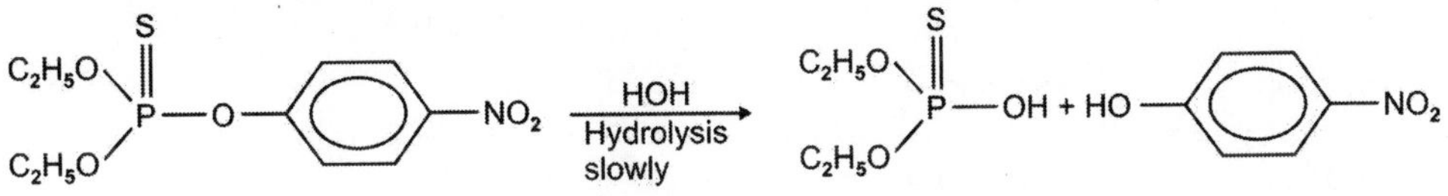

Diethyl thio-phosphoric acid
(alkali)

p-Nitrophenol

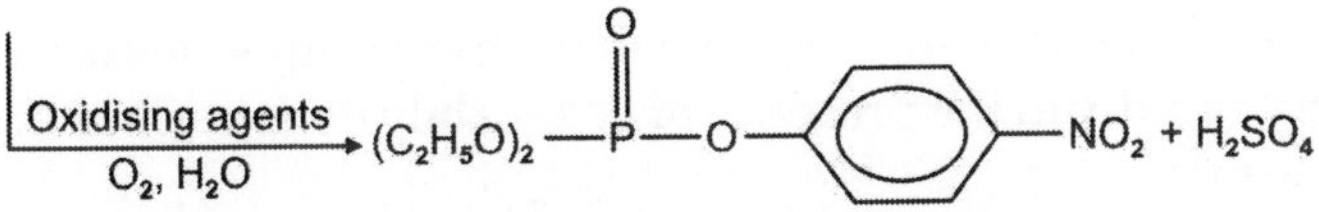

$O-O$-diethyl-O-nitrophenyl phosphate (paraoxon)

Other thiophosphoric acid derivatives:

Diazinon, Dursban, Methyldemeton, Demeton, Fenitrothion (Sumithion), Chlorothion, Metasystox

Derivatives of dithiophosphoric acid

Malathion

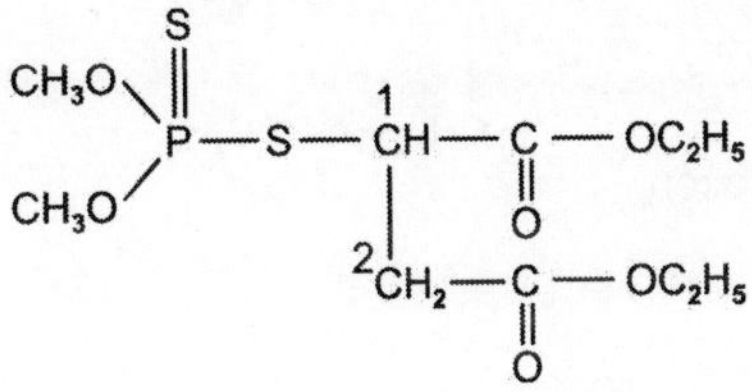

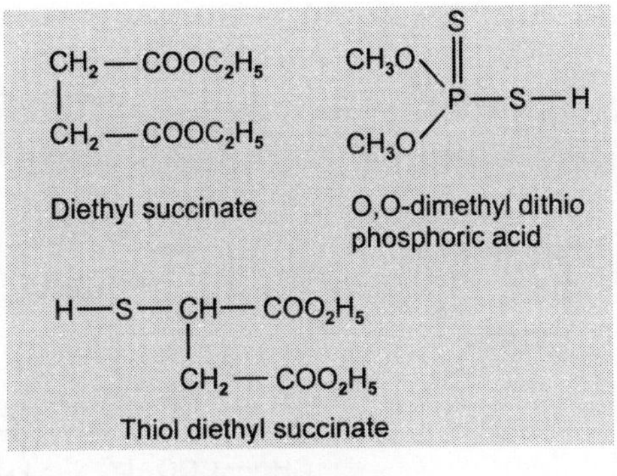

Diethyl succinate

O,O-dimethyl dithio phosphoric acid

Thiol diethyl succinate

O,O-dimethyl-S-1,2-dicarboethoxy ethyl-dithiophosphate
or
O,O-dimethyl dithiophosphate of diethyl mercapto succinate

Synthesis:

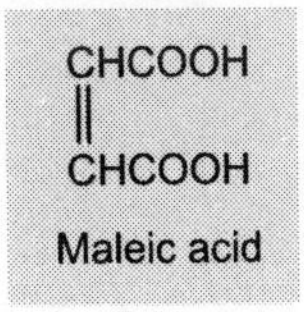

Maleic acid

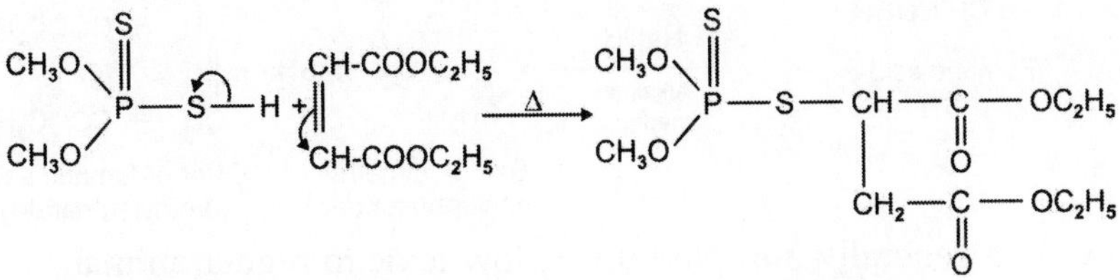

Dimethyl dithio-phosphoric acid

Maleic acid ester (ethyl maleate)

Malathion

Mechanism

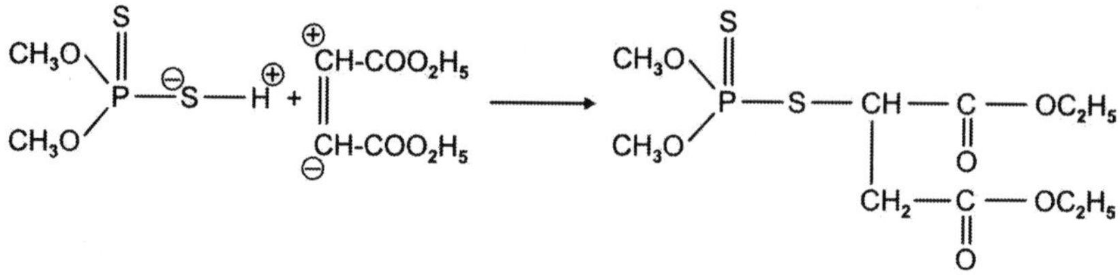

Additive type reaction, because no atom in the two compounds is lost. The reaction takes place very rapidly in the presence of base catalysts in various organic solvents or without solvents.

Properties:

i. Pure malathion is a colourless liquid boiling at 120 °C.
ii. It is sparingly soluble in water but highly soluble in most organic solvents with the exception of saturated hydrocarbons.
iii. Malathion on prolonged heating at 150 °C is isomerised and goes over to the thiolo-isomers.

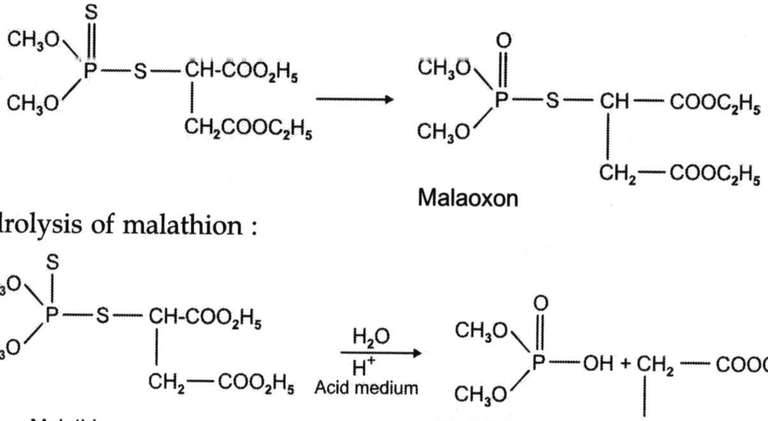

Malaoxon

iv. Hydrolysis of malathion :

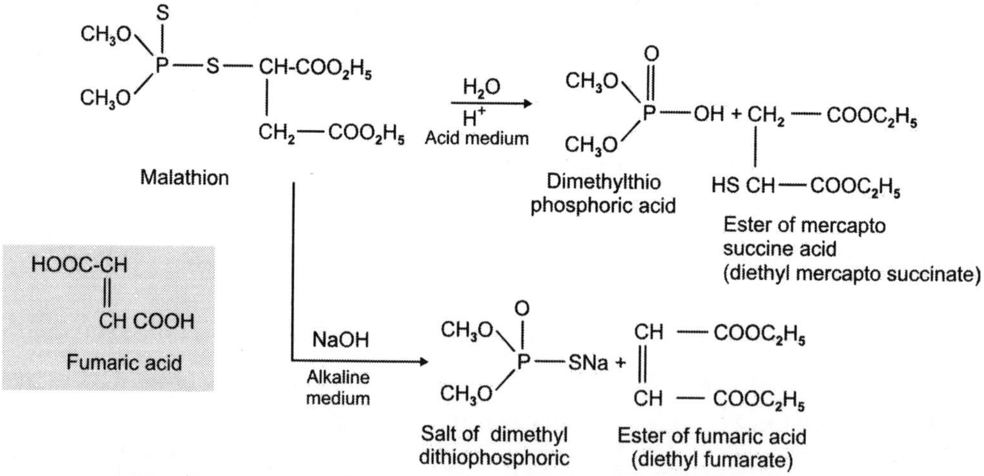

v. It is generally non-phytotoxic, low toxic to higher animal.
vi. It is highly toxic to number of insects and mites and best for stored grain pest as there is no residual effect.

Formulation: 50% EC, 25% W.P., 5% dust and 10% granule.

Others dithiophosphoric acid derivatives:

Thimet (Phorate)

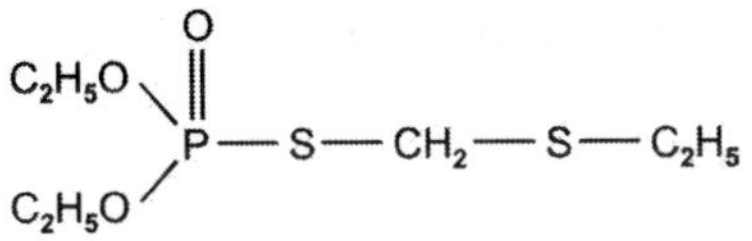

Dimethoate (Roger)

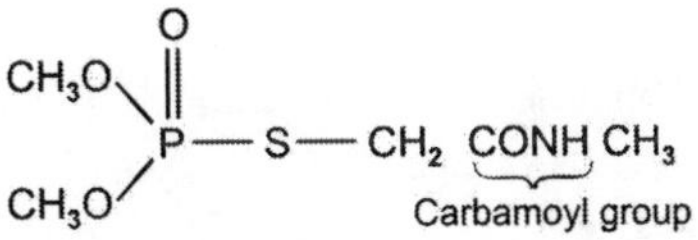

O,O dimethyl-S(N-methyl carbamoyl-methyl)
dithiophosphate

Ethion

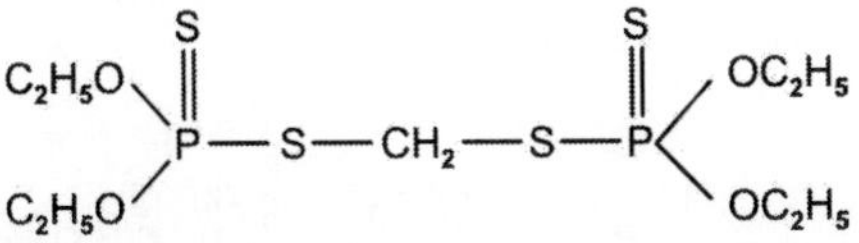

Derivatives of Pyrophosphoric Acid

TEPP (Tetra ethyl pyro phosphate)

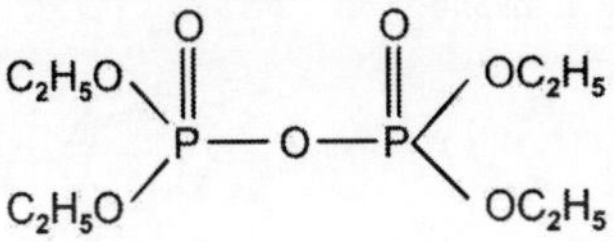

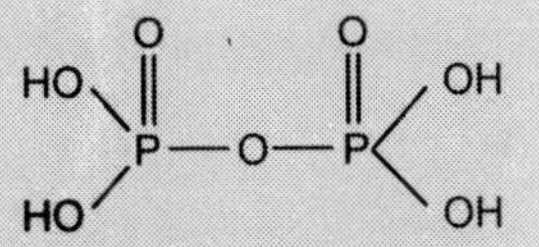

Phosphoric acid anhydride
(Pyrophosphoric acid)

Synthesis:

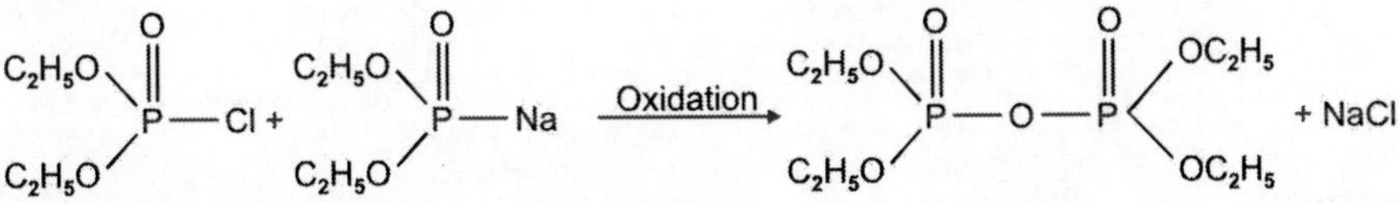

Phosphorochloridate   Sodium diethyl phosphite   TEPP

Properties:

i. TEPP is readily soluble in water, but is easily hydrolysed to non-toxic diethyl phosphoric acid (both for animals and insects). Hence the problem of toxic residues does not arise

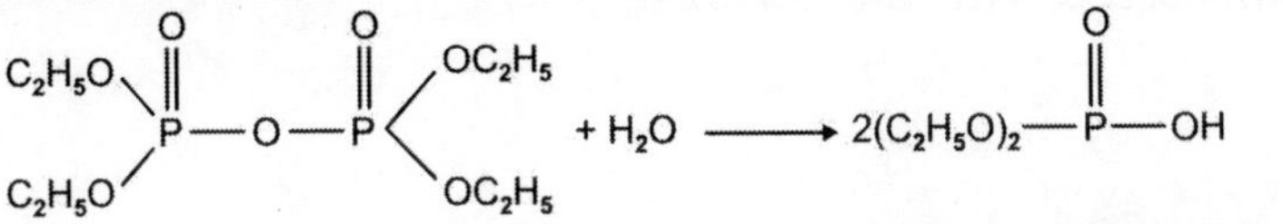

Diethyl phosphoric acid

ii. It is incompatible with alkaline pesticides, but compatible with chlorinated hydrocarbons and sulphur.

Others pyrophosphonic acid derivative:

OMPA (octamethyl pyrophosphoramide)

Derivatives of Phosphonic Acid

EPN

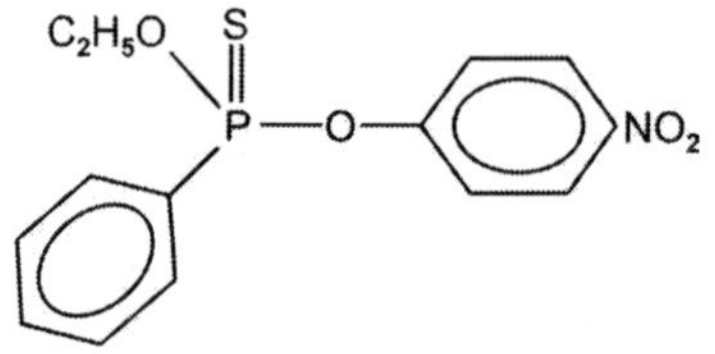

O-ethyl-O-(4-nitrophenyl)-phenyl phosphonothionate

Synthesis:

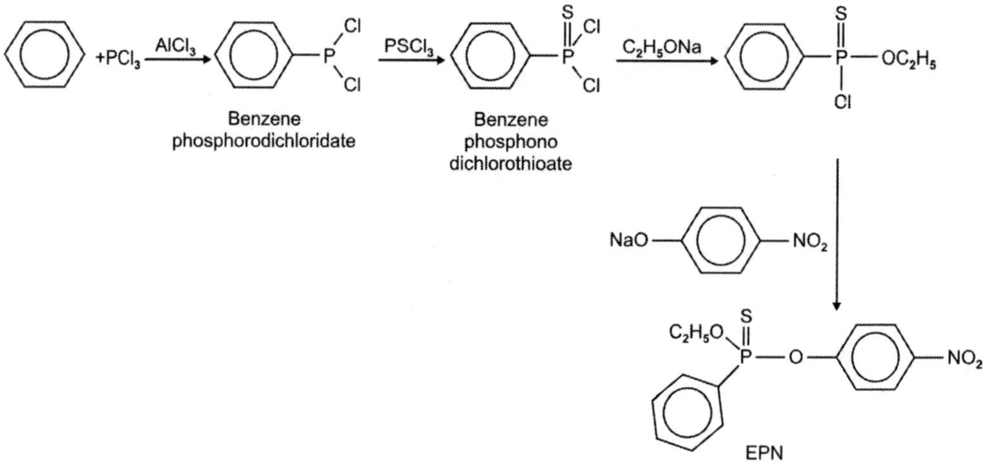

Benzene phosphorodichloridate

Benzene phosphono dichlorothioate

EPN

Properties:

i. It is powerful acaricide besides being toxic to some insects.

ii. It is relatively hydrolysed in alkaline medium, but not in acid and neutral media, EPN is more stable.

iii. It is highly toxic to warm-blooded animals.

Formulations: 35% W.P. and 5% dust

Miscellaneous organophosphatic compounds

Isopestox

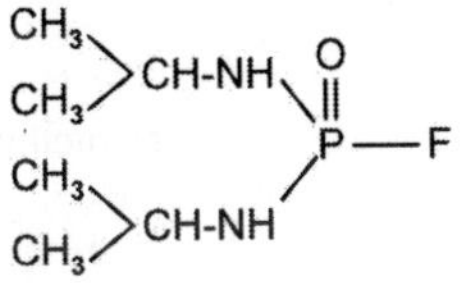

bis(isopropylamide) fluro phosphate

or

N,N'-di-isopropyl-phosphoro diamidic fluoride

i. Odourless white crystals (m.p. 60 °C) compound

ii. Its solubility in water is 8% and it is soluble in polar organic solvents.

Dimefox

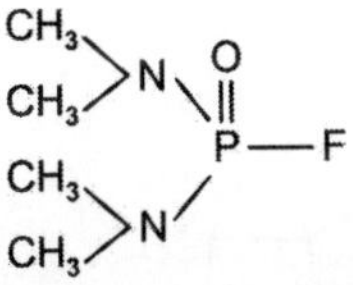

bis(dimethyl amide) fluro-phosphate

or

N,N,N',N'-tetramethyl-phosphoro-diamidic fluoride

Properties:

i. Colourless liquid, b.p. 67 °C.

ii. It is completely miscible with water and is stable in neutral solutions.

iii. It has a short residual effect in view of its volatile nature.

4.3.3 Carbamate Insecticide

Carbamic acid

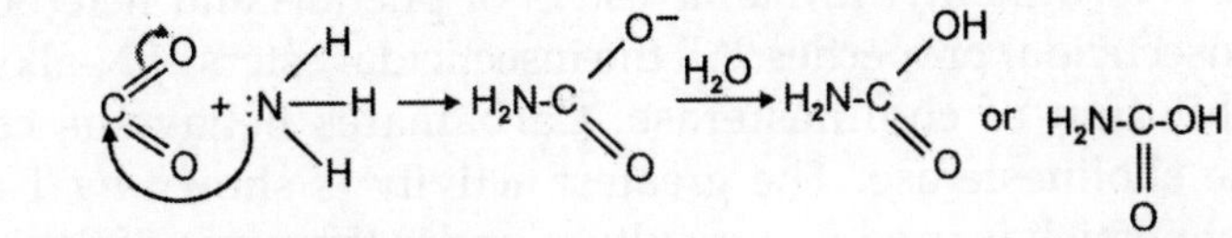

Acidic oxide base
(Nucleophile)
donate an electron pair to
carbon in an org. molecule

Carbamic acid

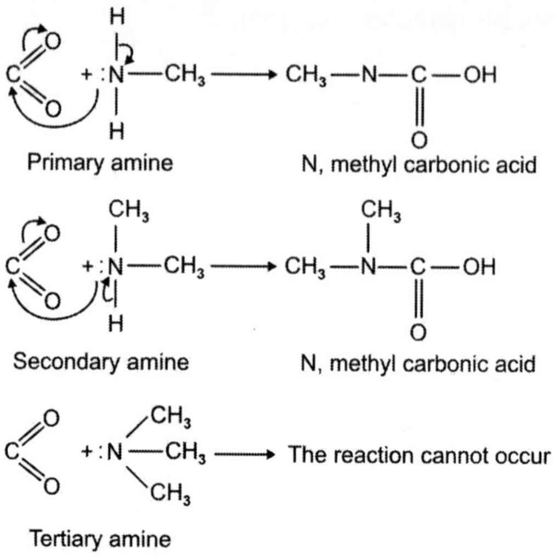

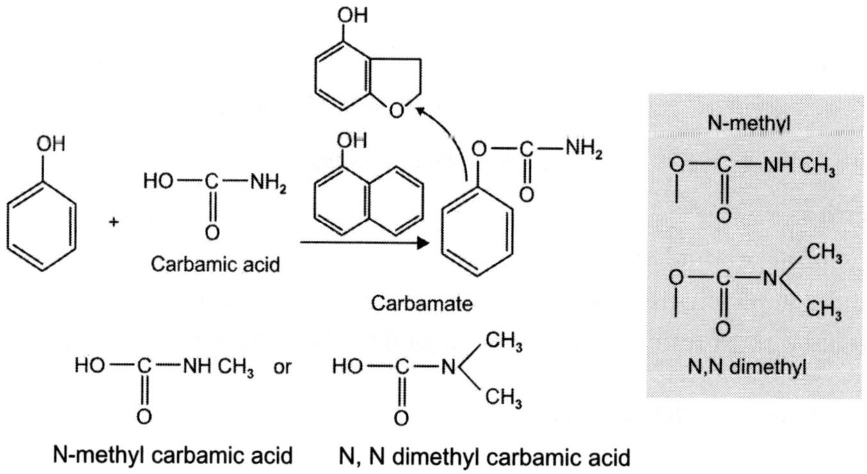

Primary amine   N, methyl carbonic acid

Secondary amine   N, methyl carbonic acid

Tertiary amine   The reaction cannot occur

OH

Carbamic acid

Carbamate

N-methyl

N,N dimethyl

HO—C—NH CH$_3$ or   HO—C—N$\diagup$CH$_3$$\diagdown$CH$_3$

N-methyl carbamic acid   N, N dimethyl carbamic acid

N-methyl and N,N-dimethyl carbamic esters of phenols and heterocyclic enols possess useful insecticidal properties. All the insecticidal esters of N-alkyl carbamic acids cause inhibition of cholinesterase. Carbamates behave as competitive inhibitors of the cholinesterase. The greatest activity is shown by 1-napthyl-N-methyl carbamate which is used in agriculture under the name of Sevin, Carbaryl and Naphthylcarbamate.

Definition:

Carbamates are derivatives of carbamic acid and have an, $-O-\underset{\underset{O}{\|}}{C}-N\langle$ group in the

molecule.

1. Heterocyclic Carbamates
Isolan

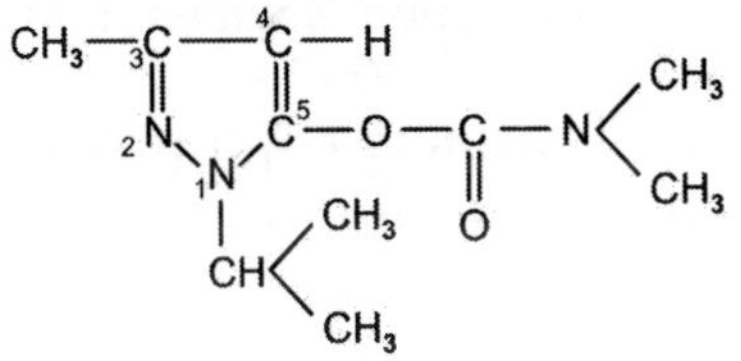

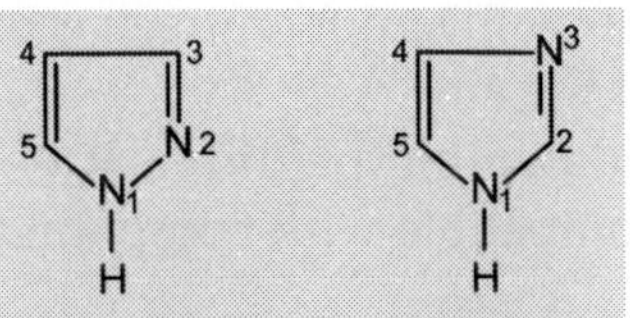

Pyrazole
(1,2 diazole)

Imidazole
(1,3 diazole)

1-Isopropyl-3-methyl-pyrozolyl-(5)-N,N-dimethyl carbamate

Synthesis:

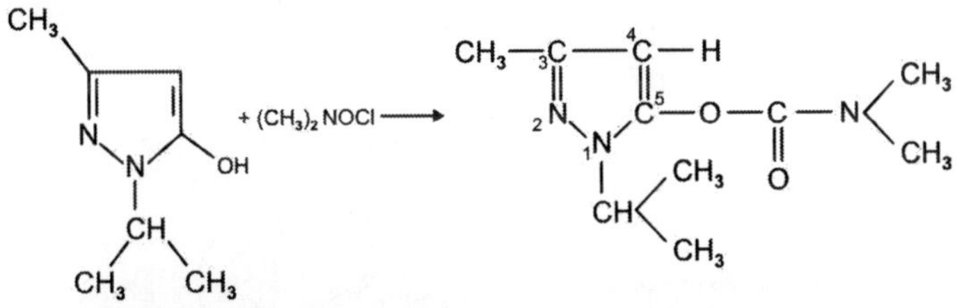

1-isopropyl 3-methyl pyrazolone   isolan

Properties:
  i. Colourless liquid, b.p. 105°–107 °C
  ii. It is soluble in water, acetone and alcohol
Isolan is an aphicide with systemic action.

2. Phenyl Carbamates
Carbaryl (Sevin)

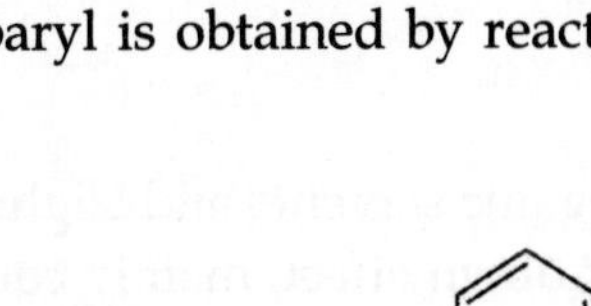

1-naphthyl-N-methyl carbamate

Synthesis:
Pure compound of carbaryl is obtained by reacting 1-naphthol with methyl isocyanate (MIC)

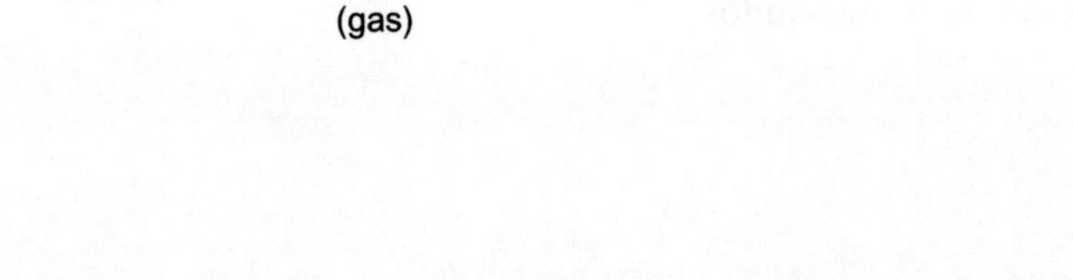

1 Naphthol   MIC
                    (gas)   carbaryl

Properties:
  i. Carbaryl is a white crystalline compounds, m.p. 142 °C.
  ii. At room temperature, it is resistant to the action of water, light and oxygen of the air.
  iii. In alkaline medium, it is rapidly hydrolysed and therefore it is not compatible with compounds of alkaline nature, e.g. Bordeaux mixture.

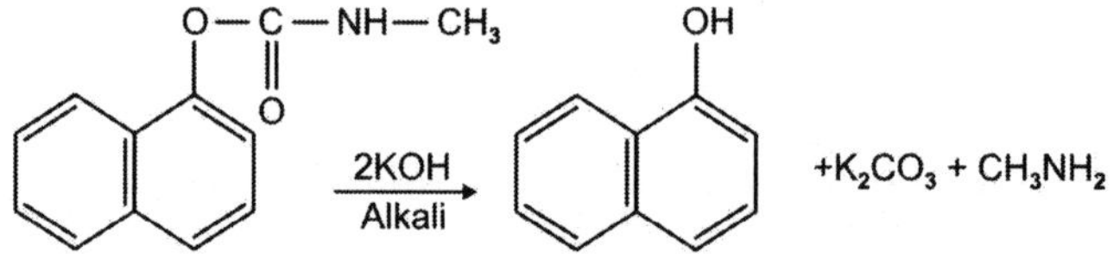

1-Naphthol

Baygon (Propoxur, Bayer 39007)

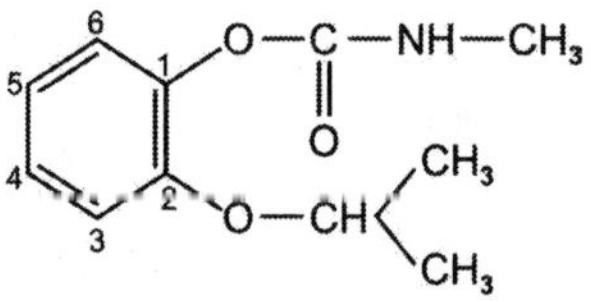

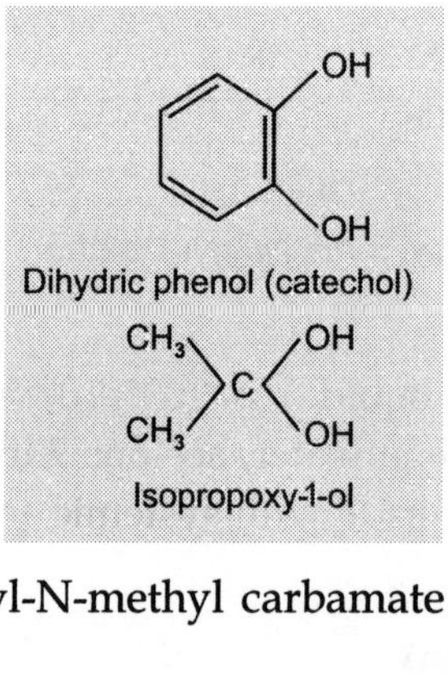

Dihydric phenol (catechol)

Isopropoxy-1-ol

2-isopropoxy-phenyl-N-methyl carbamate

Synthesis:

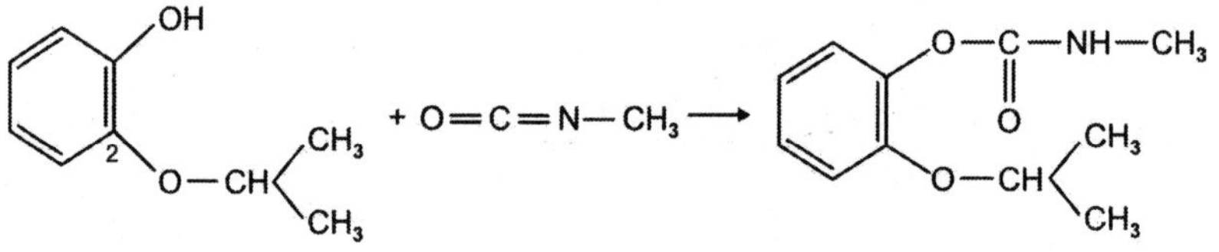

2 Isoproproxy phenol   Baygon

Properties:
  i. It is highly soluble in organic solvents and slightly soluble in water.
  ii. It produces rapid knock-down effect, mainly contact action.

Formulation: 20% EC, 50% W.P. and Dusts

Baygon is particularly effective against insects affecting man and animals such as cockroaches, flies, mosquitos.

Carbofuran (Furadan)

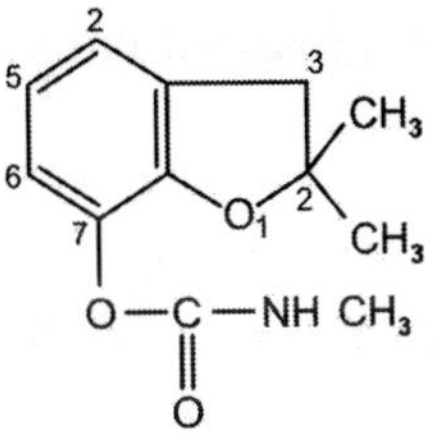

2,3-Dihydro-2,2-dimethyl-7-benzofuranyl-N-methyl carbamate

Synthesis:

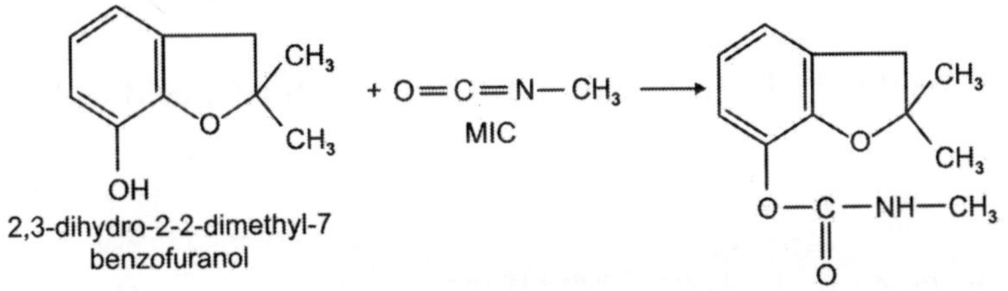

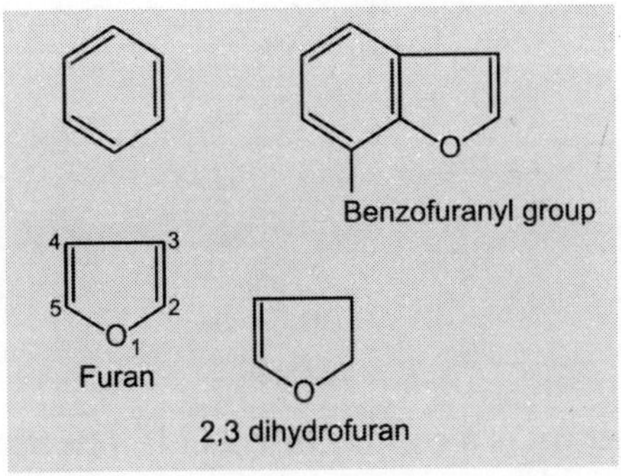

OH
2,3-dihydro-2-2-dimethyl-7
benzofuranol

+ O=C=N—CH$_3$
MIC

Benzofuranyl group

Furan

2,3 dihydrofuran

i. Carbofuran is a systemic carbamate insecticide, nematicide and acaricide of broad spectrum.

ii. White crystalline, 153–154 °C m.p.

iii. It is stable in acid and neutral media, but unstable in alkaline medium.

Formulation: 3% Granule

4.3.4 Synthetic Pyrethroids

Production cost of natural pyrethrum flower dusts are very high. The synthetic pyrethroids possess the same properties as the natural powder (e.g. low mammalian toxicity, good knock-down effect, etc.) and are very popular to the user. They have extremely high insecticidal activity at extremely low doses and are biodegradable in nature. Synthetic pyrethroids treated crops give increased yields of better quality. The first synthetic pyrethroid, allethrin appeared on the market as long as 1950.

Pyrethroids are good inhibitors of Ca-Mg and Co-ATPase enzyme systems in insect nervous system, which in turn disturb Na-Ca exchange and calcium pumping which are necessary to maintain gradient across cellular membranes in the nervous system.

Allethrin

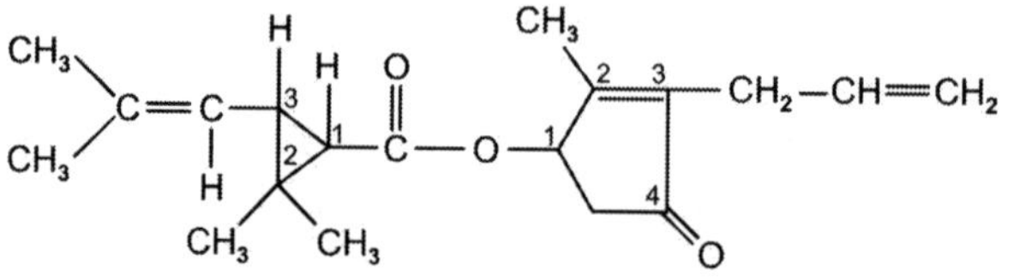

2-Methyl-4-oxo-3-(2-propenyl)-2cyclopenten-1yl

Synthesis:

Allethrin is synthesized by esterification of ± chrysanthemic acid with the alcohol, allethrolone

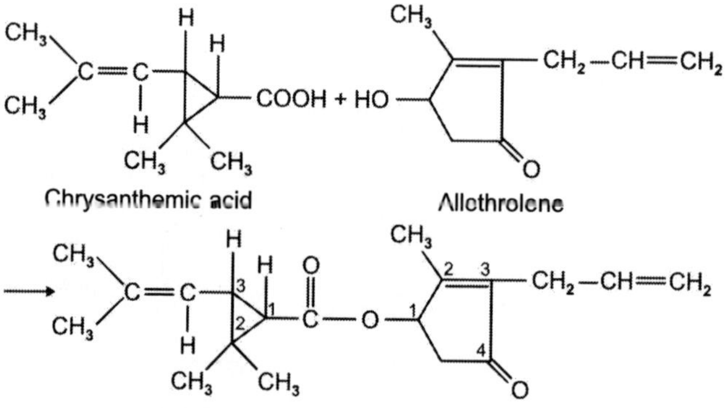

Chrysanthemic acid   Allethrolene

Allethrin

Use: Allethrin is a contact insecticide, effective against household pests.

Fenvalerate

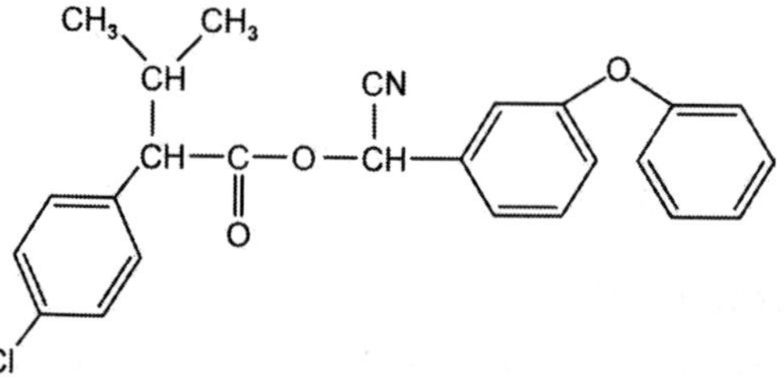

(R,S)-α-Cyano-3 phenoxybenzyl (R,S)-2-(4-chlorophenyl)-3-methylbutyrate

Fenvalerate is a viscous yellow liquid.

Use: Fenvalerate acts both as a contact and stomach poison. It uses in the control of pests in cotton, vegetables and fruits.

Deltamethrin/Decamethrin

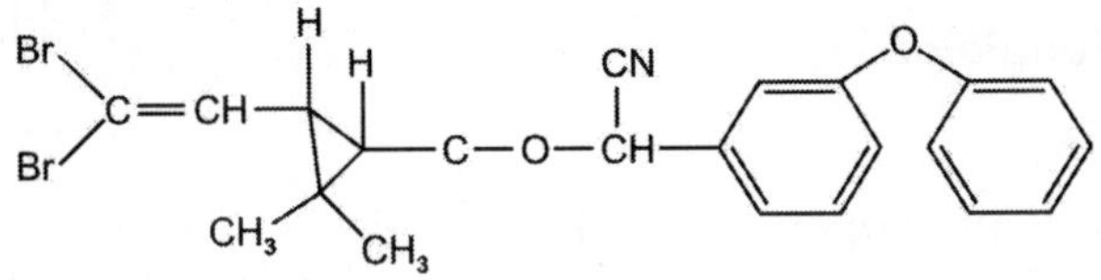

(S)-α-Cyano-3-phenoxybenzyl(1R,3R)-3(2,2-dibromovinyl)
-2,2-dimethyl cyclopropane carboxylate.

Properties:

i. Colourless crystalline powder

ii. m.p. 98–101 °C

iii. Toxicity is very low; it is used at low dosages of 12 g/ha for control of pests.

Use: Deltamethrin is both contact and stomach poison and used in wide range of pests of fruits, vegetables, cotton and stored products.

Cypermethrin

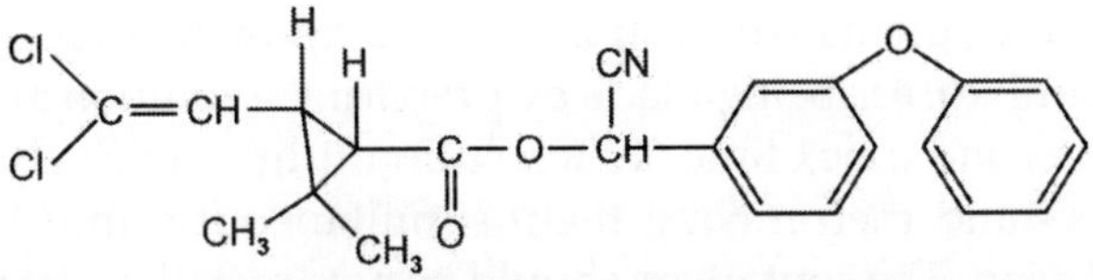

α-Cyano-3-phenoxy benzyl(1RS)-cis,trans-3(2,2-chlorovinyl)
-2,2-dimethyl cyclopropane carboxylate

Properties:

i. White, colourless and waxy solid

ii. m.p. 81–83°C

Use: Cypermethrin is a stomach and contact poisoning insecticide, effective against broad range of pests of cotton, fruit and vegetable crops.

Permethrin

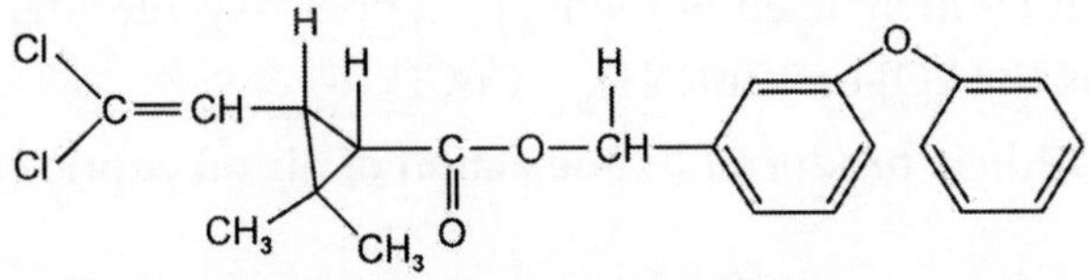

3-Phenoxy benzyl (1RS) cis,trans-3(2,2-dichlorovinyl)
2,2-dimethyl cyclopropane carboxylate

Properties:

i. White, odourless, crystalline solid

ii. m.p. *cis*-isomer : 54–56 °C and *trans*-isomer : 45–46 °C.

Use: Permethrin is a contact insecticide; use to control the pests of cotton, fruits, vegetables and tobacco.

4.4 FUNGICIDE

4.4.1 Copper Fungicide

Bordeaux Mixture

Various compounds of copper are used as fungicide. Copper sulphate has been used for more than 150 years as fungicide on growing plant in the form of so called Bordeaux mixture.

Preparation

The mixture is produced by precipitation of basic copper sulphate with lime from a 1% solution of copper sulphate. To prepare Bordeaux mixture, 1kg of copper sulphate is dissolved in 90 litres of water and to the solution obtained is added with through stirring 10 litres of freshly prepared 10% milk of lime.

$$4CuSO_4 + 3Ca(OH)_2 \rightarrow [Ca(OH)_2]_3 \cdot CuSO_4 + 3CuSO_4$$

Bordeaux mixture

Basic copper sulphate settles out in the form of a gelatinous precipitate that covers the foliage and fruit of plants well and is retained on their surface for a long time. In India Bordeaux mixture is being made by preparing a solution of copper sulphate (1% solution, 9 litre) and quick lime (10% solution, 1 litre) in finely ground form in separate containers and then mixing them simultaneously into a third container with constant agitation. The containers should be non-metallic, like wooden, plastics and earthen vessels. Bordeaux mixture should always be prepared fresh.

The fungicidal action of Bordeaux mixture is more protective than eradicative. It is effective against leaf blights and fruit falls or rots associated with large number of diseases, notable exceptions being apple scab and powdery mildews.

Copper oxychloride

(Basic chlorides of copper, Blitox-50, Fytolan, Blue copper 50)

To avoid the cumbersome preparation of Bordeaux mixture which has always to be used fresh, many fixed copper compounds have been tried as substitutes. The most important and widely used of them are copper oxychloride, or

$$[3C_4(OH)_2 \cdot CuCl_2, H_2O] \text{ or } 3Cu(OH)_2 \cdot CuCl_2$$

Copper oxychloride is produced by the action of air on cupric chloride solution or scrap copper

$$4Cu + O_2 \rightarrow 2Cu_2O$$
$$Cu_2O + 2HCl \rightarrow 2CuCl + H_2O$$
$$CuCl_2 + Cu \rightarrow 2CuCl$$
$$4CuCl_2 + 3CaCO_3 + 3H_2O \rightarrow 3Cu(OH)_2 \cdot CuCl_2 + 3CaCl_2 + 3CO_2$$

Formulation: 50% and 90% copper oxychloride (W.P.).

Copper oxychloride formulations can be used both as dust and spray. Dust formulations may contain 6–35% Cu.

Copper Oleate

$$[CH_3(CH_2)_7CH = CH(CH_2)_7COO]_2Cu$$

Synthesis:

$$CH_3(CH_2)_7CH = CH(CH_2)_7COOH \xrightarrow{CuSO_4/CuCO_3} + H_2CO_3/H_2SO_4$$

Oleic acid

$$[CH_3(CH_2)_7CH = CH(CH_2)_7COO]_2Cu$$

Copper oleate may be used as a fungicide in place of Bordeaux mixture and owing to its low phytotoxicity, may be applied widely through the whole growth period. It also serves as a wood preservative.

Use: Use against powdery mildews, *Phytophthora* spp. and bacterial diseases.

4.4.2 Mercury Fungicides

HgCl$_2$

Mercuric chloride was used as bactericide during the early nineteenth century. It decomposes in the presence of hydroxides including sodium, calcium and potassium.

Use: (1) Generally the seed materials (potato tubers and propagative materials and other root crops) are dipped in 1 : 2000 or stronger solution of mercuric chloride for a few minutes and then planted. (2) Sterilisation of seed beds with mercuric chloride has been widely practiced.

In view of the availability of organomercurials and the toxicity of mercury, the use of these compounds have declined.

Agalol (Ceresan, Aretan)

$$CH_3-O-CH_2-CH_2-Hg-Cl$$
Methoxy ethyl mercuric chloride

Synthesis:

It is produced by precipitation with chloride salts from solution of methoxy ethyl mercuric acetate

$$CH_3-O-CH_2-CH_2-Hg-O-\overset{\displaystyle O}{\underset{\displaystyle \|}{C}}-CH_3 + NaCl \rightarrow CH_3-O-CH_2-CH_2-Hg-Cl + CH_3COONa$$

Methoxy ethyl mercuric acetate   Agalol

Properties:

i. When agalol comes in contact with the skin, it causes painful burns.

ii. The compound is relatively stable in neutral and weekly alkaline media. It is decomposed by acids with evolution of ethylene:

$$CH_3-O-CH_2-CH_2-Hg-Cl + HCl \rightarrow HgCl_2 + CH_3OH + CH_2{=}CH_2$$

Use: It is an effective seed disinfectant for grains, beets and other crops and is marketed in preparation containing 2.5% and 3.5% Hg.

4.4.3 Organic Sulphur Compounds

Dithiocarbamates

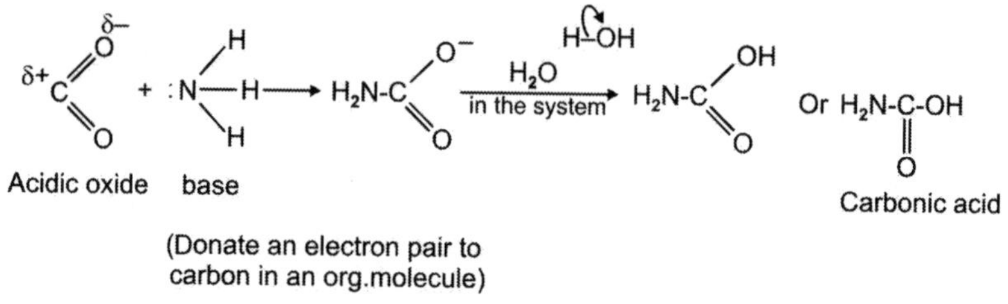

Acidic oxide   base

(Donate an electron pair to
carbon in an org.molecule)

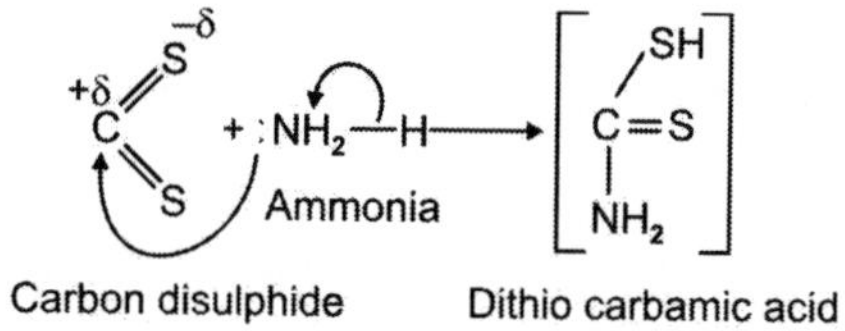

Carbonic acid

Carbon disulphide   Dithio carbamic acid

Dithiocarbamic acid is not known to exist in the free state. But the salt of dithiocarbamic acid, such as K/Na-dithiocarbamate can be prepared. Thus, instead of taking NH_3, we can take methylamine or dimethyl amine (primary and secondary aliphatic and aromatic amines) and react with CS_2 (carbon disulphide) in the presence of aq. NaOH or KOH to get desire salts.

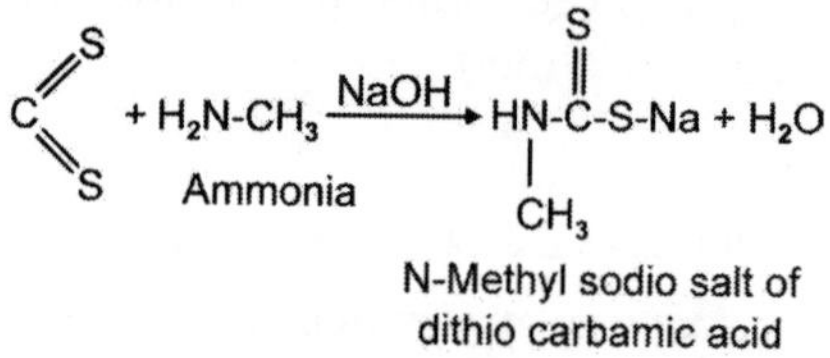

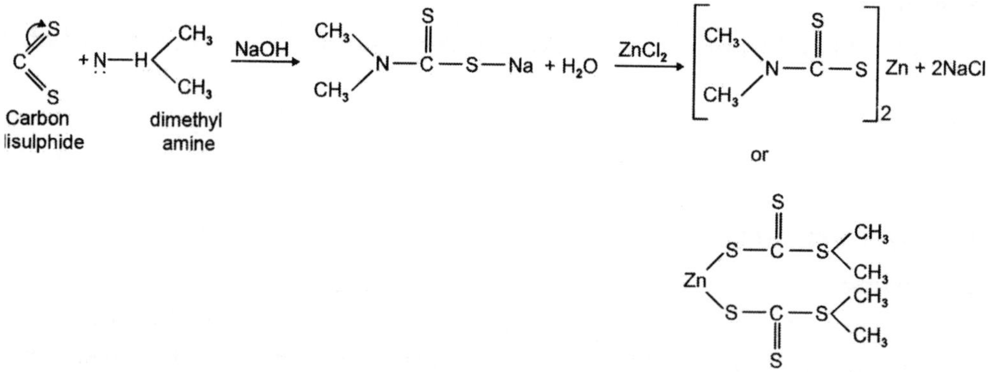

N-Methyl sodio salt of
dithio carbamic acid

Carbon   dimethyl
lisulphide   amine

or

General methods of preparation of salt of dithiocarbamic acid:

(1) 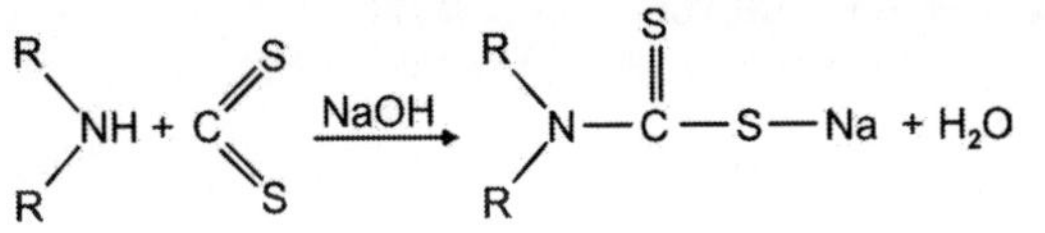 $\underset{R}{\overset{R}{\diagdown}}NH + C\underset{\diagdown S}{\overset{\diagup S}{}} \xrightarrow{NaOH} \underset{R}{\overset{R}{\diagdown}}N-\overset{\overset{S}{\|}}{C}-S-Na + H_2O$

> Na salts are water soluble; Zn and Hg salts are water insoluble

(2) 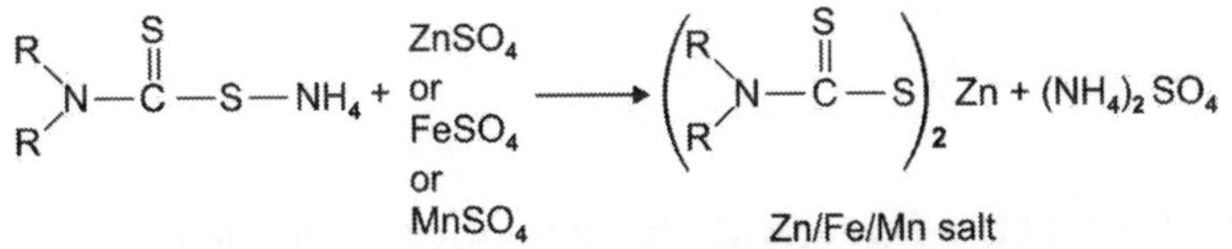 $\underset{R}{\overset{R}{\diagdown}}N-\overset{\overset{S}{\|}}{C}-S-NH_4 + \underset{\begin{array}{c}\text{or}\\\text{FeSO}_4\\\text{or}\\\text{MnSO}_4\end{array}}{ZnSO_4} \longrightarrow \left(\underset{R}{\overset{R}{\diagdown}}N-\overset{\overset{S}{\|}}{C}-S\right)_2 Zn + (NH_4)_2 SO_4$

Zn/Fe/Mn salt
of dithiocarbamic acid

(3) 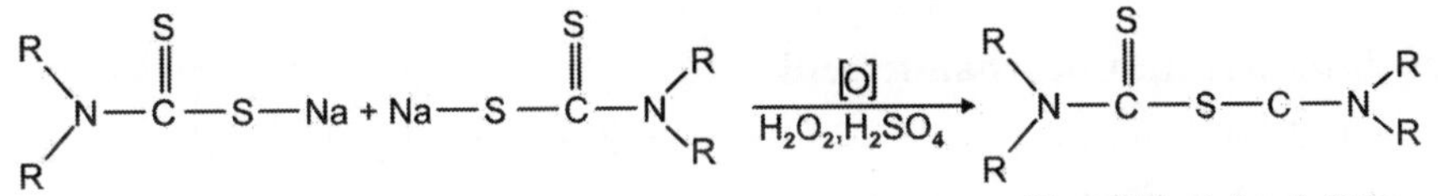 $\underset{R}{\overset{R}{\diagdown}}N-\overset{\overset{S}{\|}}{C}-S-Na + Na-S-\overset{\overset{S}{\|}}{C}-N\underset{\diagdown R}{\overset{\diagup R}{}} \xrightarrow[H_2O_2, H_2SO_4]{[O]} \underset{R}{\overset{R}{\diagdown}}N-\overset{\overset{S}{\|}}{C}-S-C-N\underset{\diagdown R}{\overset{\diagup R}{}}$

Disulphide salts of dithio
carbamic acid

Vapam

Salt of methyl dithiocarbamic acid

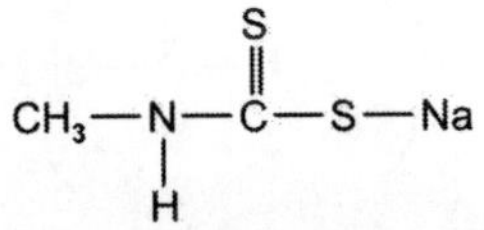

$$CH_3-N-\overset{\overset{S}{\|}}{C}-S-Na$$
$$\underset{H}{\overset{|}{}}$$

Sodium N-methyl-dithiocarbamate

Synthesis:

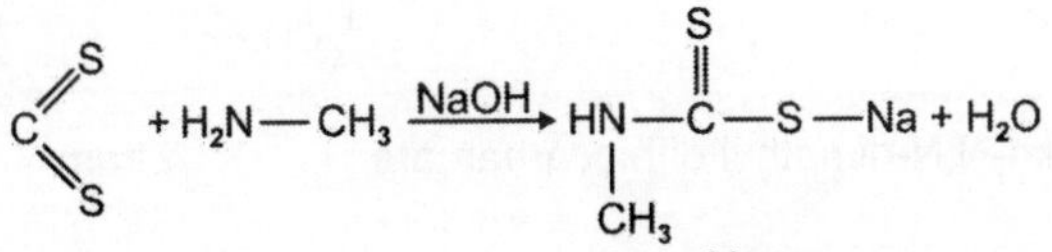

$$C\underset{\diagdown S}{\overset{\diagup S}{}} + H_2N-CH_3 \xrightarrow{NaOH} HN-\overset{\overset{S}{\|}}{C}-S-Na + H_2O$$
$$\underset{CH_3}{\overset{|}{}}$$

Vapum

Properties:

1. It is a white crystalline substance. Highly soluble in water and practically insoluble in hydrocarbon (xylene), but moderately soluble in alcohol.
2. It is unstable in storage and gradually breaks down with the formation of methyl isothiocyanate.

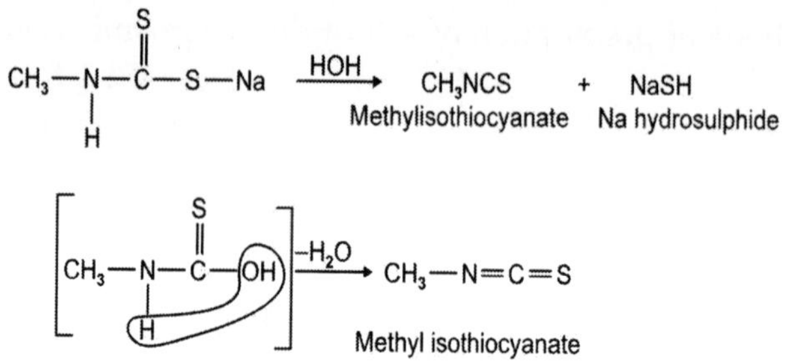

$$CH_3-N(H)-\overset{\overset{\displaystyle S}{||}}{C}-S-Na \xrightarrow{HOH} CH_3NCS + NaSH$$

Methylisothiocyanate   Na hydrosulphide

$$\left[CH_3-N(H)-\overset{\overset{\displaystyle S}{||}}{C}-(OH) \right] \xrightarrow{-H_2O} CH_3-N=C=S$$

Methyl isothiocyanate

Use: Use as soil sterilent (act as fumigant), that provides complete destruction of nematodes, fungal diseases and weeds in the soil system.

Salt of dimethyl dithiocarbamic acid

To protect plant diseases, the Zn and Fe salts of dimethyl dithio carbamic acid and on a very small-scale the Mn salts are used.

Zn Salt

Ziram, Zerlate

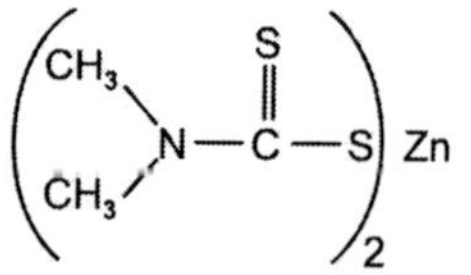

$$\left(\overset{CH_3}{\underset{CH_3}{\diagdown}} N - \overset{\overset{\displaystyle S}{||}}{C} - S \right)_2 Zn$$

Zinc *bis* (dimethyl dithiocarbamate)

Synthesis:

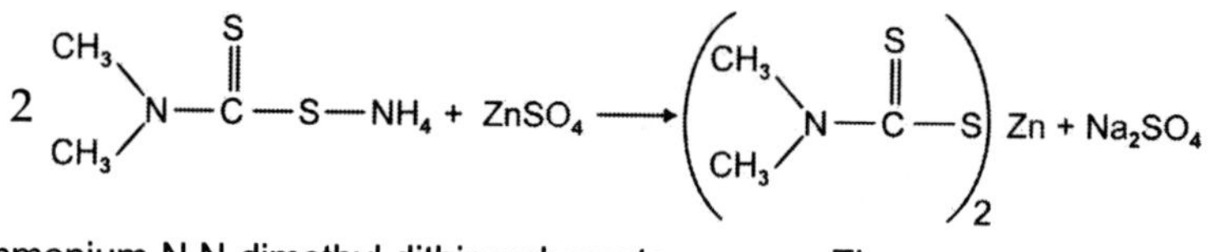

$$2 \; \overset{CH_3}{\underset{CH_3}{\diagdown}} N - \overset{\overset{\displaystyle S}{||}}{C} - S - NH_4 + ZnSO_4 \longrightarrow \left(\overset{CH_3}{\underset{CH_3}{\diagdown}} N - \overset{\overset{\displaystyle S}{||}}{C} - S \right)_2 Zn + Na_2SO_4$$

Ammonium-N,N-dimethyl dithiocarbamate   Ziram

Properties:

  i. Most stable dithiocarbamate fungicides.
 ii. Comparatively low solubility in water and insoluble in alcohol/ether.
iii. Used as 50% W.P. formulation or 0.2 to 0.3% a.i EC.

Fe Salt

Fermate, Ferbam

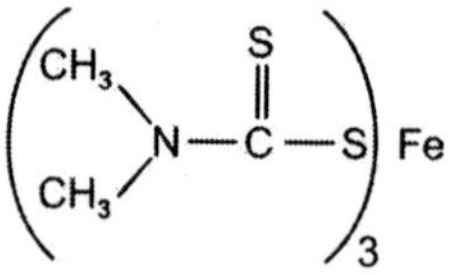

$$\left(\overset{CH_3}{\underset{CH_3}{\diagdown}} N - \overset{\overset{\displaystyle S}{||}}{C} - S \right)_3 Fe$$

Ferric dimethyl dithiocarbamate

Synthesis:

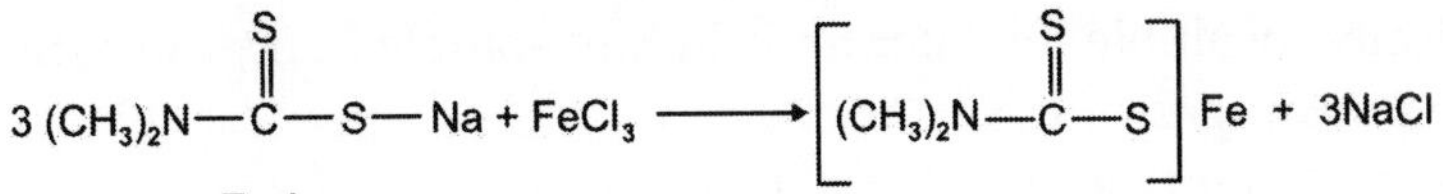

$$3 (CH_3)_2N—\overset{\overset{\displaystyle S}{\|}}{C}—S—Na + FeCl_3 \longrightarrow \left[(CH_3)_2N—\overset{\overset{\displaystyle S}{\|}}{C}—S \right] Fe + 3NaCl$$

Ferbam

It has virtually no phytotoxicity and low mammalian toxicity.

Formulation :   Dust (80% a.i.)

W.P. (50% a.i.)

Mn Salt
Marbam

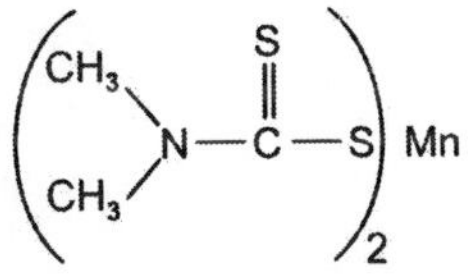

$$\left(\begin{matrix} CH_3 \\ \\ CH_3 \end{matrix} \!\! N—\overset{\overset{\displaystyle S}{\|}}{C}—S \right)_2 Mn$$

Synthesis:

$$2 \begin{matrix} CH_3 \\ \\ CH_3 \end{matrix} \!\! N—\overset{\overset{\displaystyle S}{\|}}{C}—S—Na + 2MnSO_4 \longrightarrow \left(\begin{matrix} CH_3 \\ \\ CH_3 \end{matrix} \!\! N—\overset{\overset{\displaystyle S}{\|}}{C}—S \right)_2 Zn + Na_2SO_4$$

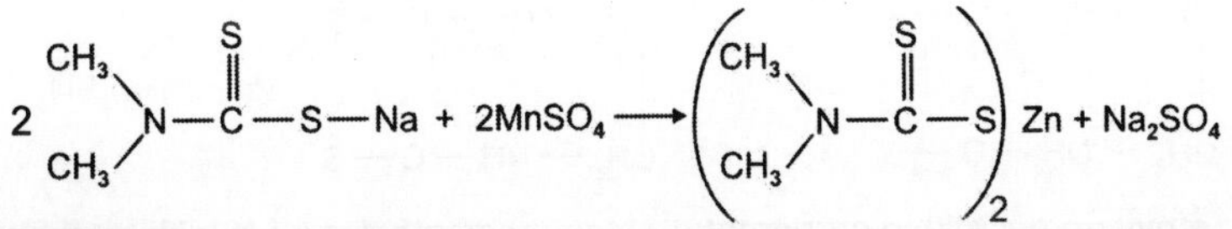

Marbam

Tetra methyl thiuram disulphide

TMTD (Thiram)

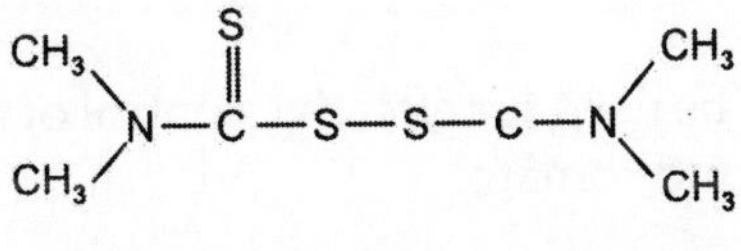

$$\begin{matrix} CH_3 \\ \\ CH_3 \end{matrix} \!\! N—\overset{\overset{\displaystyle S}{\|}}{C}—S—S—C—N \!\! \begin{matrix} CH_3 \\ \\ CH_3 \end{matrix}$$

bis (diemethyl thiocarbamoyl) disulphide

or

Tetramethyl thiuram disulphide

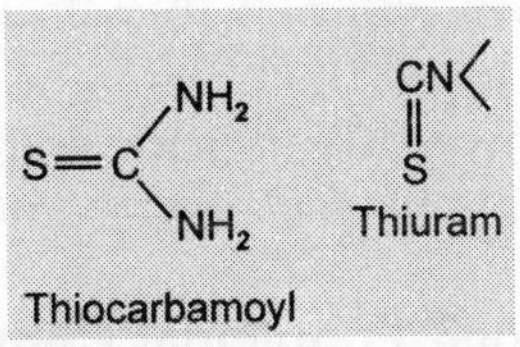

$$S{=}C \!\! \begin{matrix} NH_2 \\ \\ NH_2 \end{matrix} \qquad \overset{\overset{\displaystyle CN\langle}{}}{\underset{S}{\|}}$$

Thiocarbamoyl   Thiuram

Synthesis:

$$\begin{matrix} CH_3 \\ \\ CH_3 \end{matrix} \!\! N—\underset{\underset{\displaystyle S}{\|}}{C}—S—Na + Na—S—\underset{\underset{\displaystyle S}{\|}}{C}—N \!\! \begin{matrix} CH_3 \\ \\ CH_3 \end{matrix} \xrightarrow[H_2O_2 + H_2SO_4]{[O]} \begin{matrix} CH_3 \\ \\ CH_3 \end{matrix} \!\! N—\underset{\underset{\displaystyle S}{\|}}{C}—S—S—\underset{\underset{\displaystyle S}{\|}}{C}—N \!\! \begin{matrix} CH_3 \\ \\ CH_3 \end{matrix} + Na_2SO_4$$

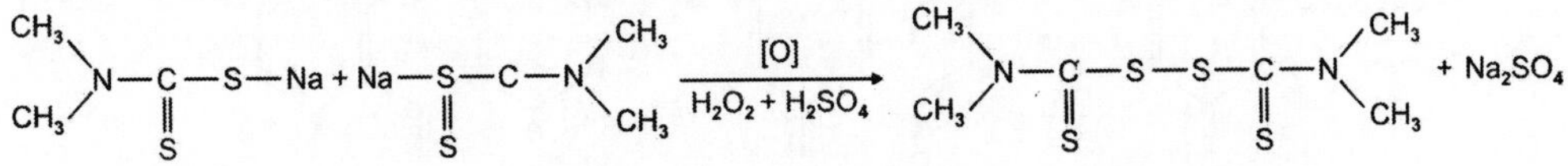

Thiram is produced in good yields by oxidation of alkali salts of dimethyl dithiocarbamic acid with H_2O_2 or other oxidizing agents like H_2SO_4.

Properties:

i. Practically insoluble in water and slightly soluble in org. solvent.

ii. Stable in storage.

Use: Seed disfectent (seeds of corn, beans etc.)

Control soil fungi and root rot diseases of plant.

Ethylene bis(dithiocarbamic) acid salts

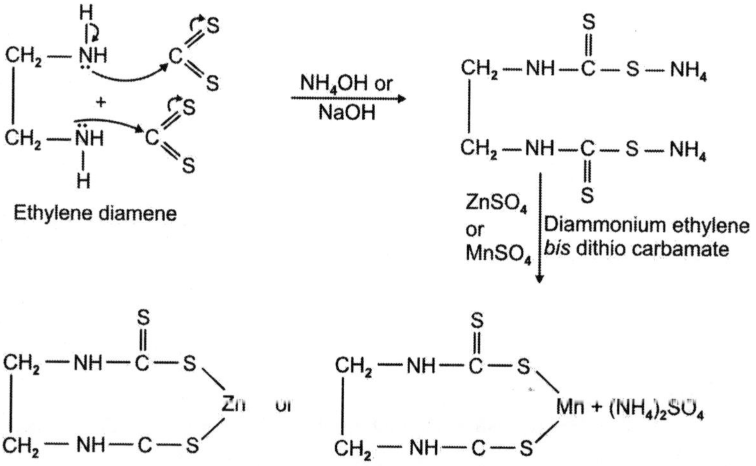

Ethylene diamene

$\xrightarrow{\text{NH}_4\text{OH or NaOH}}$

Diammonium ethylene *bis* dithio carbamate

ZnSO$_4$ or MnSO$_4$

Zinc ethylene *bis* (dithio carbamate)
Zineb

Maganese ethylene *bis* (dithio carbamate)
Maneb

i. The Na and NH$_4$ salts being phytocidal (i.e. phytotoxic) are employed only for soil treatment.

ii. These are replaced by Zn and Mn salts and they are known as Zineb and Maneb respectively.

Both are powerful fungicide and can be used for effective control of foliar diseases particularly blight diseases of potato and tomato.

4.4.4 Quinone Fungicidal Compounds

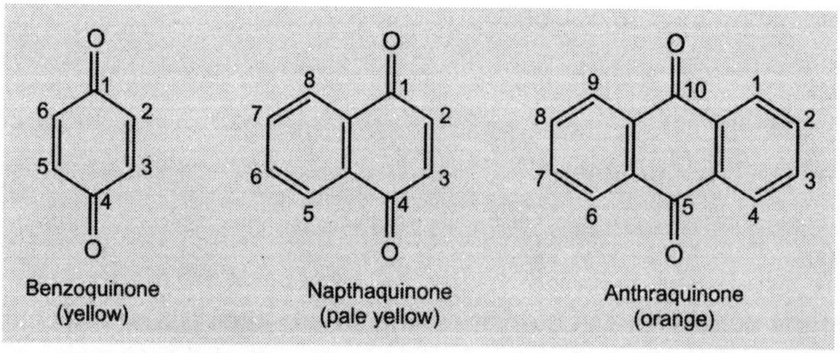

Benzoquinone
(yellow)

Napthaquinone
(pale yellow)

Anthraquinone
(orange)

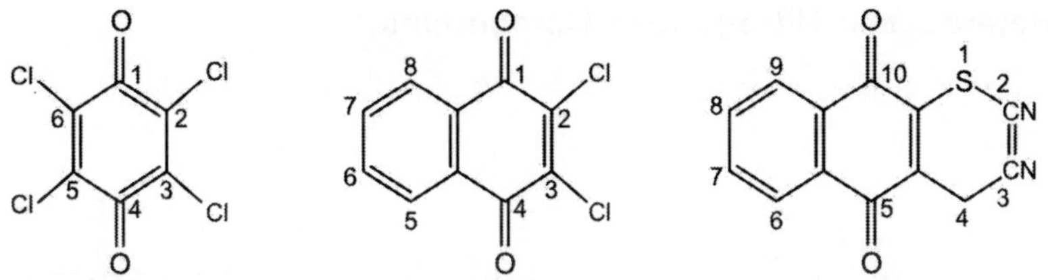

| 2,3,5,6,-Tetrachloropara p-benzoquinone (chloranil) | 2,3-Dichloro 4-napthaquinone (Phygon, Dichlone) | 2,3-Dicyano 1,4-dithio anthraquinone (Dithianone) |

1. The quinones are especially active as fungicides.
2. Benzoquinone show comparatively low fungicidal activity. But when halogens are introduced into the ring the activity is strongly increased. The order of substitution in consideration to activities are as follows: Cl > Br > I.
3. 1,4-Naphthaquinone is less active than 2-Chloro-naphthaquinone and 2,3-Dichloro-1,4-Naphthaquinone. Further addition of chlorine atoms lowers the fungicidal properties.

Properties and Use:

   i. Chloranil and Phygon are yellow crystalline substances.
   ii. Practically insoluble in water but soluble in organic solvents (xylene, chloroform and ether).
   iii. Both are unstable in the presence of alkalies.
   iv. Phygon is stable in heat, light and moisture, but chloranil degraded.
   v. Dithianon is not recommended for foliar spray due to phytotoxic in nature.
   vi. Chloranil and Phygon are generally used for seed disinfection (e.g. bean and cotton seed).

Chloranil

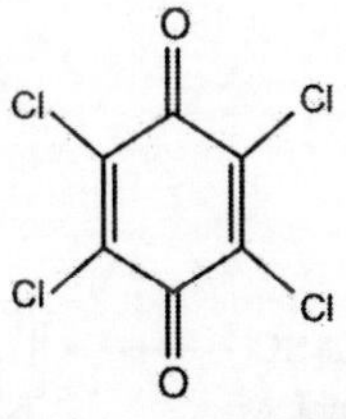

Tetrachloro-p-benzoquinone

Synthesis:

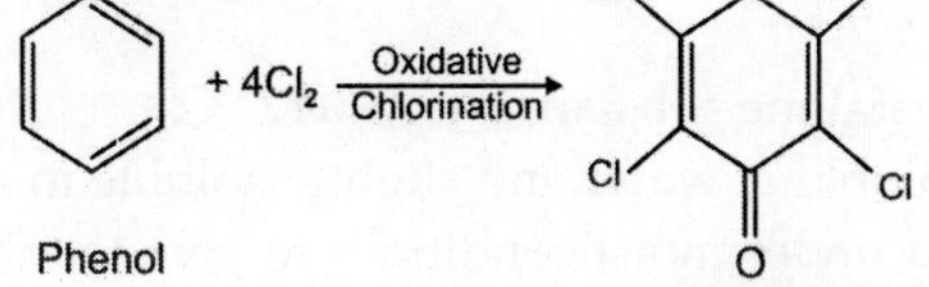

Phenol   + 4Cl$_2$ Oxidative Chlorination →   Chloronil

It is used for seed treatment against smut and diseases of vegetable seeds.

4.4.5 Heterocyclic Nitrogenous Compounds

Captan

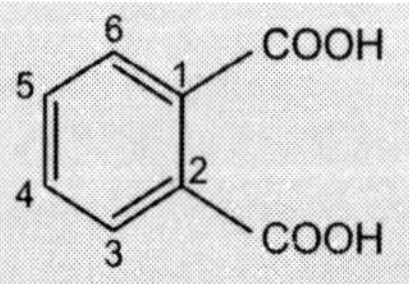

1,2,3,6 tetra hydro phthalic acid

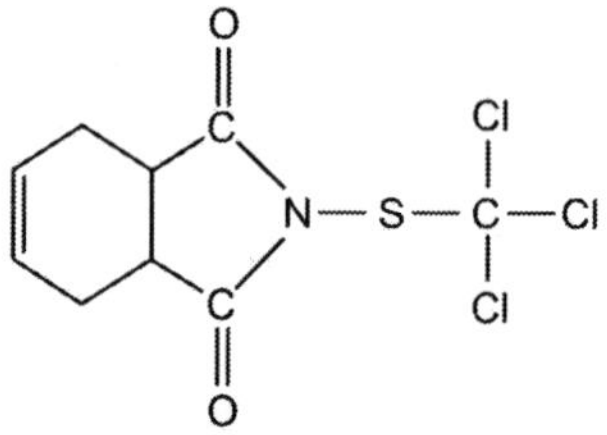

N-trichloromethyl thiotetra hydro phthalimide

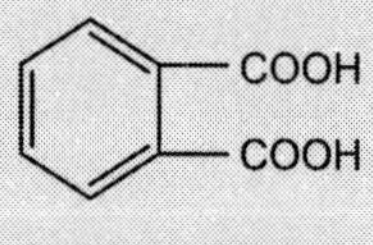

Phthalic acid

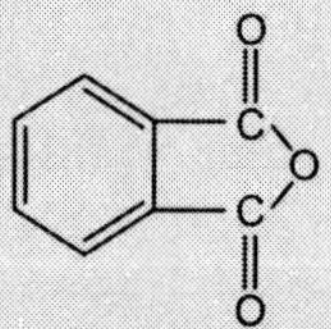

Phthalic anyhydride

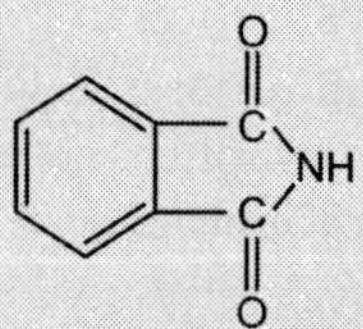

Phthalimide

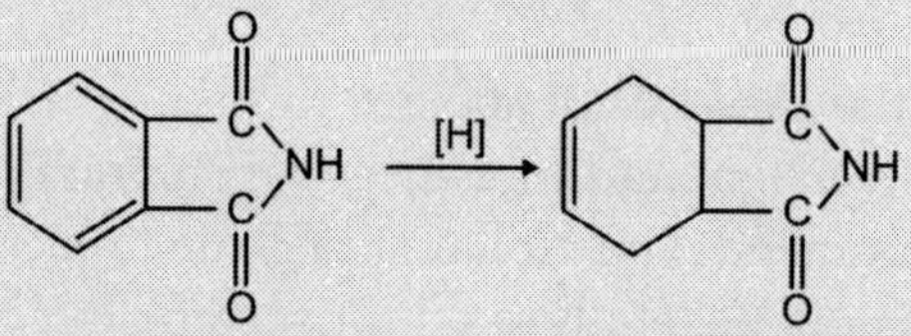

Phthalimide

Tetra hydro phthalimide

Synthesis:

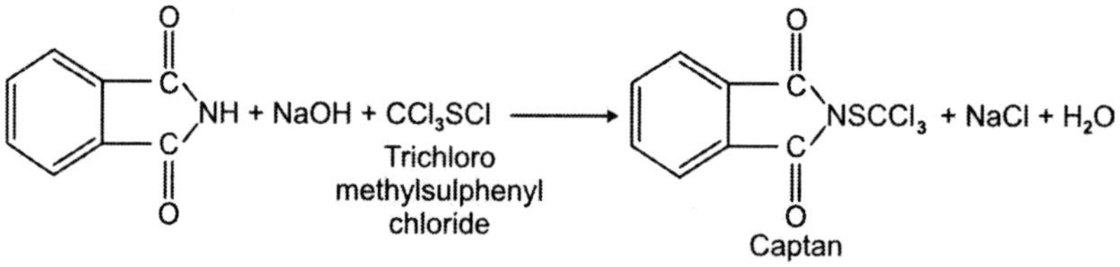

Trichloro methylsulphenyl chloride

Captan

Properties:

i. It is a white crystalline substance, m.p. 172 °C.

ii. Practically insoluble in water and slightly soluble in most organic solvent.

iii. It is hydrolysed under moist conditions to give tetrahydrophthalimide.

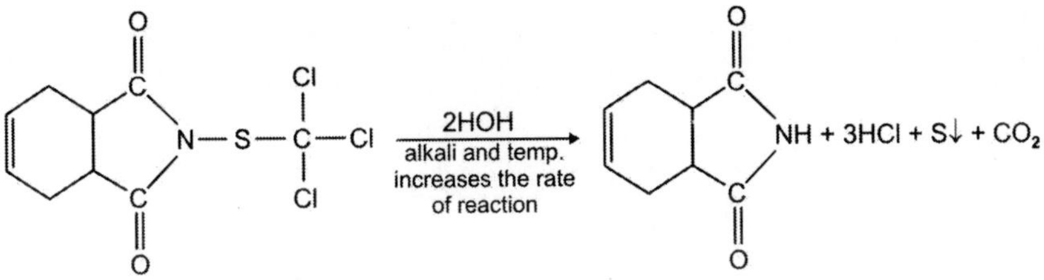

Tetrahydrophthalimide

The dissipation of captan in the environment (atmosphere) is facilitated by moist condition or even by hydrolysis by water, one can see that sulphur is precipitated (yellow colour), thereby showing an indication that hydrolysis take place. Presence of alkali and higher temperatures increases the rate of reaction.

Use: It is used for all purpose fungicides.

Formulation: 50% a.i. W.P.; 75% a.i. for seed dressing

0.5% conc. for soil drenching (control against damping-off disease)

Folpet

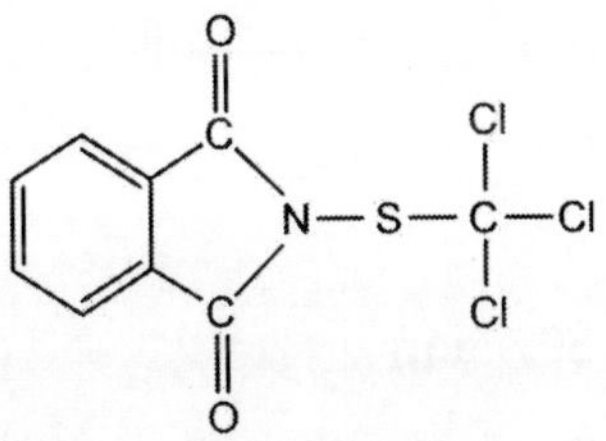

N-trichloromethyl thiophthalimide

Properties:

i. Folpet is an analog of captan.
ii. It is slightly more effective than captan against certain diseases.
iii. Like captan, it is hydrolysed by water but the rate of hydrolysis is higher than that of captan.

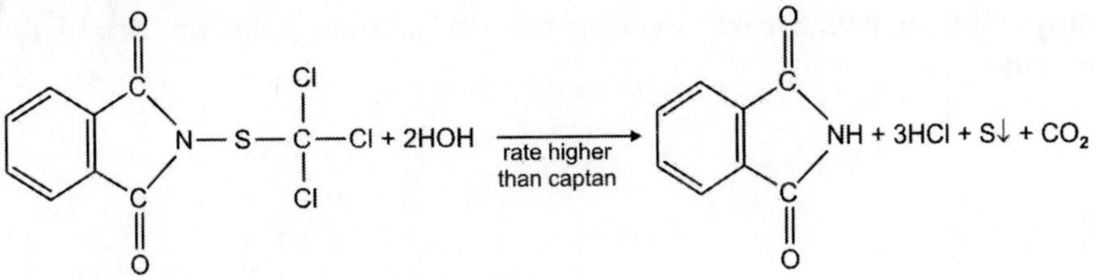

N-trichloromethyl thiophthalimide

Use: Available as W.P.

Difolatan

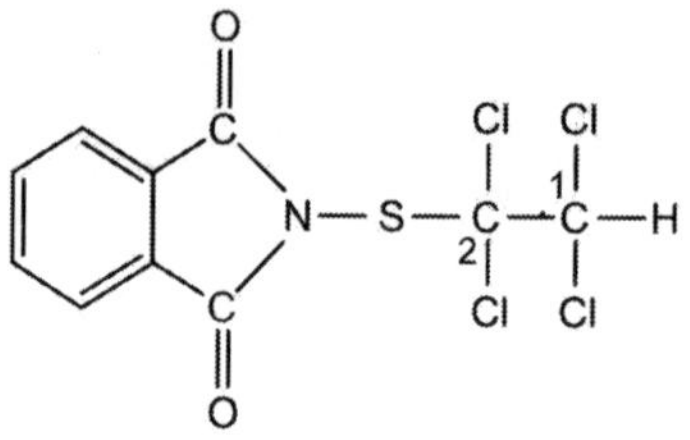

N-1,1-2,2-tetrachloroethylthiophalimide

Properties:

i. White crystalline substance, m.p. 160–161 °C
ii. slowly hydrolysed by water and more rapidly by caustic alkalies. It is more resistant to hydrolysis than captan and folpet.

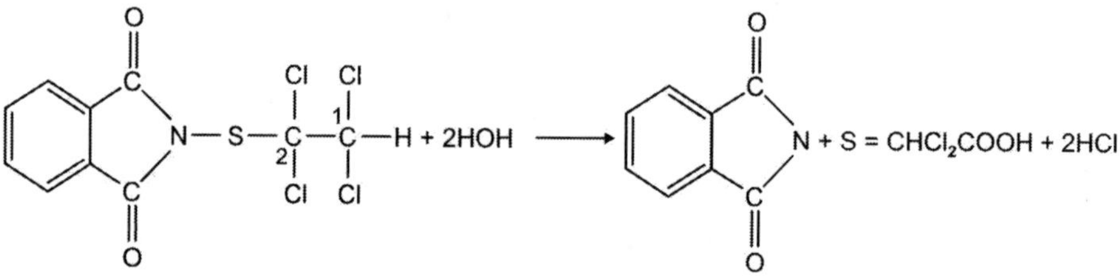

$$\text{...} + 2HOH \longrightarrow \text{...} N + S = CHCl_2COOH + 2HCl$$

Use: W.P. and E.C. (both 80% a.i.)

4.4.6 Benzimidazole Fungicides

Carbendazim

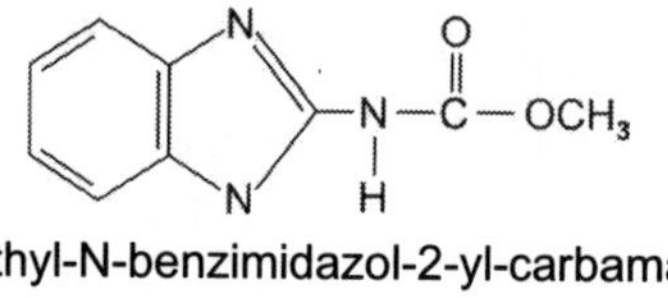

Methyl-N-benzimidazol-2-yl-carbamate

Properties & use: Slowly decomposes in alkaline solution; broad spectrum fungicide.

4.5 HERBICIDES

Types of weeds in crop

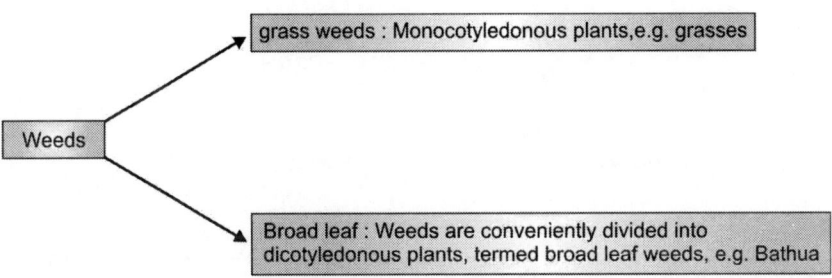

General mode of action of herbicides:

1. Inhibition of photosynthesis

   i. Disrupt the light reactions and block the photosynthetic electron transport (electron carrier e.g. plastoquinone, cytochrome, plastocyanin, ferridoxin).

   ii. Inhibition of hill reactions e.g. carbamates, ureas derivatives, 1,3,5-triazines etc.

2. Inhibition of Respiration

   i. Blocking the mitochondrial electron transport e.g. dinitrophenyl and halophenols.

   ii. Preventing coupling of oxidative phosphorylation to the electron transport chain (Respiration is not inhibited but takes place without production of energy).

3. Growth disturbances e.g. 2,4-D and its analogs, numerous benzoic acid derivatives (auxin competition).

4. Inhibition of cell and nucleus division e.g. alkyl N-aryl carbamates (cell division).

5. Disturbance of nucleic acid and protein synthesis e.g. chloro acetomide.

6. Inhibition of lipid synthesis e.g. aliphatic carboxylic acids.

4.5.1 Phenoxy Acetic Acid Derivatives or 2, 4-D and its analogs

Aryloxy alkylcarboxylic acid

$O-CH_2-COOH$

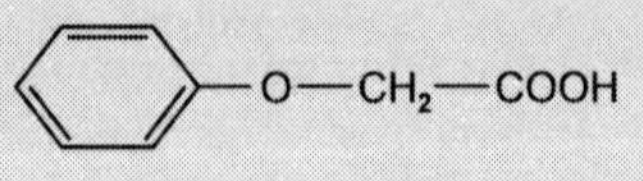

$H-CH_2-COOH$
Acetic acid

Phenoxy acetic acid

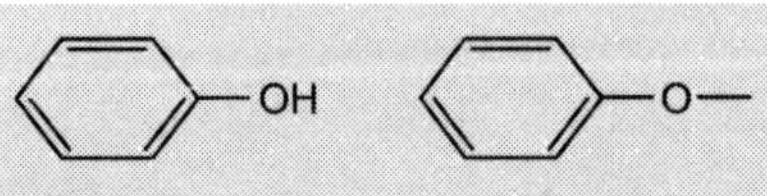

—OH
Phenol
acetic acid (2,4-D)

—O—
Phenoxy

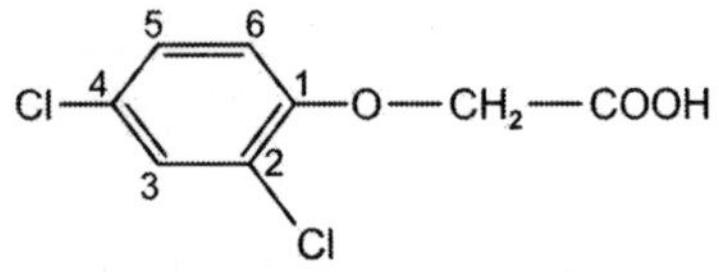

$Cl-$ ⁴⁵⁶¹²³ $-O-CH_2-COOH$, Cl

2,4-Dichlorophenoxy acetic acid (2,4-D)

The aryloxy alkyl carboxylic acids have the greatest value as herbicides and plant growth regulators.

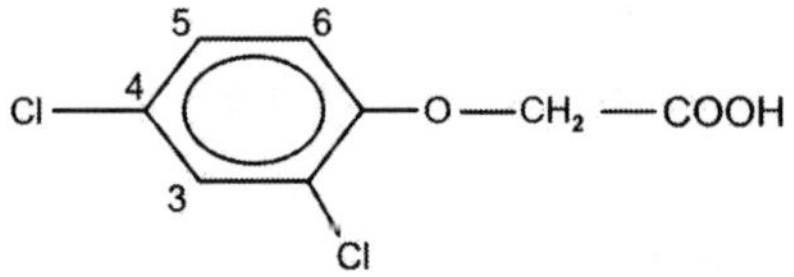

Cl — (ring 3,4,5,6) — $O-CH_2-COOH$, Cl

2,4-Dichlorophenoxy acetic acid (2,4-D)

Preparation

Condensation of salt of monochloroacetic acid with 2,4-dichloro-phenolate of the alkali metal in aqueous or anhydrous medium

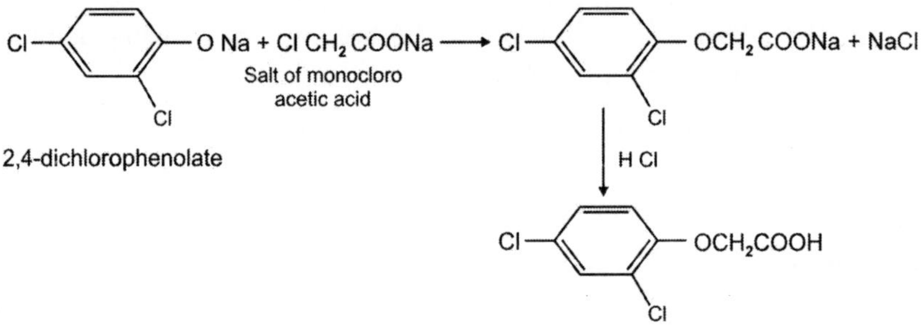

$Cl-$ —$O\,Na + Cl\,CH_2\,COONa \longrightarrow Cl-$ —$OCH_2\,COONa + NaCl$
Salt of monocloro
acetic acid

2,4-dichlorophenolate

$\downarrow$ H Cl

$Cl-$ —OCH_2COOH, Cl

2,4-D

If excess of sodium 2,4-dichlorophenolate is used, the yield of the product increased.

Physical properties:

i. Pure 2,4-D is a white crystalline substance, m.p. 141 °C.
ii. Practically has no odour, but the technical grade compounds smell more or less like dichlorophenol.

iii. 2,4-D is highly soluble in ethyl alcohol, ether, toluene, benzene, carbon tetrachloride, acetone, etc.

Chemical properties:

i. With inorganic and organic bases it forms stable salts.

ii. On prolonged boiling of 2,4-D with HBr or HCl decomposition may occur.

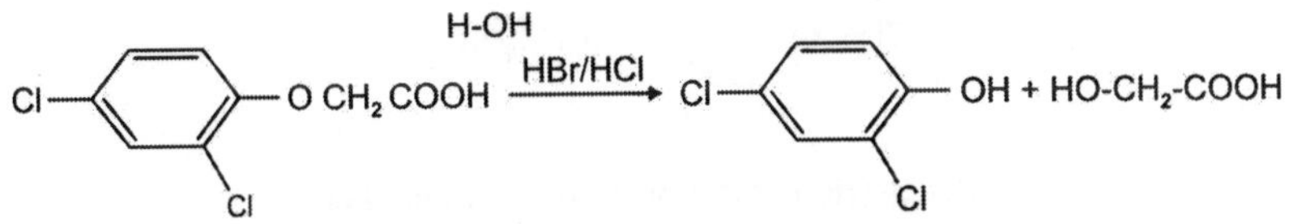

$$\text{Cl} - \langle \text{ring} \rangle - \text{O CH}_2\text{COOH} \xrightarrow[\text{HBr/HCl}]{\text{H-OH}} \text{Cl} - \langle \text{ring} \rangle - \text{OH} + \text{HO-CH}_2\text{-COOH}$$

Use: 2, 4-D as such is not used as herbicide, because of its very little solubility in water. But as it is acid, it can form alkali salt, amine salt, esters which are very much effective as herbicides, e.g.

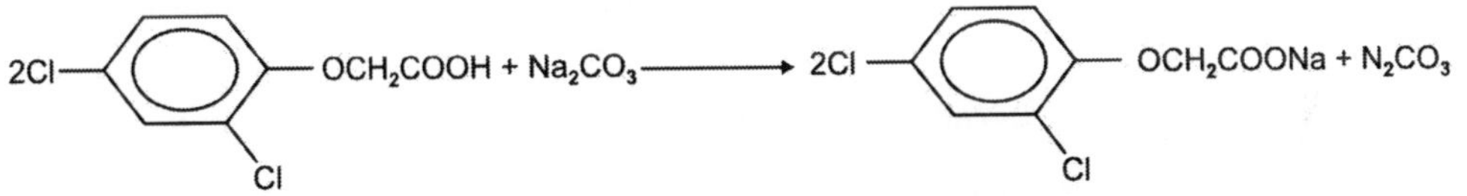

$$2\text{Cl} - \langle \text{ring} \rangle - \text{OCH}_2\text{COOH} + \text{Na}_2\text{CO}_3 \longrightarrow 2\text{Cl} - \langle \text{ring} \rangle - \text{OCH}_2\text{COONa} + \text{N}_2\text{CO}_3$$

Na-salt of 2,4-D
(water soluble)

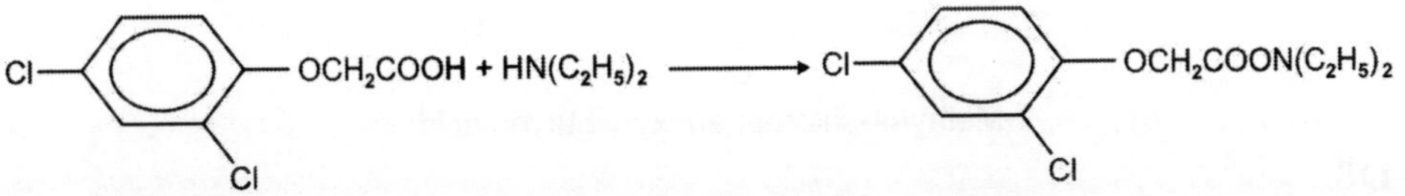

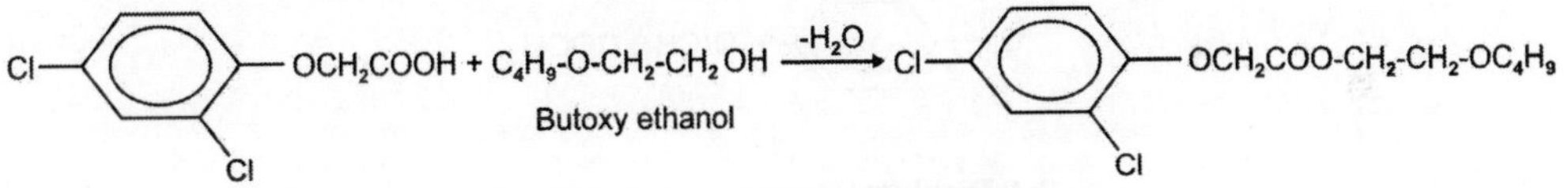

$$\text{Cl} - \langle \text{ring} \rangle - \text{OCH}_2\text{COOH} + \text{HN(C}_2\text{H}_5)_2 \longrightarrow \text{Cl} - \langle \text{ring} \rangle - \text{OCH}_2\text{COON(C}_2\text{H}_5)_2$$

$$\text{Cl} - \langle \text{ring} \rangle - \text{OCH}_2\text{COOH} + \text{C}_4\text{H}_9\text{-O-CH}_2\text{-CH}_2\text{OH} \xrightarrow{-\text{H}_2\text{O}} \text{Cl} - \langle \text{ring} \rangle - \text{OCH}_2\text{COO-CH}_2\text{-CH}_2\text{-OC}_4\text{H}_9$$

Butoxy ethanol

Ester of 2,4-D
(not highly water soluble)

The lower alkyl esters of 2,4-D (ethyl, isopropyl) are comparatively volatile and their vapours may damage crops. With an increase in molecular weight, the volatility of the esters decreases, and that is why the high molecular weight esters are preferable.

2,4-D is a selective herbicide normally applied as a post-emergence treatment.

Analogs of 2,4-D

2,4,5-T

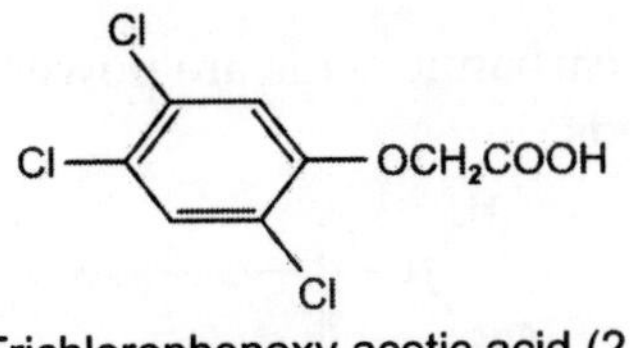

$$\text{Cl} - \langle \text{ring} \rangle - \text{OCH}_2\text{COOH}$$

2,4,5-Trichlorophenoxy acetic acid (2,4,5-T)

2,4,5-T is similar to 2,4-D in herbicidal properties. Mixtures of 2,4-D and 2,4,5-T are sold as brush killers. It is particularly effective against woody plants besides the weeds which are normally controlled by 2,4-D.

2,4,5-TP (Silvex)

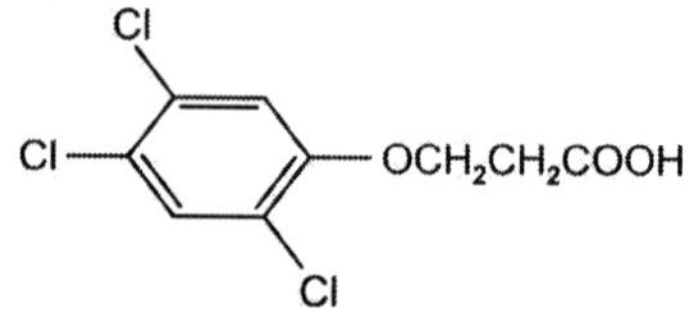

2,4,5-Trichlorophenoxy-α-propionic acid

MCPA (Agroxone, Methoxane)

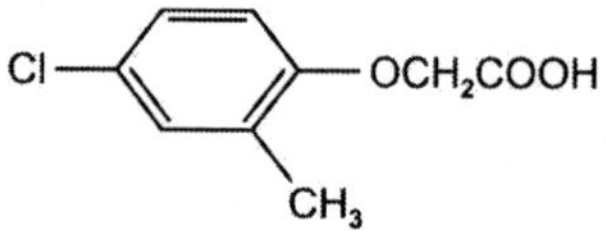

2-Methyl-4-chlorophenoxy acetic acid

MCPB

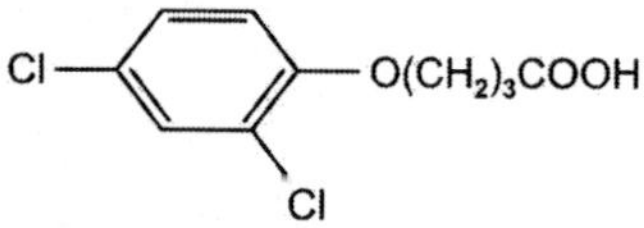

2-Methyl-4-chlorophenoxy-γ-butyric acid

2,4-DB

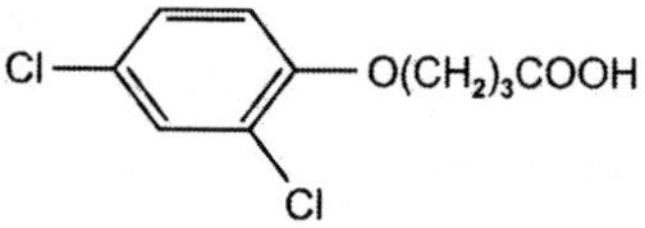

2,4-Dichlorophenoxy-γ-butyric acid

4.5.2 Carbamate Herbicides

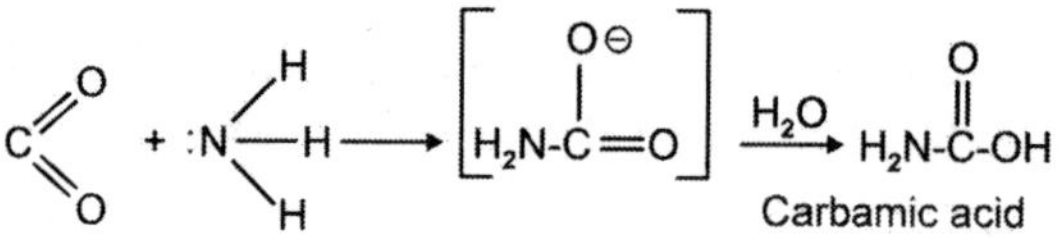

Pure carbamic acid is not stable and quickly decomposes to give NH_3 and CO_2 but its derivatives are stable and have been used as insecticides, fungicides and herbicides.

The alkyl esters of N-aryl carbamic acids are powerful herbicides for the control of monocotylendonous weeds.

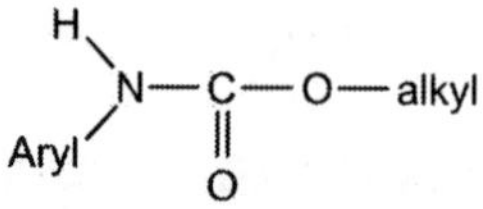

Propham (IPC)

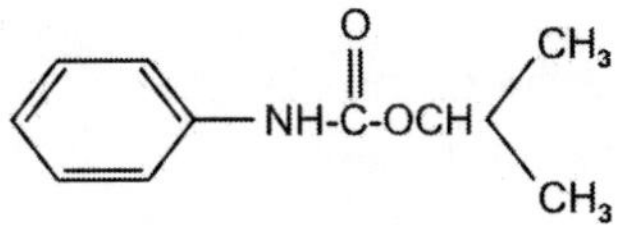

Isopropyl-N-phenylcarbamate

Synthesis:

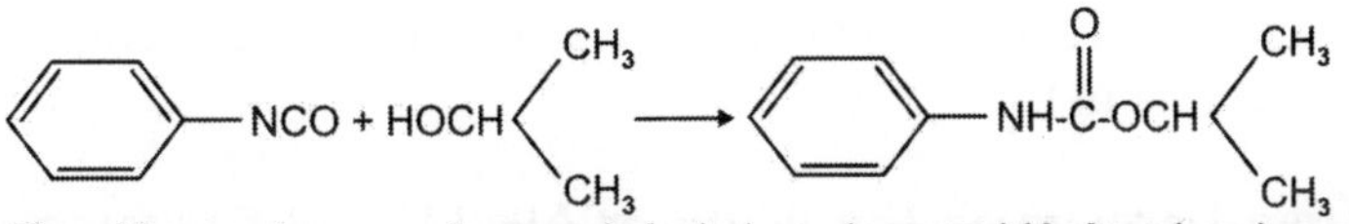

Phenyl isocynate   Isopropyl alcohol   Isopropyl-N-phenyl carbamate

The phenyl isocyanate is added gradually with stirring to an excess of absolute isopropyl alcohol.

Properties:

i. In the pure form it is a white crystalline compound, m.p. 80–90°C.

ii. It is highly soluble in alcohol, acetone, benzene, ethyl acetate, etc., and other org. solvents (xylene).

Uses:

i. IPC is sensitive towards monocotyledons plant.

ii. Soil applications have been found to give better results than foliage application, but it gets easily decomposed in the soil by soil microorganisms, hence we prefer chloroderivatives.

Chloroderivatives of IPC

CIPC

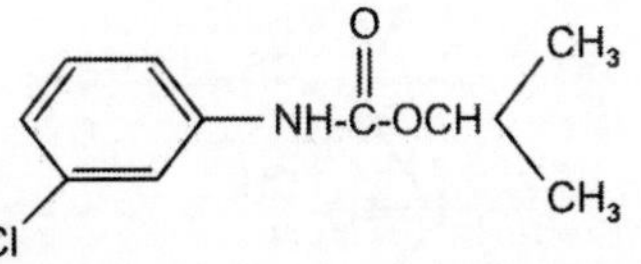

Isopropyl-N-3(chlorophenyl) carbamate (CIPC)

Uses:

i. CIPC is safe for many dicotyledonous plant.

ii. CIPC is usually not effective on emerged weeds, effectively used for pre-emergent treatment in cotton, soybean, pea, sugar beet, etc.

Swep

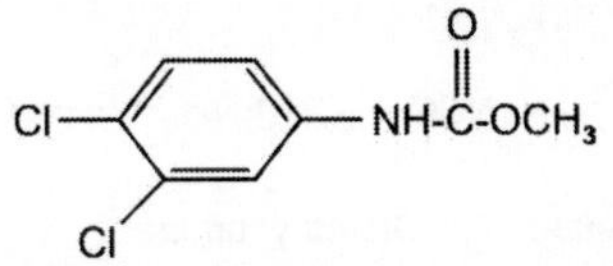

Methyl-N-(3,4 dichlorophenyl) carbamate

Synthesis:

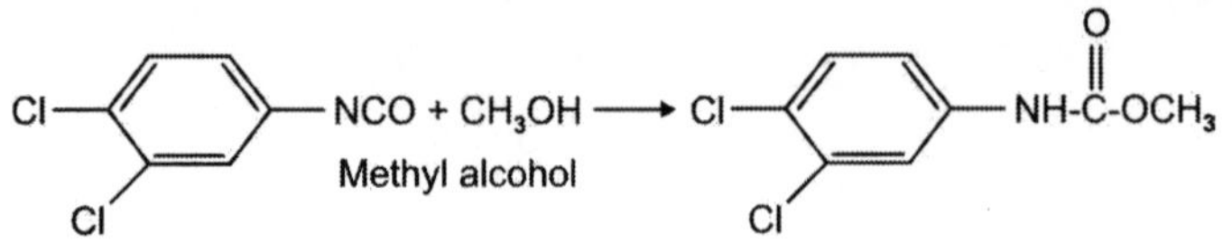

$$Cl-\langle\text{C}_6\text{H}_3\rangle-NCO + CH_3OH \longrightarrow Cl-\langle\text{C}_6\text{H}_3\rangle-NH-\overset{\overset{\displaystyle O}{\|}}{C}-OCH_3$$

Methyl alcohol

3,4 dichlorophenyl isocyanate   Swep

Use: Widely used in pre-emergence herbicide for the control of weed in the soybean and rice field.

4.5.3 Urea Derivatives Herbicide or Alkyl-N-aryl Carbamate Derivatives or Aliphatic Organic Nitrogen Derivatives

Urea is used as a fertilizer in agricultural field. Practically all plants are tolerated the use of large doses of urea, without any injury. But simple urea derivative bi-ureate has appreciably phytocidal effect.

$$\underset{\text{urea}}{(NH_2)_2CO} \qquad \underset{\text{cyanic acid}}{NH_3 + HNCO} \xrightarrow{(NH_2)_2CO} \underset{\text{biuret}}{NH_2CONHCONH_2}$$

Urea derivatives have shown toxic effects on plant. A large majority of derivatives of urea having herbicidal properties belong to aryl dialkyl urea group.

The diamide of carbonic acid is called as urea $CO(NH_2)_2$	$C=C=O$ with NH_2, NH_2	$C=O$ with N—alkyl group, alkyl group, H, N—aryl group
Urea		Urea derivative herbicide

Fenuron or Fenidim

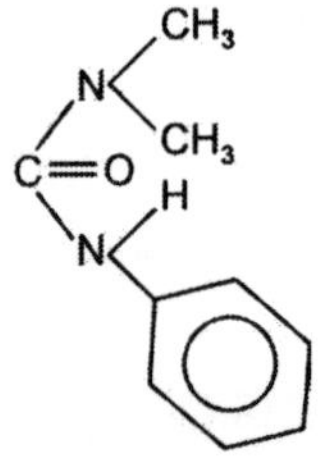

N-Phenyl-N',N'-dimethyl urea

Synthesis:

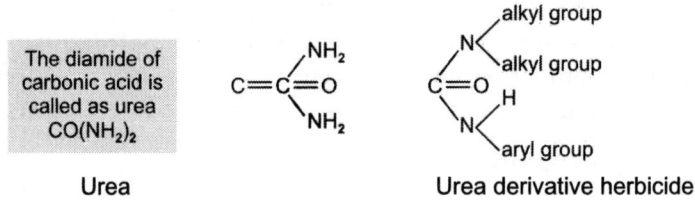

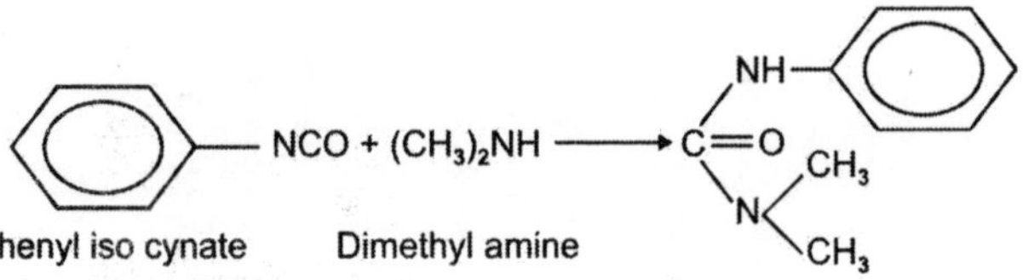

Phenyl iso cynate   Dimethyl amine

Fenuron

Properties:

  i. It is a white crystalline substance, m.p. 136 °C.

  ii. It is slightly soluble in water (0.29%) and highly soluble in alcohols, ketones, halogenated hydrocarbons and sparingly soluble in saturated hydrocarbons.

  iii. Upon boiling with caustic alkalies and mineral acids it breaks down with the formation of amines or their salts.

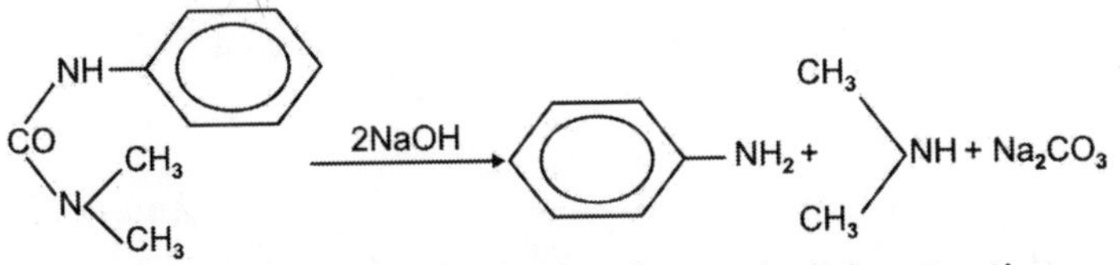

Use: Used as soil treatment to kill woody plants. As it is an active root herbicide, it is used for eradicating annual vegetation.

Monuron or Chlorofenidim

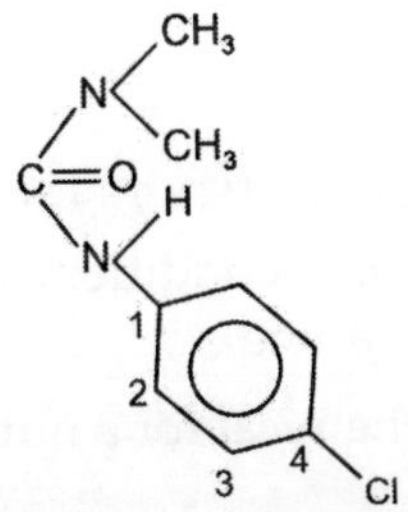

N-(4-chlorophenyl) N',N'-dimethyl urea

Synthesis:

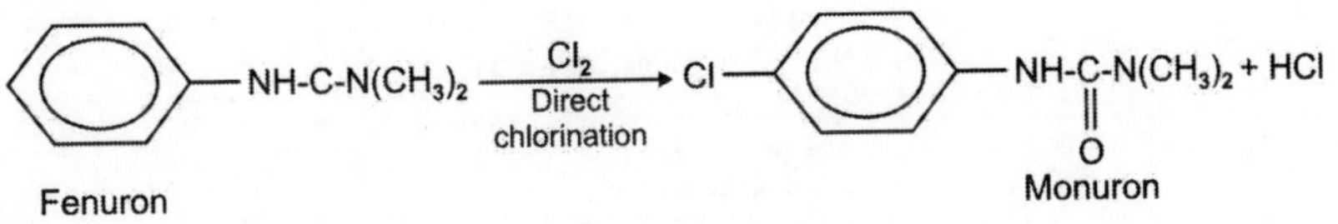

Fenuron   Monuron

Properties:

  i. It is a white crystalline substance, m.p. 176–177 °C.

  ii. Poorly soluble in water, more soluble in halogenated hydrocarbon.

  iii. Monuron is more or less stable at ordinary condition, but boiling with alkali, its hydrolysis to amine.

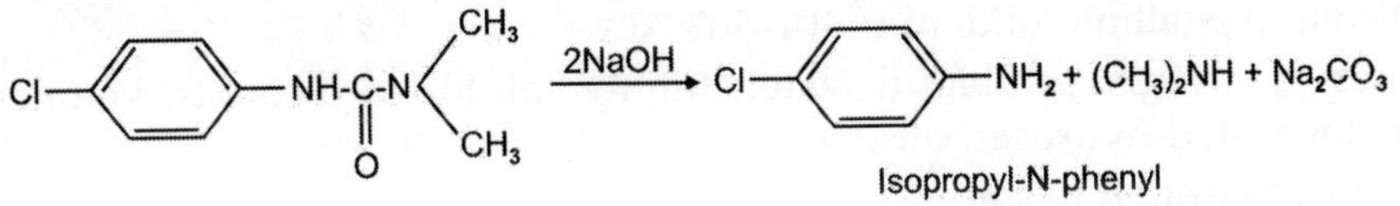

Isopropyl-N-phenyl

Use: Widely used for the control of weed in the cotton and sugarcane field.

Diuron or Karmax

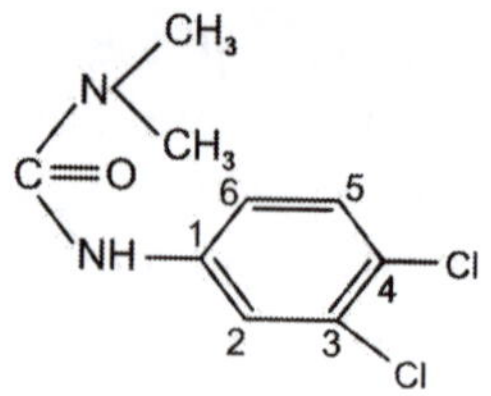

N-3,4-Dichlorophenyl-N',N'-dimethyl urea

Synthesis:

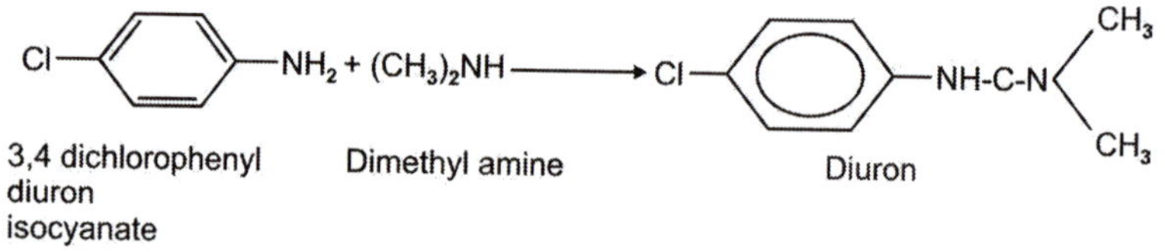

3,4 dichlorophenyl diuron isocyanate + Dimethyl amine ⟶ Diuron

Properties:

i. White crystalline substance, m.p. 158–159 °C.

ii. More or less stable in ordinary condition, hydrolysed with alkali with the formation of corresponding amine.

Use: Excellent pre-emergence chemical for a number of crops (cotton, sugarcane, pineapple, grapes etc.).

Neburon

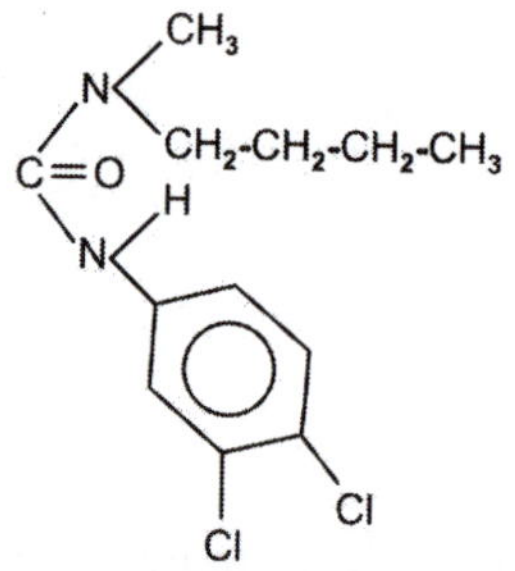

N-(3,4-dichlorophenyl)-N'-butyl-N'-methyl urea

Properties:

i. White crystalline solid, m.p. 101–103 °C.

ii. Very sparingly soluble in water, highly soluble in alcohols, ketones and halogenated hydrocarbons.

iii. Low absorption in soil.

Use: Pre-emergence herbicide.

Isoproturon

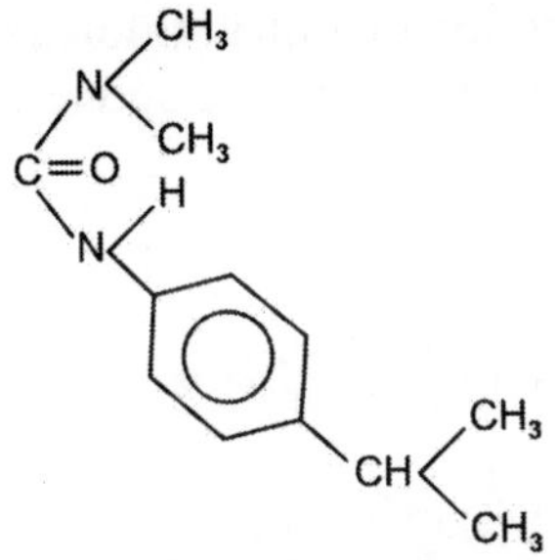

N-(p-isopropylphenyl)-N',N'-dimethyl urea

Isoproturon is used to control annual grass weeds in wheat, rye and barley.

4.5.4 Triazine Herbicides or Heterocyclic Nitrogen Derivatives

The herbicides belonging to this group of compounds have heterocyclic ring structure composed of nitrogen and carbon atoms. 6-membered heterocyclic compounds with three N-atoms in the ring are called triazines.

[If it is 5-membered, then azole]

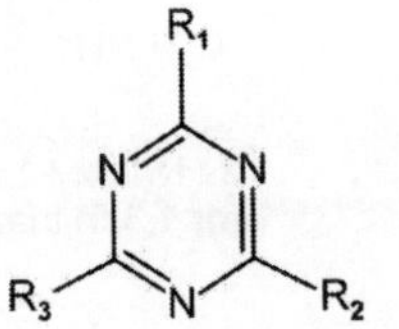

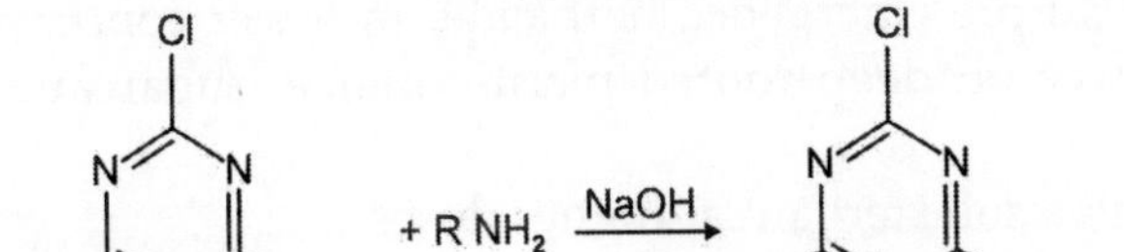

Cyanuric chloride
(basic compound)

R may be ethyl/methyl/propyl and so on

Simazine

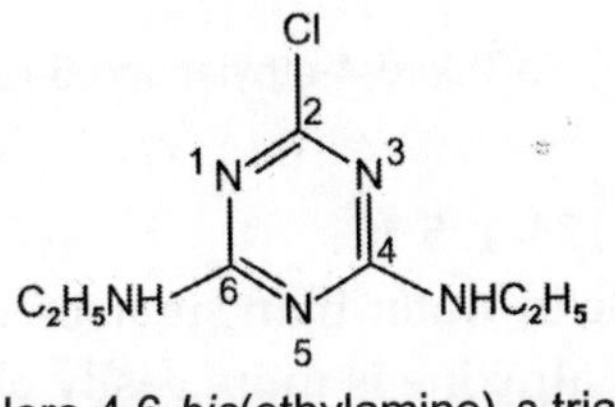

2-Chloro-4,6-*bis*(ethylamino)-s-triazine
2-Chloro-4,6-*bis*(ethylamino)-1,3,5-triazine

Synthesis:

Simazine is produced by reacting cyanuric chloride with ethylamine and sodium hydroxide in aqueous medium or in organic solvents.

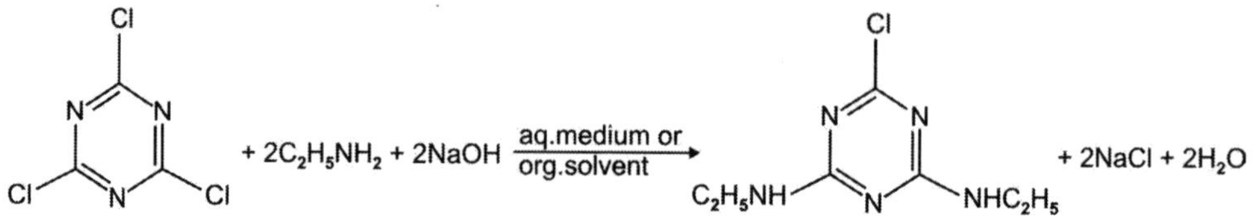

$$+ 2C_2H_5NH_2 + 2NaOH \xrightarrow{\text{aq.medium or}}{\text{org.solvent}} \quad + 2NaCl + 2H_2O$$

Properties:

i. White crystalline substance, m.p. 227–228 °C.

ii. Sparingly soluble in water but is more soluble in organic solvents, like methanol and chloroform.

iii. When simazine is heated with caustic alkalies, the chlorine is replaced by the hydroxyl and 2-hydroxy-4,6-bis(ethylamino)-1,3,5-triazine is formed.

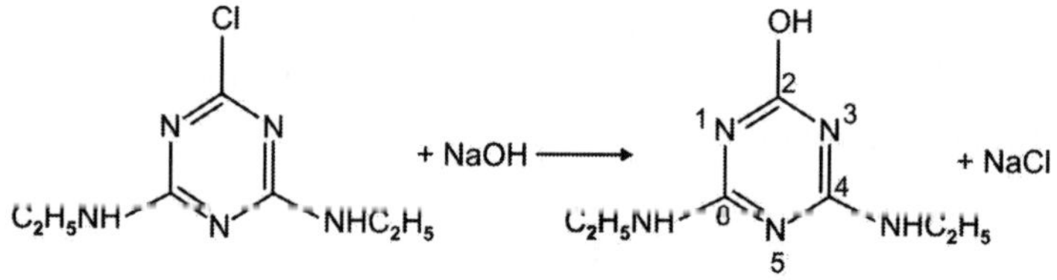

$$+ \text{NaOH} \longrightarrow \quad + \text{NaCl}$$

2-Hydroxy-4,6-bis(ethylamino)-S
(or 1,3,5) triazine

Uses:

1. It is a non-selective pre-emergence herbicide; in lower concentration being virtually ineffective on deep rooted plants (maize, sugarcane, pineapple, grapes, etc.).

2. It is also an effective soil sterilant at higher doses.

Atrazine

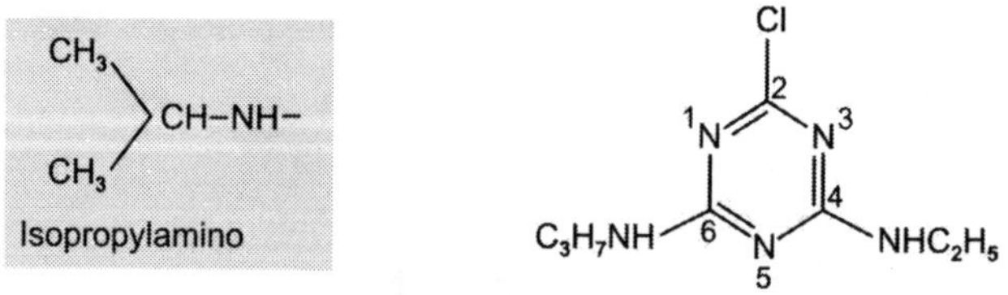

Isopropylamino

2-Chloro-4-ethylamino-6-isopropylamino triazine

Properties:

i. White crystalline, m.p. 173–175 °C.

ii. Atrazine is more soluble in water than simazine.

iii. Compared to simazine, atrazine is more easily absorbed through the foliage.

Use: Both as pre-emergent herbicide and post-emergent herbicide.

Propazine

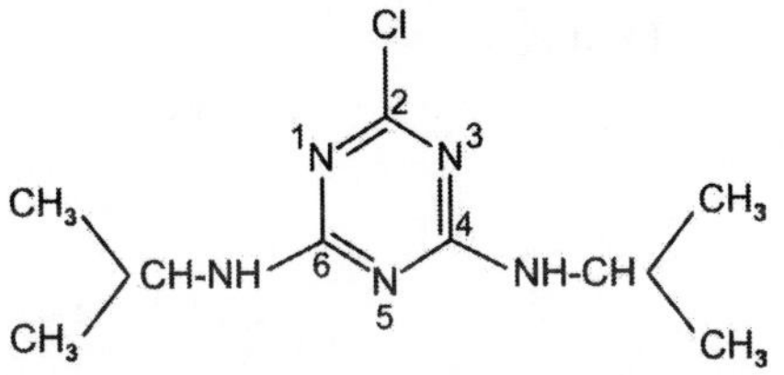

2-Chloro-4,6-*bis* (isopropylamino)-*s*-triazine

Properties:

i. White crystal, m.p. 210–212 °C.

ii. At room temperature, propazine is stable and as in the case of simazine, heating with caustic alkalies convert it to the corresponding hydroxy derivatives.

Use: Propazine has been proposed for the control of weeds in umbelliferous crops.

4.5.5 Substituted Phenols

The physiological activity of phenols is considerably greater than that of alcohols. They are more powerful insecticides, fungicides, bactericides and herbicides. The pesticidal properties is increased when various substituents, for example, halogen, nitro, thiocyano alkyl and other groups are introduced into the aromatic radical.

Pentachlorophenol (PCP)

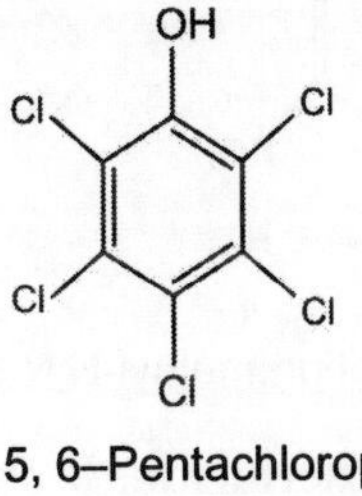

2, 3, 4, 5, 6–Pentachlorophenol

Properties:

i. m.p. 190–191 °C.

ii. Water solubility is very little. The solubility in organic solvent depends greatly on the natures of the solvent. Highly soluble in methanol.

Use: PCP and its sodium salt are used as contact and pre-emergent treatments on a variety of crops. It is applied as a fine powder fortified with oils for general contact pre-emergent weed control.

Dinitrophenols

DNOC

Dinitrophenol

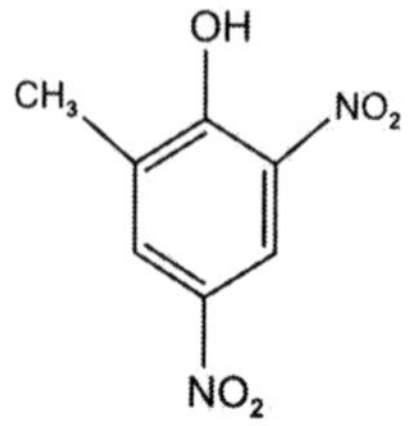

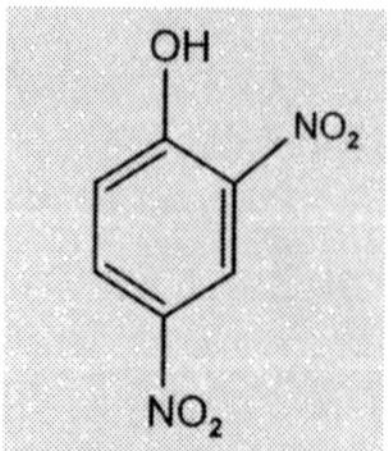

2,4-Dinitro-6-methyl phenol; Dinitro-*o*-cresol

i. It is a yellow crystalline substance, m.p. 86.4 °C.
ii. Water solubility is very poor, soluble in organic solvents.
iii. Reducing agent convert it to amines (primarily one -NO_2 group).

4.5.6 Dinitroaniline Herbicide

Trifluralin

Dinitroaniline

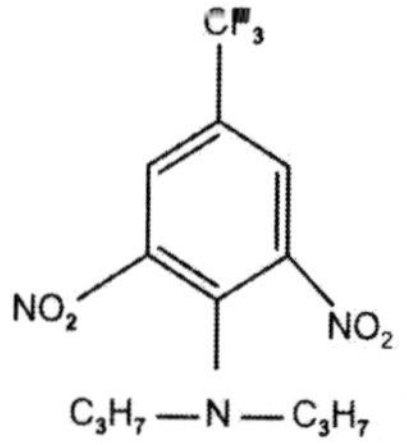

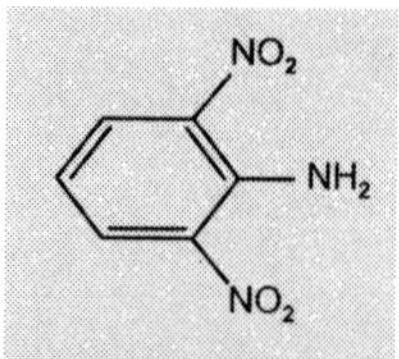

2,6-Dinitro-4-triflurometyl-N,N-dipropyl-aniline

It is a selective pre-emergence herbicide. It should be incorporated at 5–10 cm depth within four hours of application. It is absorbed on clay colloids and organic matter and does not stay active in soil for more than 4–6 months.

Pendimethalin (Stomp)

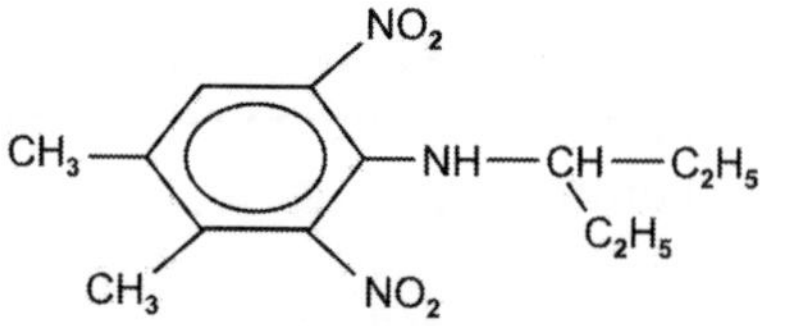

N-(1-ethyl-propyl)-3,4-dimethyl, 2,6-dinitro aniline

Stomp is mainly used for control of grasses in maize, cereals, rice, cotton and soybeans.

Others:

Butachlor

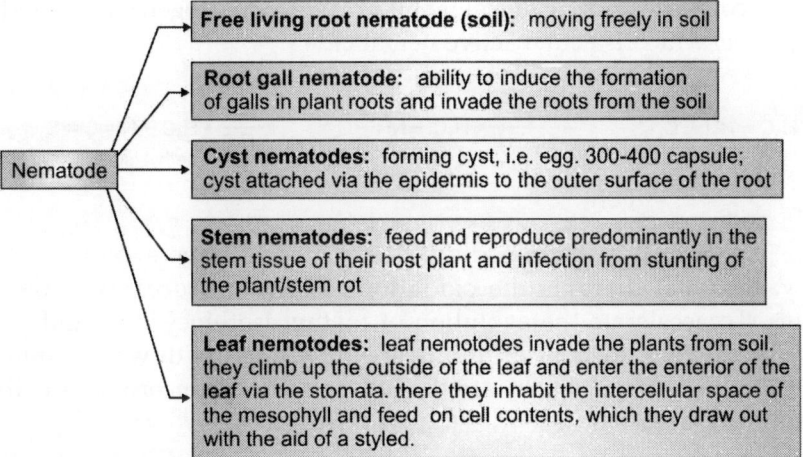

2-Chloro-2',6'-diethyl-N-butoxymethyl acetanilide

Butachlor controls most of the annual grasses and some broad leaved weeds in transplant and direct seed rice.

4.6 NEMATICIDES

Classification of pathogenic nematodes:

Nematode:

Free living root nematode (soil): moving freely in soil

Root gall nematode: ability to induce the formation of galls in plant roots and invade the roots from the soil

Cyst nematodes: forming cyst, i.e. egg. 300-400 capsule; cyst attached via the epidermis to the outer surface of the root

Stem nematodes: feed and reproduce predominantly in the stem tissue of their host plant and infection from stunting of the plant/stem rot

Leaf nemotodes: leaf nemotodes invade the plants from soil. they climb up the outside of the leaf and enter the enterior of the leaf via the stomata. there they inhabit the intercellular space of the mesophyll and feed on cell contents, which they draw out with the aid of a styled.

General principles of nematode control

1. Of all the phytopathogenic nematodes the group of root parasitic species (root gall nematodes, and cyst nematodes) are the most significant in terms of economic losses. Furthermore, as the stem and leaf nematodes only appear on aerial plant parts, their control is much easier than that of root nematodes. They are usually killed by insecticides, particularly those with systemic properties.

2. Under the term nematicide, one therefore understands a chemical agent that kills the so called soil nematodes (i.e. the root-parasitic species).

3. A nematicide must be able to distribute well in the soil. Distribution can take place via the air or water-capillary systems in the soil. Nematicides are therefore divided into fumigants and water-soluble agents.

Nematicidal Agents

4.6.1 Fumigants

One great drawback to the fumigants is their high phytotoxicity. They can only be used when the harvest has been gathered from the fields to be treated. The most important fumigants are listed in the following:

1. Methyl bromide : CH_3Br
2. Ethylene dibromide : $BrCH=CHBr$
3. Metham-Sodium : Vapam

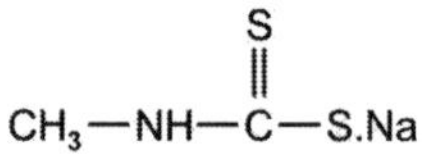

$$CH_3-NH-\overset{\overset{\displaystyle S}{\|}}{C}-S.Na$$

N-methyl dithiocarbamate

or

Sodium salt of methyl dithio carbamic acid

Vapam decomposes slowly in soil by hydrolysis to hydrogen sulfide and methyl isothiocyanate, which is actual active nematicide

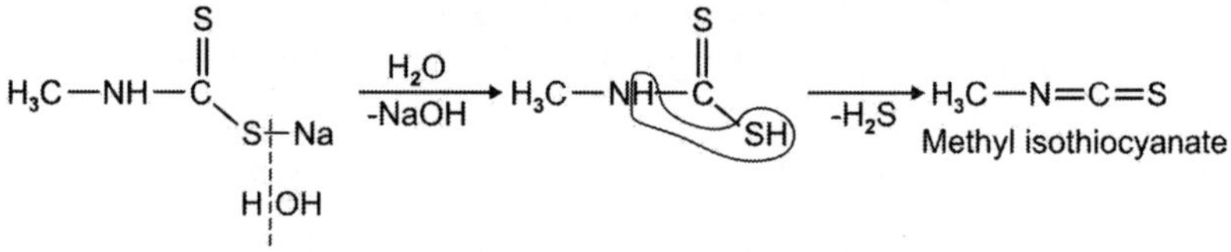

$$H_3C-NH-\overset{\overset{\displaystyle S}{\|}}{C}\underset{S+Na}{} \xrightarrow[\text{-NaOH}]{H_2O} H_3C-N\overset{\overset{\displaystyle S}{\|}}{\underset{SH}{C}} \xrightarrow[\text{-H}_2\text{S}]{} H_3C-N=C=S$$

$$\underset{H|OH}{}$$

Methyl isothiocyanate

The toxic action of metham-sodium is explained by the evolution of methyl isothiocyanate that disrupts the oxidation-reduction processes in the cells of organisms. To accelerate the evolution of methyl isothiocyanate and ensure its uniform distribution, metam-sodium is greatly diluted with water (upto a 2–3% concentration) when introduced into the soil, and after its incorporation, the soil is abundantly irrigated.

Bunema

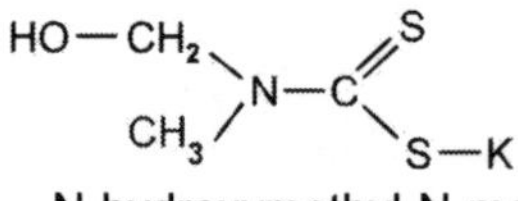

$$\underset{CH_3}{\overset{HO-CH_2}{}}N-\overset{\overset{\displaystyle S}{\diagup}}{C}\diagdown_{S-K}$$

Potassium – N-hydroxymethyl-N-methyldithio carbamate

Bunema also releases methyl isothiocyanate in the soil.

4.6.2 Water-soluble Agents

Chemical compounds that spread via the water-capillary system of the soil are taken up by the roots (systemic action) and poison, the so-called soil nematodes are termed water-soluble nematicides. The most active agents have been found among the insecticidal organophosphates and carbamates. Both the phosphate and carbamate types of nematicides are inhibitors of cholinesterase.

1. Nemacide/Dichlofenthion

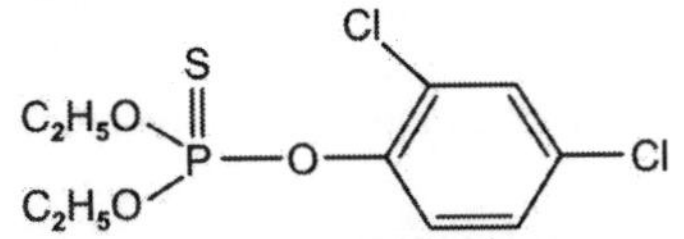

O,O-diethyl-O,2,4 dichlorophenyl-thiophosphate

or

O-2,4-dichlorophenyl O,O-diethyl phosphorothioate.

This compound was the first organophosphate to be used against soil nematodes. Apart from its nematicidal effect, dichlofenthion has a certain insecticidal action.

2. Ethoprophos/Mocap

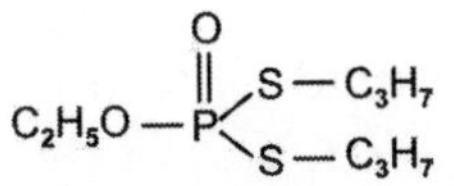

O-Ethyl S,S-dipropyl phosphorodithioate

3. Diamidafos/Nellite

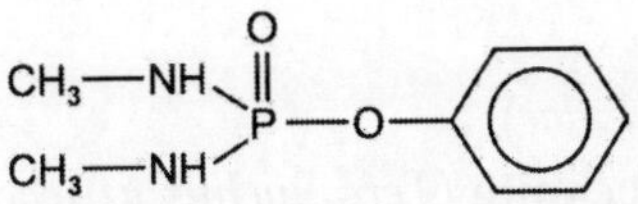

Phenyl N,N'-dimethyl phosphorodiamidate

4. Phorate

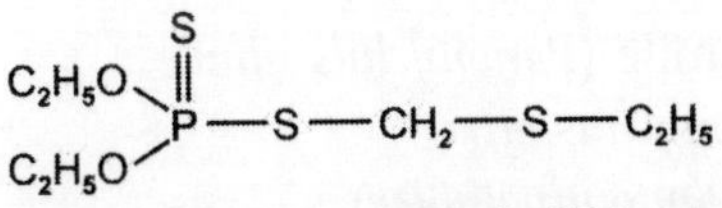

O,O-Diethyl-S-(ethyl-thio-methyl)-dithio phosphate

5. Carbofuran

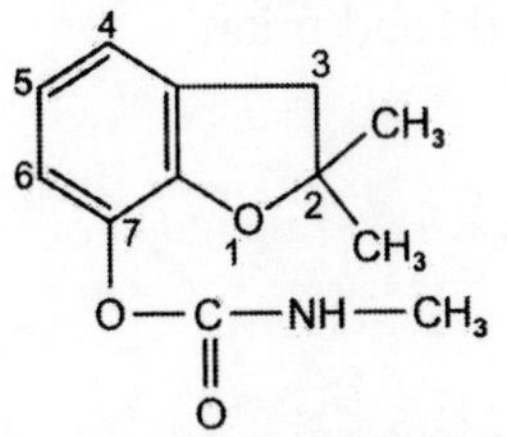

2,3-Dihydro-2,2-dimethyl-7-benzofuranyl methyl carbamate

Highly active insecticide, nematicide and acaricide

6. Aldicarb

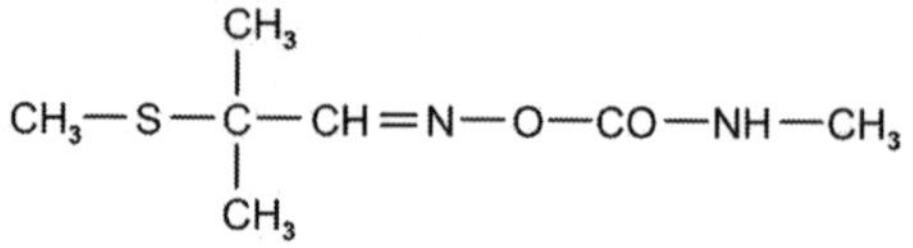

$$CH_3-S-\overset{\overset{\displaystyle CH_3}{|}}{\underset{\underset{\displaystyle CH_3}{|}}{C}}-CH=N-O-CO-NH-CH_3$$

2-Methyl-2(methyl thio) propanal-O-(methyl amino)-carbonyl-oxime

Aldicarb is a systemic insecticide and nematicide

Nematodes have nervous system similar to insects. All these organophosphates and carbamates inhibit the nervous transmitter enzyme, cholinesterase resulting in paralysis and ultimately death of the affected nematode.

Biological Control

1. Non-edible oil cakes: Neem, Mahua and Karanj oil cakes control nematode population.
2. Marigold (*Tagetis erecta* L): The nematicidal principles of root exudates of marigold have been identified as terthienyl and substituted bisthienyl compound.

4.7 ACARICIDES

Classification of phytophagus mites:

Class of mite	Host plant
1. Spider mites (*Tetranychidae*)	
e.g. Common red spider mite (*Tetranychus utricae*) :	Fruit, vegetables, roses and greenhouse crops
Tea mite (*Tetranychus kanzawai*)	: Tea
Fruit tree red spider mite (*Panonychus ulmi*)	: Lichi
Citrus red mite (*Panonychus citri*)	: Citrus fruit
2. False spider mites (*Phytoptipalpidae*)	
e.g. *Brevipalpus oudemansi*	: Greenhouse crops
3. Soft-bodied mites (*Tarsonemidae*)	
e.g. *Hemitarsonemus latus* (broad mite)	: Cotton and tea
4. Gall mites (*Eriophyidae*)	
Phyllocoptruta oleivora	: Citrus rust mite

ACARICIDAL AGENTS

4.7.1 Sulphur Powder

Finely divided form (wettable sulphur) is generally used in grape vine as a fungicide with potential acaricidal effect.

4.7.2 Organochlorinated Compounds

Dicofol (Kelthane, Chloroethanol)

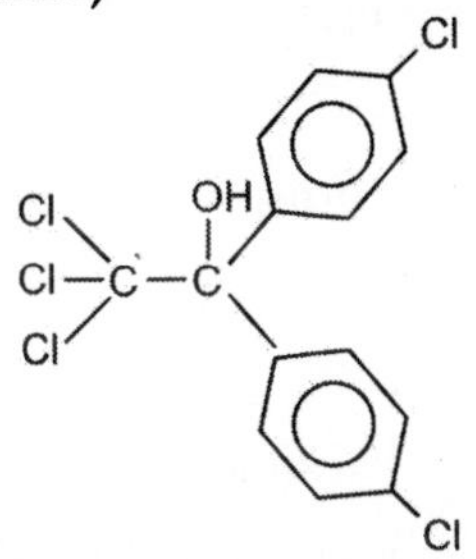

1,1-bis(chlorophenyl)-2,2,2-trichloroethanol

Synthesis: Chlorination of chlorfenethol (acaricide)

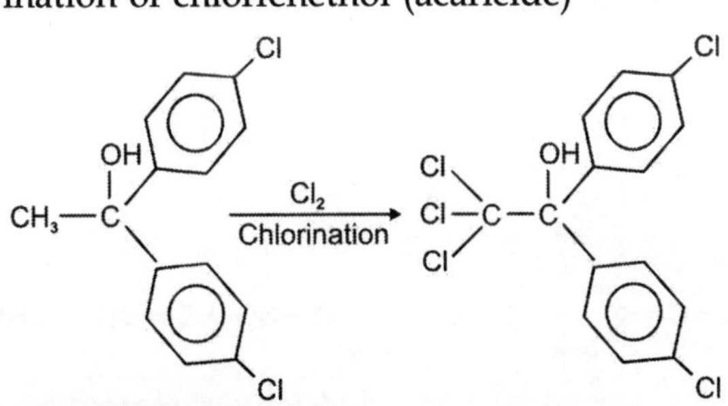

1,1-bis(4-chlorophenyl)ethanol   Dicofol
chlorfenethol

Chlorfenethol (dimite) is also acts as an acaricide

Properties:
   i. Dicofol, organochlorinated acaricide is a solid, m.p. 78.5–79 °C.
  ii. Insoluble in water, well soluble in organic solvents.
 iii. Stable in water and an acid medium, but under the action of alkalies, it readily decomposes (dehydrochlorination, like lindane) with the formation of non-toxic products.

Formulation: EC(20%) and WP(18.5%)

4.7.3 Sulphur-containing Compounds

They are contact acricides.

Tetrasul (Animert)

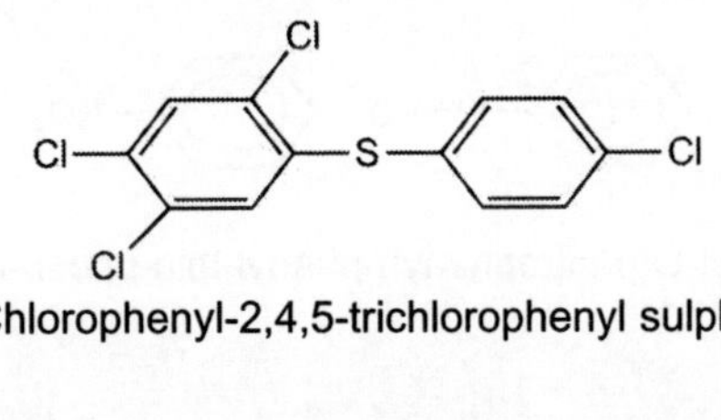

4-Chlorophenyl-2,4,5-trichlorophenyl sulphide

Tetrasul is highly selective, not being a hazard to beneficial insects or to wild life. It controls various spider mites species that hibernate in the egg stage and must be applied during hatching of these eggs.

Properties:

Tetrasul oxidized to sulfone (tetradifon) on prolonged exposure to sunlight.

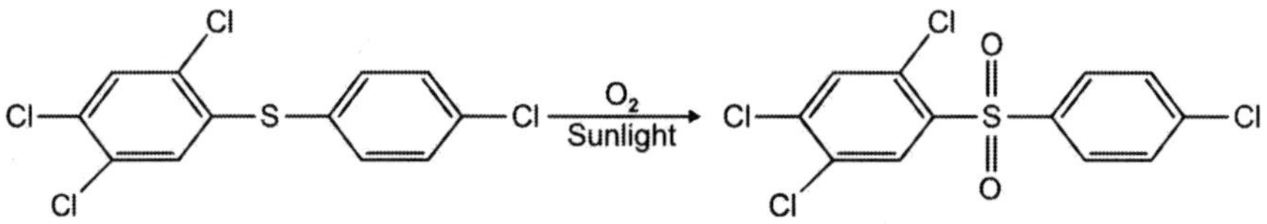

Tetrasul
LD_{50} : 6810 mg/kg female rats

Tetradifon (also acaricide)
LD_{50} : > 15 mg/kg rats

Propargite (Omite)

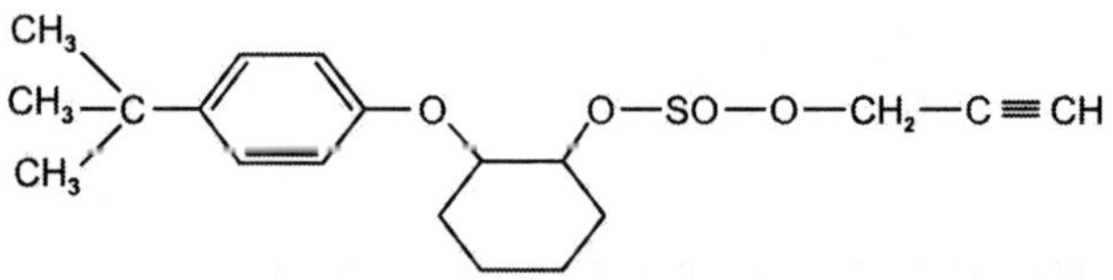

2-[4-(1,1-Dimethyl ethyl) phenoxyl] cyclohexyl-2-propynyl sulfite

Propargite does not affect bees and is less harmful to predatory mites than any other acaricide.

4.7.4 Organophosphates

Most of the organophosphate insecticides also have acaricidal properties. But, the problem of use of organophosphate as acaricide is that the spider mites strains develop resistant very rapidly to this class of pesticides. The organophosphates having acaricidal activity are demeton (systox) methyl demeton (metasystox), ethion, dimethoate, omethoate, carbophenothion, etc. The highly potential organophosphate acaricides are EPN and dimefox.

EPN

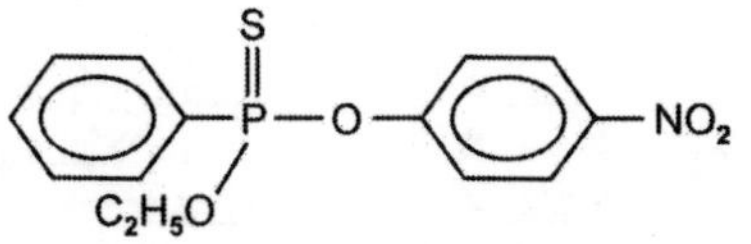

O-ethyl-O(p-nitrophenyl)-phenyl-thio-phosphonate

Dimefox

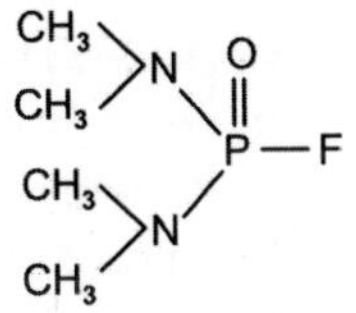

bis(dimethyl amide) fluro-phosphate

Dimefox is used for soil treatment to control hops and spider mites.

4.7.5 Carbamates

Some insecticidal N-methyl carbamates have also shown acaricidal properties.

Carbofuran (Furadan, Curaterr)

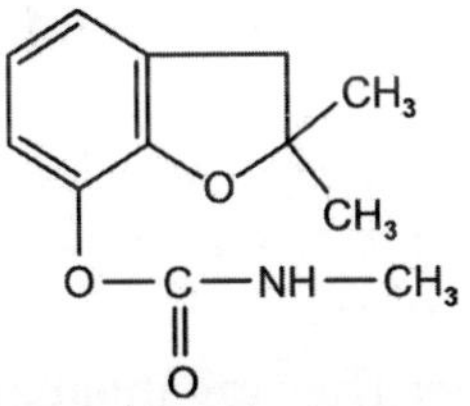

2,3-Dihydro-2,2-dimethyl-7-benzofuranyl methyl carbamate

Highly active insecticide, acaricide and nematicide

Aldicarb

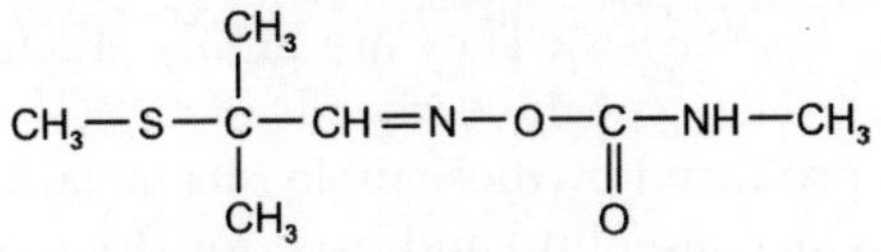

2-Methyl-2-(methylthio)-propanol O-(methyl carbonyl) oxime

Aldicarb is used as insecticide, acaricide and nematicide in granular formulation (extremely toxic and absorbed through skin).

4.8 RODENTICIDE

Rats and mice are pests because:

i. They consume food in field as well as store house.
ii. They destroy qualities of food (through feces, hair, urine).
iii. They act as a vectors for disease (e.g. typhus, amebic dysentery).

Greater losses of crops through rodents are caused by contamination than by direct consumption. Urine feces hair spoil stored products. Mouse feces are difficult to separate from grain owing to their similarity in size. In most cases the germs of various diseases distributed by rodents (e.g., typhus, amebic dysentery) are transferred to foodstuffs by such contaminants or by direct contact with paws and fur.

General classes of rodents:

1. **Brown or Norway rat** (*Rattus norvegicus*): They prefers near water, often walks great distances for food and can swim for long periods and dive and thus penetrate into inhabited areas via the sewer system. They are found in channels, drains, they do not store food. Brown rat accounts for more than 95% of all the existing rats and is known worldwide as the largest spp.

2. **House mouse** (*Mus musculus*): Apart from its dietary preferences, the house mouse behaves completely differently from the rats, it is strictly non-nomadic. Usually one male lives with several females in a small territory often only a few meters in cross section.

3. **Black rat or Indian house rat** (*Rattus rattus*): They prefer a dry warmer environment and lives in store house. It always settles near the source of food. It is found in rural as well as urban areas in warehouses and godowns near the source of food.

4. **Indian field mouse** (*Mus booduga*): They live generally in fields and farms in villages. They secure their food from the field as well as grains stored in the food chamber of other spp. of rat.

5. **Indian gerbils or White rats:** They are inhabitants of sandy areas. They make their burrows near the field crops. Burrows made by them are deeper, but shorter than those made by other sp. (mole rats). Openings of these burrows are hidden under bushes or vegetation. Apart from the plant parts, they also feed on insects. They make small burrows which do not have any side branches.

6. **Mole rat** (*Bandicota bengalensis*): They are highly efficient in making burrows where it stores food. They cut the earheads of cereals and store them in their burrows. Burrows produced by these mole rats usually have 12 openings and 2-5 lanes some of which are blind and used for storage of food and breeding.

Chemical control of rodents

Acute poisoning rodenticides

Fumigation : The control of rodents, particularly mole rats and others which form burrows in the field may be achieved by the process of application of toxicant in gaseous form. Fumigation for rodent control can be carried out in the open field (not building structure) in the dry season.

$$\text{Aluminium phosphide} \xrightarrow{\text{HOH}} 2PH_3 + Al_2(OH)_3$$

Celphos (tablet): Al_3P_2 (aluminium phosphide)

This is particularly useful for the control of field rats (mole rat) in the paddy fields. Tablets containing aluminium phosphide (Al_3P_2) and ammonium carbonate [$(NH_4)_2CO_3$] are placed inside the burrows and openings are sealed with mud. Phosphine gas (toxic gas) is released which kills the rats.

Mode of action of chronic poisoning rodenticide (anticoagulants)

The chronically acting or multiple dose, rodenticides are inhibitors of blood platelet coagulation that reach their full effect only after the consumption of several sublethal doses. As competitive antagonists of vitamin K_1, even small quantities of anticoagulant displace the former from its role in the formation of prothrombin which is necessary for blood coagulation. Anticoagulation is intensified by repeated doses and eventually the blood can no longer coagulate. As the anticoagulants also have toxic capillary side effect, internal bleeding occurs in organs and tissues, leading to death.

Physiological nature of anticoagulant rodenticide:

i. Anticoagulant properties (continuous flow of blood).

ii. Interfere the action of vitamin K_1, and reduce the coagulating powers of blood, so that small injuries cause fatal haemorrhanges.

iii. Tasteless, odourless, colourless and fatal properties.

Anticoagulant rodenticide

Two types of anticoagulant rodenticides, viz. indandione and coumarin.

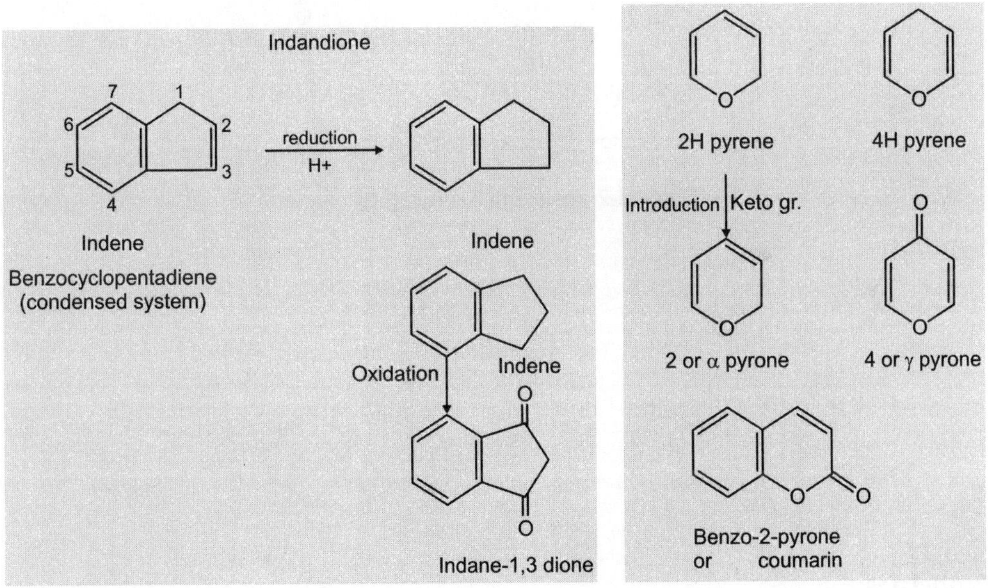

Indandione

reduction
H+

Indene

Benzocyclopentadiene
(condensed system)

Indene

Oxidation

Indene

Indane-1,3 dione

2H pyrene

4H pyrene

Introduction Keto gr.

2 or α pyrone

4 or γ pyrone

Benzo-2-pyrone
or coumarin

Coumarin (Dicourmarol)

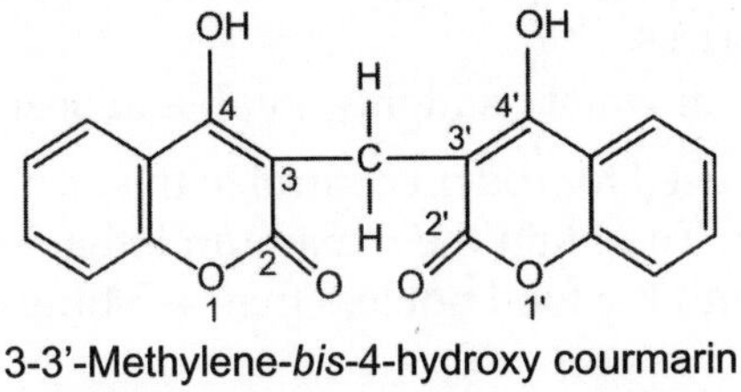

3-3'-Methylene-*bis*-4-hydroxy courmarin

Synthesis:

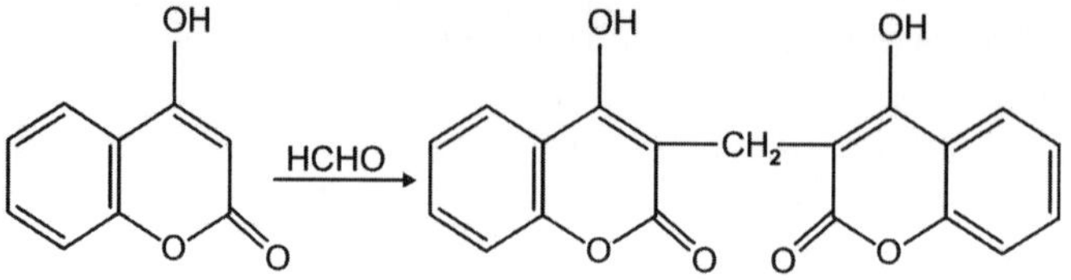

4-hydroxycoumarin   Dicoumarol

It is a white crystalline substance, m.p. 285°–293 °C. It is one of the least toxic compounds of this series for rodent.

These compounds are used in very low concentration in the bait (0.001–0.05%).

Warfarin, Compound 42; W.A.R.F.-42

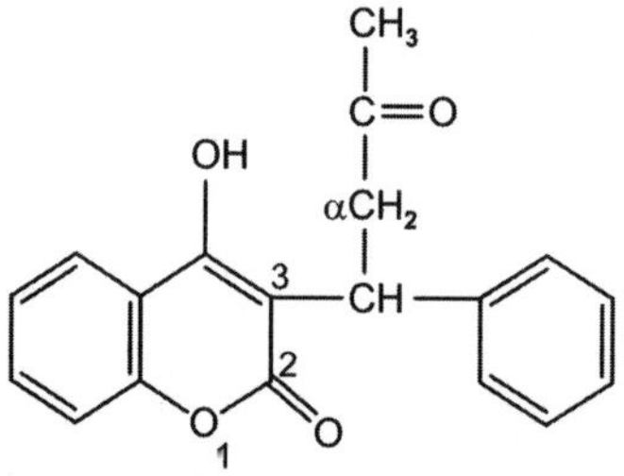

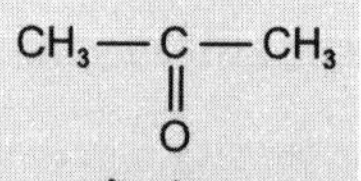

3-(α-Acetonylbenzyl)-4-hydroxycoumarin
or
3-(1-Phenol-2-acetylethyl)-4-hydroxy coumarin

Synthesis:

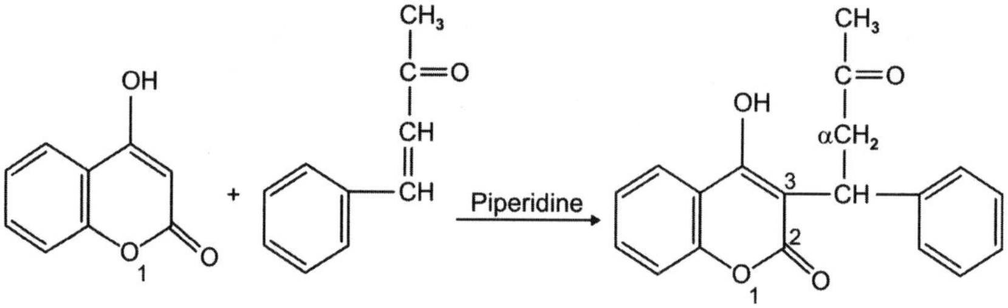

Warfarin

Properties:

i. Warfarin is a white crystalline substance, m.p. 159°–161 °C.
ii. Tasteless and odourless.
iii. If does not dissolve in water, is highly soluble in acetone, alcohol.

Use: The compound is used for rodent control in the form of food baits containing 0.5–1% active ingredient. To obtain the maximum lethal effect, the animal should receive the compound with the food not less than 4–5 times in the course of several days.

Coumachlor or Tomorin

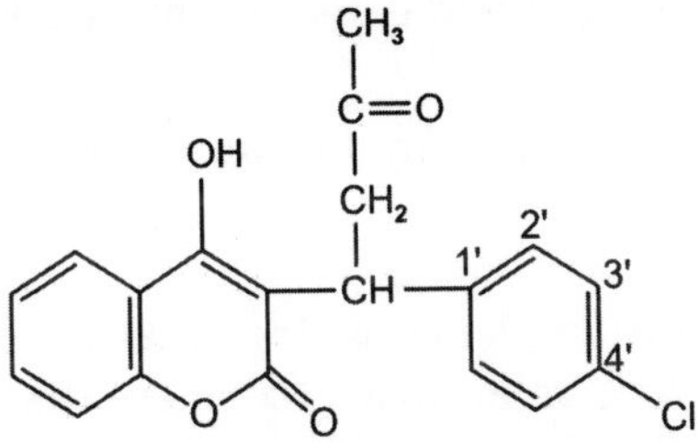

3-(α-Acetonyl-4'-chlorobenzyl)-4-hydroxycoumarin

Properties:

i. Colourless, crystalline substance, m.p. 169°–171 °C.

ii. Practically insoluble in water, more soluble in alcohols, acetone and chloroform.

It is closest derivative of warfarin and is similar to warfarin in both chemical and toxicological properties.

Pival or Pindone

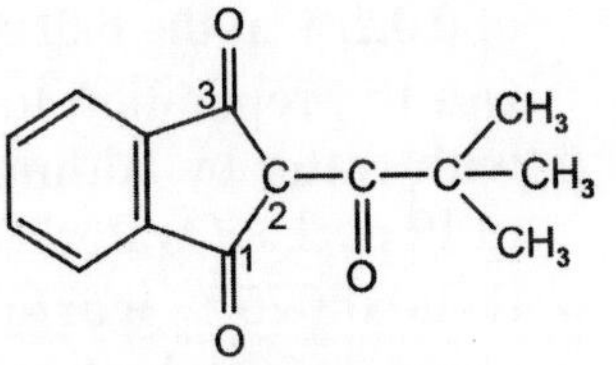

2 Pivalyl-1,3 indandione

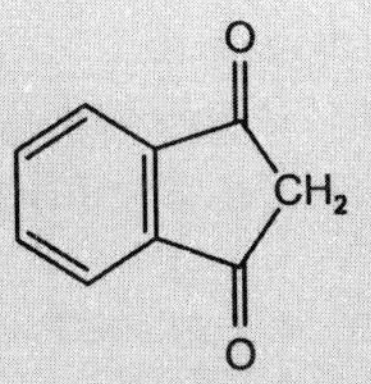

1,3 indandione

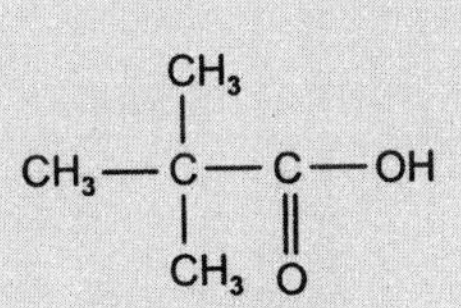

Trimethyl acetic acid
(pivalic acid)

Synthesis:

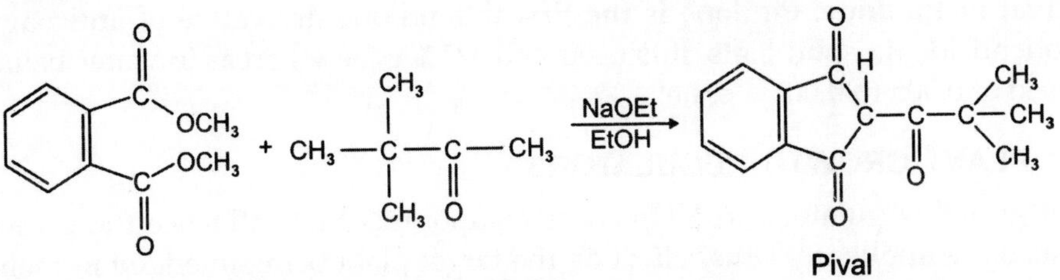

Pival

It has many of same physiological properties as warfarin. It is further reported that this compound has the insecticidal and fungistatic action. Thus prevent insect, fungi infestion in bait.

Pival = 0.5% a.i. available for mixing the bait preparation.

Prolin or Banarat

Prolin is an anticoagulant rodenticide having warfarin and equivalent amount of sulphua-quinoxaline which is an antibacterial agent that retards the production of vitamin K in the intestine producing bacteria in rodents.

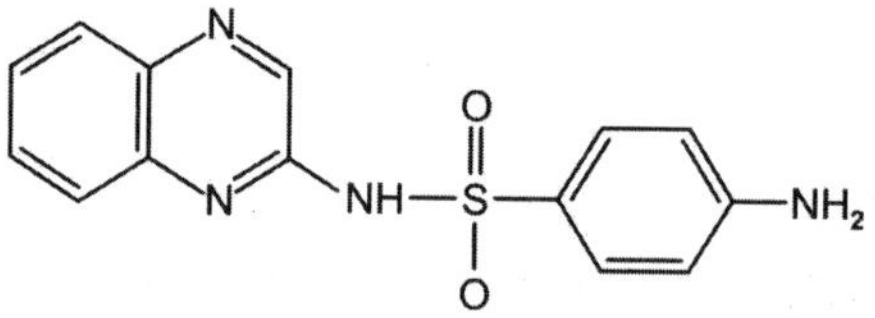

Comparative benefit of the use of different anticoagulant rodenticides.

Application methods of anticoagulant rodenticide:

1. Warfarin

Formulation		Use
1. Warfarin 'C' containing 0.5% warfarin	:	It is mixed wide bait material in the ratio 1:19 to get final concentration of 0.025% in the bait
2. Warfarin 'S' sodium salt of warfarin	:	Use to preparation to liquid baits with water by adding 1 part of it to 19 parts of water 0.025% in bait
3. Warfarin 'R' in wax blocks	:	It is 0.025% warfarin-treated ready-to-use bait embedded in paraffin wax. It is ideal for moist conditions like paddy and sugarcane crop

2. Coumachlor:
  i. ready to use bait containing 0.025 to 0.05% a.i.
  ii. ready to use tracking powder containing 1.0% a.i.
  iii. concentrates containing 10% a.i.

3. Pival or Pindone: Pindone is the first indandione derivative of anticoagulant rodenticide. In solid baits, it is used at 0.025% cone whereas in water baits, it is used at 0.005 to 0.006% cone.

4.9   PLANT GROWTH REGULATORS

Plant growth regulators are defined as compounds that influence the growth of plants but without any lethal effect on the target plant being intended in their use.

Classes of plant growth regulators:

I. Naturally occurring Growth Regulators (Phytohormones);

II. Commercial or synthetic Growth Regulators.

I. Naturally Occurring Growth Regulators

1. Auxins

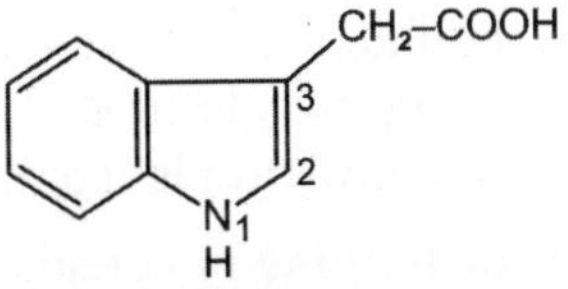

Indole-3-acetic acid (IAA)

Biological effects: Growth promotor; necessary for longitudinal growth in all plant parts including the roots; stimulates ethylene synthesis at higher concentrations.

2. Abscisic acid (ABA)

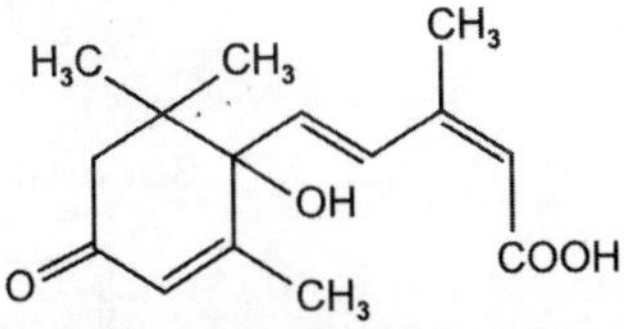

ABA

Biological effects: Growth and development inhibitor (phytotranquilizer); partial antagonistic activity towards IAA and GA_3; accelerates ripening and senescence.

3. Ethylene

$$CH_2=CH_2$$

Biological effects: Promotor of ripening and senescence "chaotropic hormone"; accelerates ripening of fruit, degradation of chlorophyll and leaf drop; inhibits growth.

4. Gibberellins

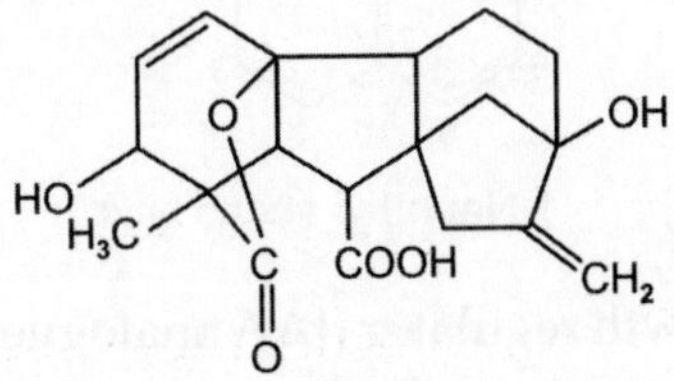

GA_3

Biological effects: Growth promotor; initiates enzyme synthesis in germinating seeds; normalizes growth of dwarf mutants; promotes longitudinal and foliar growth; induces flowering.

II. Commercial or Synthetic Growth Regulators
1. Ethephon or Ethrel (Planofix)

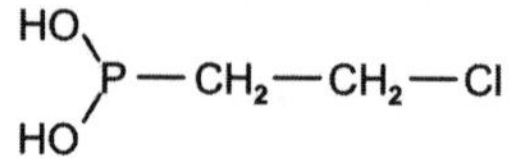

$$\text{HO} \backslash \atop \text{HO} \diagup P - CH_2 - CH_2 - Cl$$

(2-Chloroethyl)-phosphonic acid

Biological effects: Growth regulator releases the endogenous ripening hormone ethylene, stimulates flowering, accelerates ripening of pineapple, tomato, apple, cherry, stimulates latex flow in Hevea; harvest aid in walnut.

Use: It is used to prevent the lodging of cereals in a dose of 1.5–2 kg a.i/ha in a solution of 150–300 litres (the lower internodes became shorter).

2. IBA

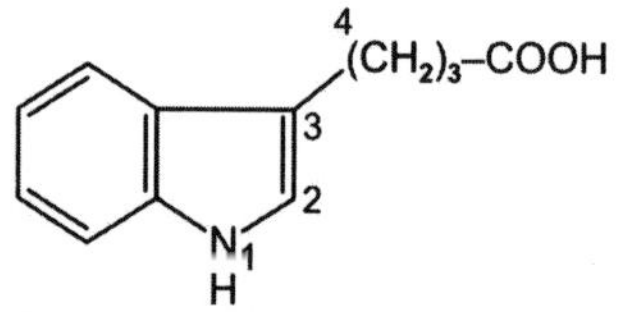

$(CH_2)_3–COOH$

4-(indol-3yl)-butyric acid
indole-3-butyric acid (I BA)

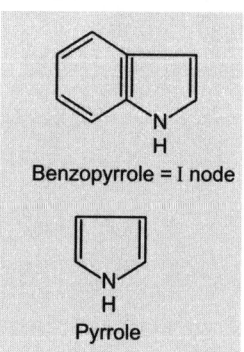

Benzopyrrole = I node

Pyrrole

Biological effects: Auxin (is metabolized to IAA), for rooting of cuttings (commercial product: seradix).

3. NAA

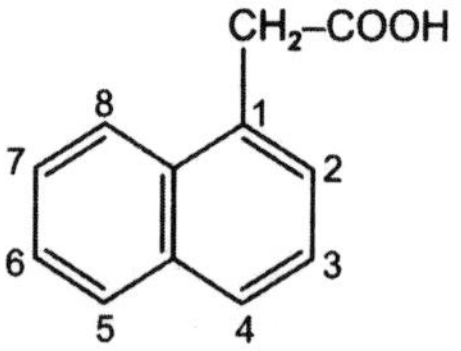

$CH_2–COOH$

1-Naphthyl acetic acid

Biological effects: Growth regulator (IAA analogue) for thinning of apple, pear, induction of flowering in pineapple, prevention of pre-harvest fruit drop, stimulation of rooting of cuttings.

4. Cycloheximide

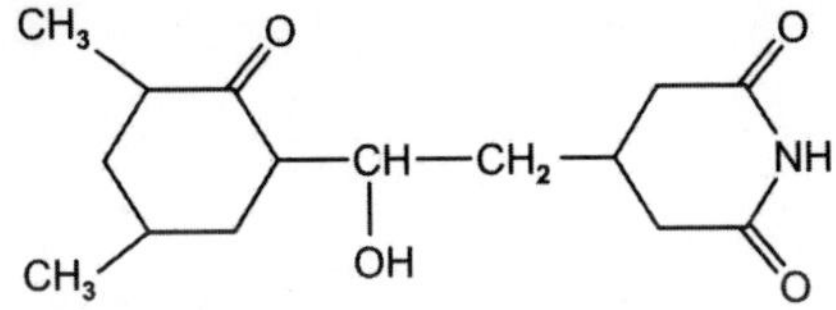

Biological effects: Growth regulator and fungicide inhibits protein biosynthesis; promotes abscission of orange and olive (harvest aid).

5. MH (Maleic hydrazide)

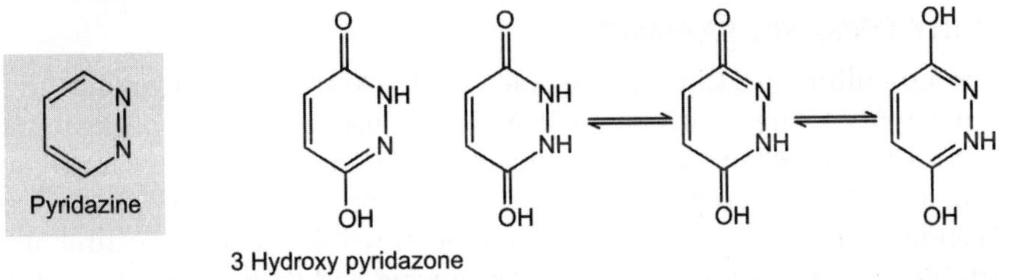

Pyridazine

3 Hydroxy pyridazone

MH can exist in three isomeric forms.

Biological effects: Growth regulator inhibits cell division but not extension, translocated for prevention of sucker development in tobacco.

Double role (herbicide and growth regulator) agrochemicals are: MH, endothal, 2-4-D (high dose, low dose) etc.

5

Organic Farming

5.1 WHY ORGANIC FARMING?

Organic agriculture is a safe, sustainable farming system producing healthy crops without damage to the environment. It avoids the use of artificial chemical fertilizers and pesticides on the land, relying instead on developing a healthy, fertile soil and growing a mixture of crops. In this way, the farm remains biologically balanced with a wide variety of beneficial insects and other wildlife to act as natural predators for crop pests and a soil full of micro-organisms and earthworms to maintain its vitality. The avoidance of artificial chemicals means organic farmers minimize health and pollution problems.

Principles of Organic Farming

In principle, organic farming is based on the use of materials and practices that enhance the ecological balance of natural system and integrate the farming system by maintaining the ecological balance, health and productivity of soil life, plants, humans and animals. This system avoids or largely excludes the use of synthetic compounds like inorganic fertilizers, herbicides, pesticides, growth regulators and other chemicals and relies upon crop rotation, crop residues, organic manures, green manures, bio-pesticides and biofertilizers to maintain soil productivity, to supply plant nutrients, and to control insects, weeds and other pests.

Organic farming aims to encourage building up the microorganism population particularly aerobic bacteria and fungi in the topsoil. Enrichment of the organic carbon content of the soil is further encouraged in basic concept of organic farming that is why generally ploughing is restricted to top six inches soil.

Organic farming is the form of agriculture that relies on crop rotation, green manure, compost, biological pest control, and mechanical cultivation, etc., to maintain soil productivity and control pests, excluding or strictly limiting the use of synthetic fertilizers and synthetic pesticides, plant growth regulators, livestock feed additives, and genetically modified organisms.

5.2 PERMITTED AND RESTRICTED INPUTS FOR ORGANIC FARMING

Based on the principles of organic farming certain inputs have been identified by IFOAM as permitted and some as restricted for the use in fertilization and soil conditioning. The lists of permitted and restricted inputs are mentioned. A clear-cut policy decision about the permitted and restricted inputs for fertilization and soil conditioning based on the availability and use under Indian perspective for organic agriculture is to be framed. Wealth of information is available about the effect of different organic sources on specific crop and feasibility of nutrient supplementation in soil system under organic farming.

Crop and vegetable residues, mulch, green manure, straw, mushroom waste, humus from worms and insects, urban composts from separated sources that are monitored for contamination, plant preparations and extracts, worms and microbiological preparations based on naturally occurring organisms, farmyard manure, biodynamic preparations, limestone, gypsum, chalk, sugar beet lime, calcium chloride, calcified seaweed, magnesium rock, epsom salt (magnesium sulphate), clay (e.g. Bentonite, perlite, vermiculite, zeolite), sodium chloride, sulfur and compost made from ingredients listed below under restricted use category:

Slurry, urine, vermicastings, blood meal, hoof and horn meal, meat, meat meal, bone, bone meal, feather meal, fish and fish products, wool, fur, hair, dairy products, biodegradable processing by-products of microbial, plant or animal origin, e.g. by-products of food, feed, oilseed, brewery, distillery or textile processing. Sawdust, wood shavings, wood ash, wood charcoal from untreated wood, seaweed and seaweed products, basic slag, calcareous and magnesium amendments, mineral potassium (e.g. sulphate of potash, kainite, sylvanite, patentkali), natural phosphates, pulverized rock, stone meal and trace elements.

5.3 NUTRIENT SUPPLEMENTATION AND CROP PROTECTION STRATEGY IN ORGANIC FARMING

The basic idea of nutrient supplementation in organic farming module is to replenish the requirement of nitrogen by using permitted inputs. A large number of fast growing nitrogen fixing crops like dhaincha (*Sesbania* sp.), sunhemp (*Crotolaria* sp.) and cowpea (*Vigna* sp.) may be used as green manure that can fix N to the extent of 60–100 kg/ha. Biofertilizers are very important components in organic agriculture which converts and fix unavailable sources of elemental N, bound phosphates and decomposed plant residues into available forms and at the same time produces growth promoting substances. The legume – *Rhizobium* association can fix N ranges from 40–120 kg/ha under optimum conditions. Vegetable crops in general give good response to *Azotobacter*, a free-living heterotropic N fixing bacteria. Besides *Azotobacter*, other microorganisms like *Azopirilla*, P-soubilizers like *Aspergillus, P. striata, B. polymixa* and AM are also found to be very effective. In general, the application of 5–10 tonnes/ha of locally available any organic sources like compost, FYM, biogas slurry, pressmud, carpet waste, vermicompost coupled with the inoculation of bio-fertilizers like *Rhizobium, Azotobacter/Azospirillum*, PSM and green manuring in alternate years can take care the nutrient requirement for most of the vegetable crops. The nutrient composition of some organic nutrient sources and its equivalent amount of available nutrients (kg/ha) are presented (Table 5.1).

Table 5.1:   Range of nutrient content in some organic nutrient sources

Source	N %	P_2O_5 (%)	K_2O (%)	Zn (ppm)	Cu (ppm)	Fe (ppm)	Mn (ppm)
FYM	0.7–0.3	0.3–0.9	0.4–1.0	100–150	140–260	156–362	180–220
Pressmud	0.8–1.2	0.9–1.4	0.2–0.4	400–480	240–300	4500–5500	450–490
Vermicompost	1.1–1.8	0.3–0.7	0.2–0.6	720–800	110–150	4000–5000	230–280
Carpet waste	12.5	0.05	0.05	90	20	20	20
Digested sludge	1.75	0.40	0.3	760	130	4740	250
Compost	0.5–1.0	0.4–0.8	0.8–1.2	185	150	400	275
Cattle manure	0.4–1.5	0.3–0.9	0.3–1.9	225	100	450	230
House ash	0.5–0.7	1.6–4.2	2.3–11.0	30	25	50	40
Sheep dung	0.7–1.5	0.4–0.6	0.3–1.0	–	–	–	–
Sheep urine	1.5–1.7	Nil	1.8–2.0	–	–	–	–
Cattle dung	0.3–0.4	0.1–0.2	0.1–0.3	210	90	420	250
Poultry manure	1.0–1.8	1.4–1.8	0.8–0.9	285	160	600	300
Grean manure							
Dhaincha (dry wt.)	2.1	0.5	2.4	–	–	–	–
Sunhemp (dry wt.)	2.16	0.46	2.2	–	–	–	–
Green gram (dry wt.)	2.0	0.44	2.5	–	–	–	–
Balck gram (dry wt.)	2.0	0.40	2.0	–	–	–	–

IFOAM have identified some inputs as permitted and some as restricted products for plant pest and disease control weed management and growth regulation, based on the principle of organic farming. These lists of products deserve special attention, particularly the inputs reflected as restricted use category. Due care and attention is warranted and at the same time based on the availability and effectiveness the inputs need to be finalized. Keeping in mind the basic principle and philosophy of organic farming a number of effective inputs particularly for the protection of crops need to be improvised. The indigenous technical knowledge, old axioms, the wealth of information on the herbs and medicinal plants can help the researchers for the development of effective natural pesticides. This area also warrants due attention. It is important to note that neem plant (*Azadirachta indica*), falls under restricted category while in tropical and subtropical countries neem and its product are the most potential source exploited for the development of pest management module under organic farming. The policy decision for finalizing these two important input categories bears a long-term impact and basic key for the success of organic agriculture in India.

5.4 COMPONENTS OF ORGANIC FARMING

5.4.1 Green Manuring

A number of green manures are major source of nitrogen, carbon and for the improvement of physical condition of soil. Generally dhaincha (*Sesbania esculenta, S. rostrata*) and sunhemp (*Crotolaria juncia*) have proved important and successful as green manure crops that are ploughed in the soil after about 6 to 8 weeks of sowing when adequate vegetative growth is attained. Green manure increases water holding capacity of soil and population of beneficial microorganism.

5.4.2 Compost

It is the traditional source of nutrients for the crops. Though it is a low source of nutrient, its special merit lies in its capacity to supply large number of essential micronutrients in addition to NPK, which are becoming deficient in the intensively cultivated areas. The supply of micronutrients particularly satisfies the hidden hunger in plants and safeguards against toxicity/injury. It improves soil physico-chemical and biological properties like soil structure, water-holding capacity, nutrient supply and the benefit to the soil microbial population. Some improved form of composts have been developed recently and grouped under:

- In order to encourage soil biological properties, regular use of Cow Pat Pit (CPP) and Cow Horn Manure (BD-500) is beneficial.
- Use of liquid manure prepared from cow dung; cow urine, leguminous leaves or vermi-wash is also effective in promotion of growth and fruiting.
- Biodynamic compost is an effective soil conditioner and is an immediate source of nutrient for a crop. Biodynamic compost can be prepared by using green leaves (nitrogenous material) and dry leaves (carbonaceous material) in 8–12 weeks.
- Use of cow dung slurry enhances the decomposition process of composting. The compost becomes ready in 75–100 days depending upon the prevailing temperature.
- NADEP compost is the most effective one for organic agriculture and is being used commercially.

5.4.3 Cow Dung

Since ancient times, human beings have recognized the importance of cows and their contribution to the society. Cow dung and urine are the important components in organic farming. Their role is summarized below:

- Cow dung cake and ghee are basic components of *Agnihotra* in *Homa* farming.
- Japan uses cow dung to get protection from atomic emissions.
- Cow dung is the best soil conditioner.
- Central Institute of Subtropical Horticulture, Lucknow has identified few *Actinomycetes* which are helpful in control of many plant diseases like gummosis, die back and anthracnose.

- Cow dung has been a regular component for plastering houses in the Indian villages.

5.4.4 Cow Urine

- Cow urine contains copper which transforms into gold in human body. Gold has power to destroy all diseases and is an antidote.
- Besides copper, cow urine contains iron, calcium, phosphorus, carbonic acid, potash and lactase.
- It contains 24 types of salts and the medicines made from cow urine are used to cure several diseases.
- Cow urine is disinfectant and prophylactic and it purifies and improves the fertility of land.

5.4.5 Vermicompost

Vermiculture technology is an aspect involving the use of earthworms as versatile natural bioreactors for effective recycling of non-toxic organic wastes to the soil. They effectively harness the beneficial soil micro flora, destroy soil pathogens, and convert organic wastes into valuable products such as bio-fertilizers, bio-pesticides, vitamins, enzymes, antibiotics, growth hormones and proteinous biomass. Earthworms participate in soil farming system in following ways:

- They influence soil pH.
- They act as agents of physical decomposition.
- They promote humus formation.
- Improve soil structure.
- They enrich soil.

5.4.6 Vermi-wash

Vermi-wash is prepared from the heavy population of earthworms reared in earthen pots or plastic drums. The extract contains major micronutrients, vitamins (such as B_{12}) and hormones (gibberellins) secreted by the earthworms. Earthworms produce bacteriostatic substances found in the vermi-wash which can protect the bacterial infections. Vermi-wash can be sprayed on crops and trees for better growth, yield and quality.

5.4.7 Biofertilizers

Biofertilizers are bacterial cultures of appropriate species that have the capability of fixing atmospheric nitrogen such as *Rhizobium* species in leguminous crops and *Azotobacter* and *Azospirillum* in non-leguminous crops. The Phosphate Solubilising Microorganism (PSM) has proven utility in making unavailable soil phosphorus available to the crops. The renewable source of nutrient supply to the crops has become popular during the last decade or so among the farmers. A great potential exists for its widespread use in all crops under all situations. *Azospirillum* has been recommended in a number of crops for increasing the production and productivity of crops. Nitrogen fixing systems offer an economically attractive and ecologically sound means of reducing external inputs and improving internal resources. Symbiotic systems such as that of *Azolla* and *Anabaena* complex and that of leguminous green manures with *Rhizobium* and *Azo-rhizobium* associations can be of particular value to wet land rice crop and renewable biological source supplementing inorganic N for cereals. At TNAU, Coimbatore significant contributions have been made on *Azolla* biofertilizer particularly on the selection of new strains of *Azolla microphylla* that is highly tolerant to high temperature and also tolerant to salinity with higher biomass producing capacity (25 t/ha). An *Azolla* hybrid was also developed by sexual hybridization and the hybrid is also highly adaptive and has higher N fixing potential.

The results from extensive field trials conducted in different agro-climatic regions of our country during the last two decades have shown that the effect of algal inoculation in terms of increased crop yield was satisfactory. Studies with algal inoculation at different levels of fertilizer nitrogen have shown that the supplementation effect is more pronounced at low level of nitrogen. This effect does not change with the soil type and rice variety. The subdued effect in acidic soils can be enhanced by the application of appropriate quantities of lime.

In long-term experiment, there was a gradual increase in organic carbon due to algal inoculation but the amount remained steady at the end of 3 years. An increase of organic matter, water-holding capacity and exchangeable Ca was reported to from medium to high level due to algal treatments of saline and alkaline soils. Algalization was also reported to increase available phosphorus in the soil, possibly because of excretion of organic acids by the blue-green algae. The blue-green algae have been found to solubilize the unavailable phosphate sources like Missouri rock phosphate.

The process of photosynthesis provides energy and carbon skeletons for nitrogen fixation. This is evidenced by evolution of oxygen under nitrogen fixing conditions. The nitrogen fixation is drastically reduced in dark because of depleting supply of photosynthates. The strains with very high rate of photosynthesis and ability to store the photosynthates will be capable of fixing nitrogen for a comparatively longer period in the dark.

It is known that under certain conditions, nitrogenase can act as ATP dependent hydrogenase systems. An understanding and enzymology of this hydrogen evolution will enable us to train this system to evolve hydrogen from water at the expense of solar energy. This is expected to reduce our dependence on the fuel energy especially in the manufacture of fertilizer nitrogen.

Another approach to achieve this can be through the development of ammonia leaking strains. *Anabaena azollae* actually makes available the nitrogen fixed by it to Azolla as ammonia. Algal mutants with the defect in the regulation of the enzyme Glutamine Synthetase can be made to liberate ammonia. The ammonia excreted into the medium can be harvested and used for various purposes.

The efficiency of inoculum can also be increased if it contains a heavy load of the perennating bodies like akinetes and hormocysts. Many species of Anabaena and Nostoc form a long chain of spores and sometimes the entire trichome gets transformed into spores. A culture containing such organisms will multiply faster when inoculated into the field. Genetic engineering can be used to clone together, the properties of growth, nitrogen fixation and spore formation in addition to the tolerance to fertilizer nitrogen and pesticides. Although, use of algae has been restricted to mainly rice especially low-level rice cultivation successful results have been reported in sugarcane, jute, vegetables, tomatoes, fruit trees, banana, etc.

5.5   CHEMICAL FARMING *VERSUS* ORGANIC FARMING

Soil Differences

Chemical Farming	Organic Farming
Cultivation and production (nutrient, pest & disease management) of crops by inorganic chemical inputs	Cultivation and production (nutrient, pest & disease management) of crops by biodegradable organic inputs
Against nature In chemically managed soil, the plant nutrients are supplied only through inorganic source, without any organic carbon source to derive food. This ultimately deprives the soil-eco system of the growth medium	**Harmony with nature** In an organic management, the focus is on food web relations and element cycling aiming to maximize the agro ecosystem's stability, sustainability and homeostasis (balanced equilibrium)
Blocks the microbial activity Due to the absence of carbon source, microbial population tends to be less or sometimes NIL in soil	**Increases the microbial life** Organics is the main source for nutrients. The soil microbes derive the food from the carbaneous source and multiply and make the soil lively, also decomposing the complex organic compounds present in the added organics
Soil structure is destroyed Non-availability of binding material of the soil particles result in disintegration and reduce the soil granulation. In the long run it may reduce the productive capacity of land to harbor the crops and become unfit for production	**Soil structure improves** Stable organic resins (humus) resulting from organic residue decomposition imparts stability to soil aggregates and corrects the permeability, i.e. crumb like structure. This structure facilitates to improve soil aeration, water-holding capacity, root penetration, while reducing the soil erosion by b aggregation of soil particles
Soil becomes dead While chemical farming satisfies only the crop nutrient requirements, it is not conducive for biological environment of the soil, finally resulting in a problematic soil loaded with inorganic salts	**Soils become fertile** Here the biological property of the soil is improved by addition of organic manure. Intensive biological activity promotes better symbiotic relationship between plant and the soil focusing on sustainable plant production and nutrient management.
Alters the soil pH Continuous use of inorganic chemicals leads to changes in the pH of the soil	**Buffering of soils (Enables neutral pH)** Presence of organic colloidal matter improves

Contd.

Contd.

Chemical Farming	Organic Farming
(either acidic or alkaline depending on the type of fertilizer used). It unbalances the nutrient availability status and in some cases creates toxicity to the plants	the buffering capacity of the soil and Cation Exchanging Capacity. It regulates the nutrient availability due to buffering action, besides checking the toxicity levels to plants and soil microbes
Nutrients are available only for shorter period Certain fertilizers in the absence of microbes permanently fix on to the soil particles and may not be available for plant root absorption. In addition, the chemical fertilizers are easily water soluble and this may lead to various types of losses through leaching, evaporation, etc.	**Nutrients available for longer period** Microbes decompose the complex organic compounds to mineral components and CO_2. Further the mineral elements are converted into available plant nutrients through mineralization process. These ions are held by organic matter and soil colloids and are slowly released as nutrients over a longer period.
Leads to erosion Absence of binding agents (organic substances) between soil particles makes the soil particles to be easily detached by water and wind. It leads to loss of top fertile soils ultimately making the land barren and unfit for farming/cultivation	**Prevents the soil erosion** Organic soil management techniques such as organic fertilization, mulching and cover cropping increases aggregation (by polysaccharide glue), improves soil structure and therefore increase the soil's water infiltration and retention capacity, substantially reducing the risk of erosion
Accumulation of hazardous material in soil Over and abuse of chemical fertilizers (nitrate) and pesticides harm the biological life of the soil. The residues such as heavy metals present in the inorganic soils may pose serious health hazards. Excessive nutrient and salt application such as nitrate, causes ground water pollution, and may be linked to certain diseases in human beings	**There is no hazardous material in soil** It doesn't leave any residues/hazardous material in the soil, since all input is biodegradable & non-toxic

Crop Differences

Chemical Farming	Organic Farming
Quick lodging of crop Most of the nutrient is leached beyond the root zone and the crop might loose much of the needed nutrient for better root anchor. Similarly chemically managed soil doesn't provide much of the structure support to the crops. The combination of above leads to lodging of crop	**Provide good anchorage to the crop** Physical (structure), chemical (nutrients transformation and mineralization) and biological activity (decomposition) favors the crop stand and growth. Liveliness' of soil provides a good growth media and support to crop growth
More chemical residues present in crops For managing fertility, pest and diseases, large quantity of synthetic chemicals are used in crops. It does not metabolize properly and leaves residues as such in the end product. It	**No chemical residues present in crop** Only decomposable materials (organic manure and biocontrol agent) are used. It does not leave any harmful residue in the crop or the soil environment

Contd.

Contd.

Crop Differences

Chemical Farming	Organic Farming
will reduce the quality of product and can turn into poison for consumption	
Crops are highly susceptible to pests and diseases Crops in fleshy condition are naturally inviting pest and diseases. A chemically grown crop does not have much resistance power against pest and diseases because of less cell wall thickness and low calcium and potassium absorption by plants	**Protects from pests and diseases** Availability of much of calcium and potassium in organically managed soils improves the uptake in crops. It provides the natural resistance to crops against pest and diseases.
Harvested produce are in low quality The conversion of source to sink, non-availability of nutrients especially potassium reduce the quality of the product.	**Premium quality** Nutrients availability in entire crop growth period increases up taking capacity and proper conversion of source to sink improves the keeping quality especially of fruits and vegetables

Health / Social Differences

Chemical Farming	Organic Farming
Cause pollution to the environment Chemically managed soils release the residues in soil and water environment leads to pollution. Sometimes it causes toxic effect to human environment	**Pollution free approach** All practices are interrelated and the end product will be decomposable one so there is no cause for environmental pollution
Provide chemical mixed/toxic food to the human life Inorganic fertilizers (nitrogen) and pesticide (synthetic compound) does not decompose properly and leave residues in plant parts, when used as feed material for animal and food for human beings may create diseases, and malformations	**Provide nutritive food to the human life** In organic farming, ideal combination of agronomical, physical and biological measures bring down the population of harmful microbes and do not release any residues in soil and crop environment. The plant parts from organically managed soils are intuitively rich and safe
Causes inborn disease to the human beings Presence of toxic substance in food materials alters the genetic characteristics of human beings. This genetic mutation cause several in-borne diseases to human beings	**It provides the immune power to the human beings** Crops are grown under balanced nutritive approach. Crop uptake nutrients as and when required in entire growing period and convert the absorbed nutrients properly in to sink when the food material from organically managed soils is consumed, natural immunity of the human beings is developed.
High investments in inputs Inorganic input materials are costly and require much technical knowledge and investment to produce and handle	**Low investments in inputs material** Organic input materials are less costly source, readily available at the door step and very easy to apply

Contd.

Contd.

Economic Differences

Chemical Farming	Organic Farming
Highly fluctuation in yield Fertilizer managed soil does not provide nutrient properly during the entire crop duration. The deficiency of one essential nutrient directly effects the growth and metabolism and act antagonistic to other nutrient absorption by crop resulting in fluctuation and loss in yield	**Satisfactory and reliable yield** The nutrients are available in entire crop period in balanced way. It provides optimal environment to the crop growth and taps the full genetic potential of crops to provide satisfactory level yield and quality
No strands to break competitiveness There is no difference in harvested product among the chemically managed farming. It reduces the offer in a competitive market. Products sold in low rate. Chemical farming products are less keeping quality as well as of low nutrient status. Therefore it offers only low rates in market.	**High efficiency to improve the competitiveness** The end product is superior in nutritive quality than chemical farming and gets higher offer in the competitive market. Offered premium price. Whereas, in organic farming products, presence of potassium improves the keeping quality and also it have more nutritive value in balanced way. It offers much premium price in market

5.6 INDIAN ORGANIC CERTIFICATION AGENCY

INDOCERT is a nationally operating, charitable trust, accredited by Government of India for certification of organic farmers, processors and traders. INDOCERT functions as a platform for training, awareness creation, information dissemination and networking in the field of organic farming. In this endeavor, INDOCERT is supported by two well reputed organizations from Switzerland: FiBL (Research Institute of Organic Agriculture) and bio-inspecta (a Swiss certification agency also accredited in EU) in the form of strong technical collaborations. The National Steering Committee has designated Agricultural and Processed Food Products Export Development Authority (APEDA), Coffee Board, Spices Board, Tea Board, Coconut Development Board, Directorate of Cashew and Cocoa Development as accreditation agencies.

Conversion / Transition period for Organic Agriculture

The process of changing an agricultural farm from conventional to organic farm needs to complete a conversion period before products can be sold as "organic". The conversion period starts with the date of signing the contract with INDOCERT. After 12 months, products can be sold with a label "in conversion to organic agriculture". Annual crops can be sold as "organic" after 24 months and perennial crops after 36 months.

The Indian Scenario

The Official Position

As per a food and agriculture organisation (FAO) study of mid-2003, India had 1,426 certified organic farms producing approximately 14,000 tons of organic food/produce annually. In 2005, as per Govt. of India figures, approximately 190,000 acres (77,000 hectares) were under organic cultivation. The total production of organic food in India as per the same reference was 120,000 tons annually, though this largely included certified forest collections.

Another side to the story

There are a number of farms in India which have either never been chemically-managed/cultivated or have converted back to organic farming because of their farmers' beliefs or purely for reason of economics. These farmers cultivating in a considerable areas are not classified as organic though they are. Their produce either sells in the open market along with conventionally grown produce at the same price or sells purely on goodwill and trust as organic through select outlets and regular specialist bazaars. These farmers will never opt for certification because of the costs involved as well as the extensive documentation that is required by certifiers.

Relevance of Organic farming to Indian agriculture: New potential areas

About 65% of India's cropped area which is mainly rain-fed, negligible amount of fertilizers are being used. Farmers in these areas often use organic manure as a source of nutrients that are readily available either in their own farm or in their locality. This particular area not irrigated and it can be safely assumed that high-input demanding crops are not grown on these lands. Fertilizer use on dry lands is always less anyway as chemical fertilizers require sufficient water to respond. Pesticide use in these lands would also be less as the economics of these hardy or "not-so profitable" crops will not permit expensive inputs. These areas are at least "relatively organic" or perhaps even "organic by default". The north-eastern region of India provides considerable scope and opportunity for organic farming due to least utilization of chemical inputs. It is estimated that 18 million hectare of such land is available in the North-East, which can be exploited for organic production. With the sizable acreage under naturally organic/default organic cultivation, India has tremendous potential to grow crops organically and emerge as a major supplier of organic products in the world's organic market. Need is for putting up a clear strategy on organic farming and its link with the markets. The report of the Task Force on Organic Farming appointed by the Government of India also observed that in vast areas of the country, where limited amount of chemicals are used and have low productivity could be exploited as potential areas for organic agriculture. Arresting the decline of soil organic matter is the most potent weapon in fighting against unabated soil degradation and imperilled sustainability of agriculture in tropical regions of India, particularly those under the influence of arid, semi-arid and sub-humid climate. Application of organic manure is the only option to improve the soil organic carbon for sustenance of soil quality and future agricultural productivity. Future of sustainable development of agriculture, next to water, depends on arresting fall in organic matter in soils.

Appendix

Fertilizer/Manure/Pesticide Industries in India

Table A.1: List of fertilizer companies engaged in fertilizer business

Company	Address	Website
Rashtriya Chemicals & Fertilizers Limited (RCF)	Madras Fertilizers Limited Manali Chennai-600 068.	www.madrasfert.nic.in
Neyveli Lignite Corporation Ltd. (NLC)	Fertilizer Factory NLC Ltd, Neyveli-607807 Tamil Nadu	www.nlcindia.com
Paradeep Phosphates Limited (PPL)	PPL Township Jagatsinghpur-754145	www.paradeep-phosphates.com
Pyrites, Phosphates & Chemicals Ltd. (PPCL)	Amjhore, Distt. Rohtas (Bihar) Saladipura, P.O. Khandela, Distt. Sikar, Rajasthan 1-AB, Ravindra Nath Tagore Marg Dehradun, Uttaranchal	www.ppclindia.com
Hindustan Fertilizer Corporation Limited (HFC)	Durgapur Mucchipara, Distt. Burdwan-713212 West Bengal Barauni, P.O. Urvarak Nagar, Distt. Begusarai-851115, Bihar Haldia, P.O. Haldia Oil Refinery, Distt. Midnapur-721606 West Bengal	www.hindustancoppes.com
Brahmaputra Valley Fertilizer Corporation Limited	Namrup, P.O. Parbatpur, Distt. Dibrugarh, Assam	www.bvfcl.com
Hindustan Copper Limited (HCL)	Khetri Acid Cum Fertilizer Plant, Khetrinagar	
FCI Aravali Gypsum And Minerals India Limited	Namrup, P.O. Parbatpur Dibrugarh-786623 Assam	www.fagmil.nic.in

Contd.

Table A.1: List of fertilizer companies engaged in fertilizer business *(Contd.)*

Company	Address	Website
Co-operative Sector		
Krishak Bharati Cooperative Limited (KRIBHCO)	Hazira, Hazira Fertiliser Complex, P.O. KRIBHCO Nagar Hazira, Surat-394515 Gujarat	www.kribhco.net
Private Sector Fertilizer Manufacturing Companies		
Gujarat State Fertilizer and Chemical limited	Fertilizernagar (Vadodara) Kosamba (Surat) Sikka (Jamnagar) Nandesari (Vadodara)	www.gsfclimited.com
Coromandel Fertilizers Limited	Vishakhapatnam Ennore, Ranipet Navi Mumbai	www.cflindia.com
Sriram Fertilizers and Chemicals	Kota, Rajasthan	http://www.dscl.com/ Business_Agree_Urea.aspx
Zuari Industries Limited-Fertilizer Limited	Goa	www.zuari-chambal.com
Southern Petrochemicals Inds. Corp. Ltd.	Tuticorin	www.spic.in
Duncans Industries Limited	Kanpur	www.duncansfertiliser.com
Mangalore Chemicals & Fertilizers Limited	Panambur, Mangalore	www.mangalore chemicals.com
Gujarat Narmada Valley Fertilisers Co. Ltd.	Bharuch, Gujarat	www.gnvfc.net
Deepak Fertilizers & Petrochemicals Ltd.	Plot K1, MIDC Industrial Area, P.O. Taloja-A.V-410 208, Dist. Raigad Maharashtra	www.dfpcl.com
Indo-Gulf Fertilizers & Chemicals Corporation Limited	P.O. Jagdishpur Industrial Area, Dist. Sultanpur-227 817 Uttar Pradesh	www.indo-gulf.co.in
Godavari Fertilizer & Chemicals Limited	Kakinada	www.gfcl.com
Nagarjuna Fertilizers and Chemicals Limited	Kakinada	www.nagarjuna.com

Table A.2: List of pesticide companies engaged in pesticide business

Aakar Exports Manufacturers	No. 401, Shantam Complex, Gurukul Road, Memnagar, Near Ageta Tennis Court, Subhash Chowk, Memnagar, Ahmedabad-380052, Gujarat	www.indiamart.com/ aakarexports/
Adhik Chemicals Pvt. Ltd	207, New Cloth Market, O/S. Rajpur Gate, Gujarat, India	www.adhikchemicals.com/
Cheminova	Cheminova 'Keshava', 7th Floor, Bandra Kurla Complex, Bandra (East), Mumbai-400051	www.cheminovaindia.in/
Chemet Chemicals Ltd	G-13/C Hemkoot building, B/H LIC office, Ashram road Ahmdabad-380009, Gujarat, India	www.chemetchemicals. indiabizsource.com/
The Dhanuka Group	Dhanuka House 861-862, Joshi Road, Karol Bagh, New Delhi-110005	www.dhanuka.com/ contact-us
EID Parry(India) Ltd.	Dare House New No. 2, Old 234, NSC Bose Road, Chennai	www.eidparry.com/
Gujarat Insecticides Limited (GIL)	Plot No.805/806, GIDC Estate Ankleshwar-393002, Dist. Bharuch Gujarat	www.gilgharda.com/ www.gilgharda.com/ Link.../contactus-new.htm
Indianeem	23, Anuradha Society, Old Nagardas Road, Andheri(E), Mumbai-400069	www.neemindia.com
Kedia Chemical Industries Limited	53 B, Mittal Court 224, Nariman Point, Mumbai	www.kedia.com
Rallis India Limited	Rallis India Limited, 156/157, 15th Floor, Nariman Bhavan, 227, Nariman Point, Mumbai-400021	www.rallis.co.in/
Shogun Organics Ltd.	106 A, Kotia Nirman, New Link Road Andheri (West), Mumbai-400 058	www.shogunorganics.com/
Vallabh Pesticides	PO Box. No. 30, Cyto Compound, Anand-Sojitra Road, Vitthal Udyognagar, Anand, Gujarat-388121	www.vallabhpesticides.com
Novartis Ltd.	Sandoz House, Shivsagar Estate Dr Annie Besant Road, Worli, Mumbai-400018	www.novartis.in/
BASF Ltd.	1st Floor, VIBGYOR Towers, Plot No. C-62, 'G' Block, Bandra-Kurla Complex, Mumbai-400051, Maharashtra	www.india.basf.com/
Bayer Crop Science Ltd.	Bayer House, Central Avenue, Hiranandani Estate ,Thane(West) 400607	www.bayer.co.in/
United Phosphorous Ltd.	UPL Limited, Uniphos House, Madhu Park, 11th Road, Chitrakar Dhurandar Marg, Khar(West), Mumbai 400 052	www.uplonline.com/
Sarthi Chem. Pvt. Ltd.	Gidc Industrial Estate, Plot No-H/254, National Highway-8-B, Kuvadava Road, Rajkot-360003, Gujarat	www.indiamart.com/sarthi-chem/

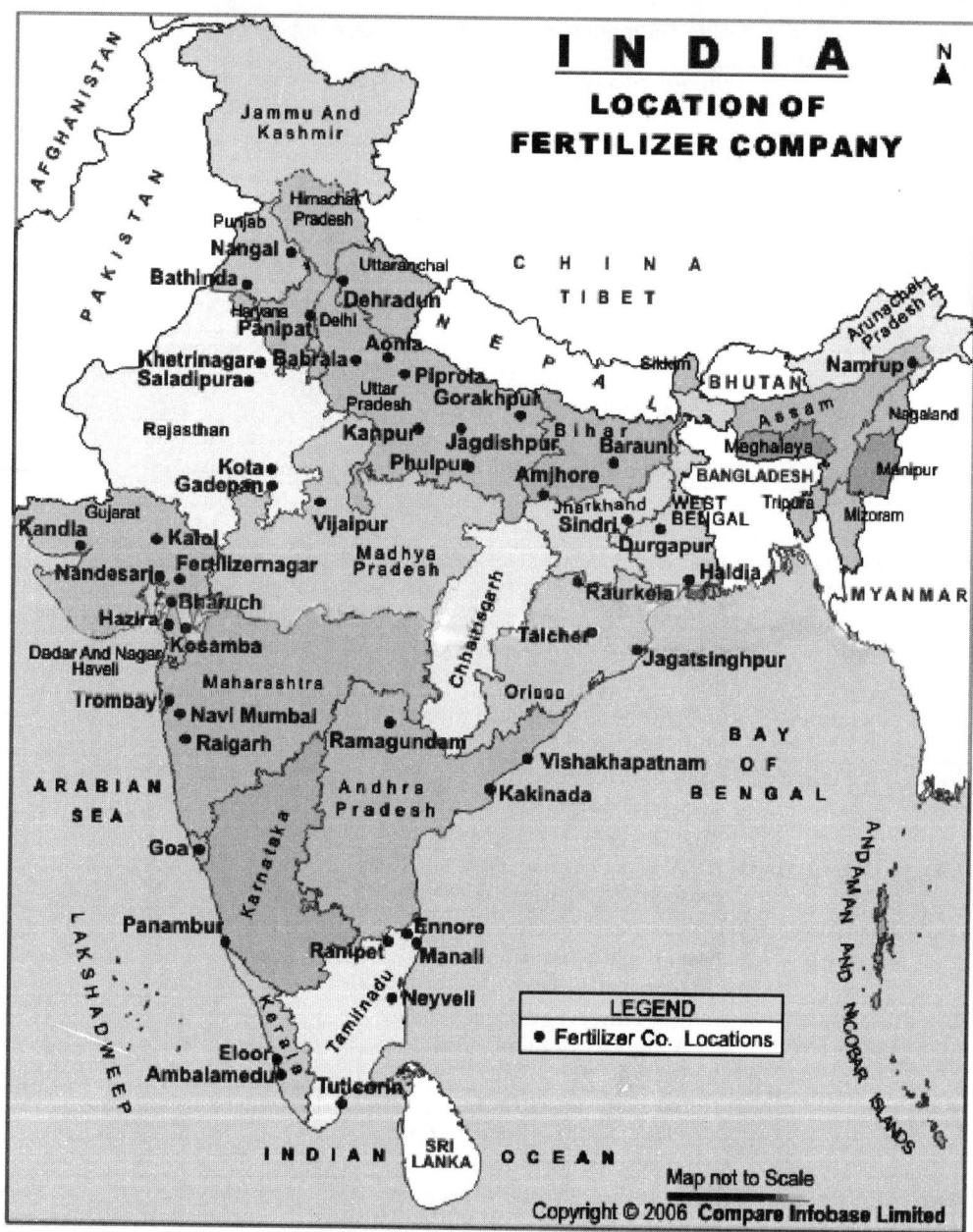

Fig. A.1: Location of fertilizer companies

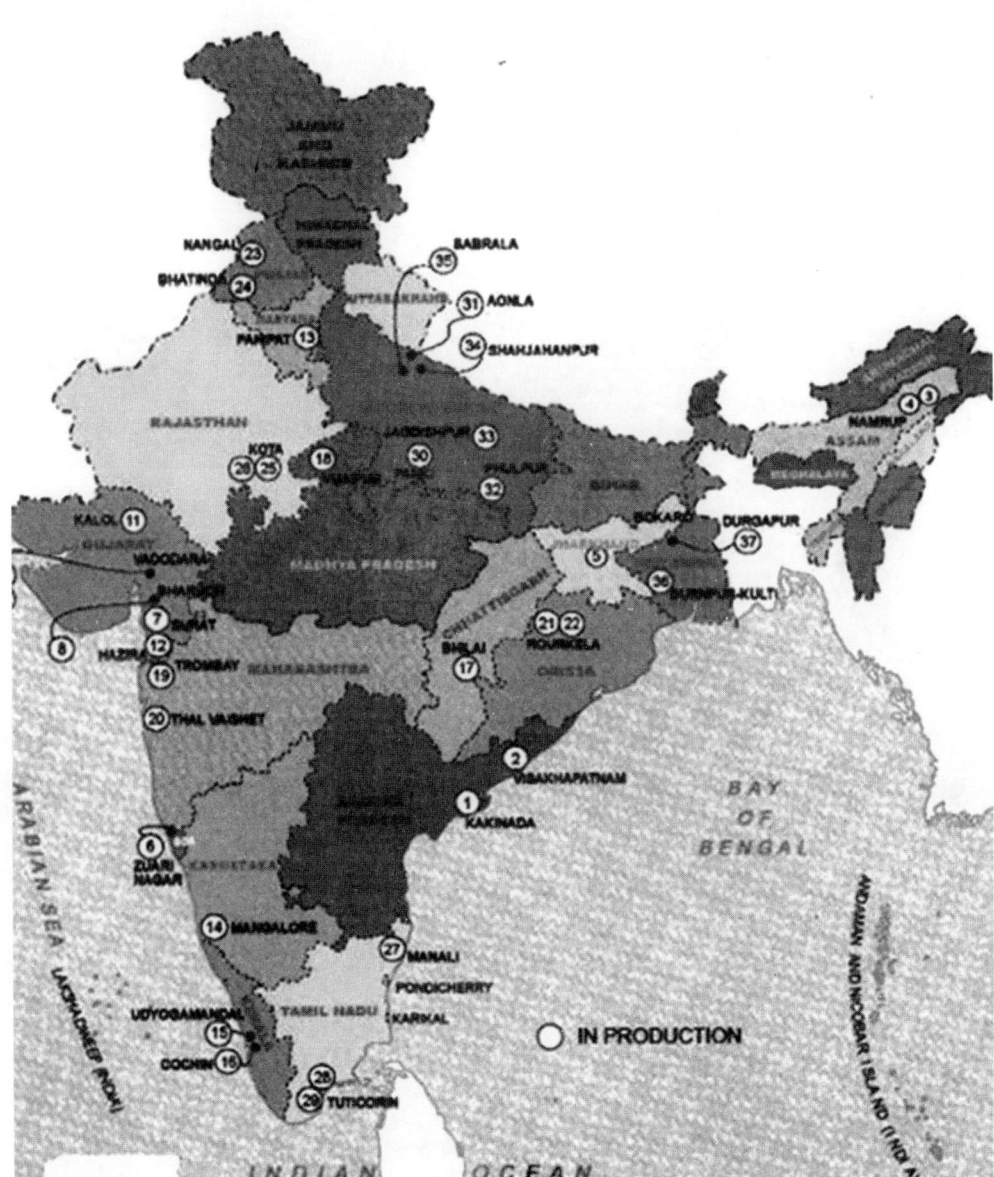

Fig. A.2: Location of straight nitrogenous fertilizer plants

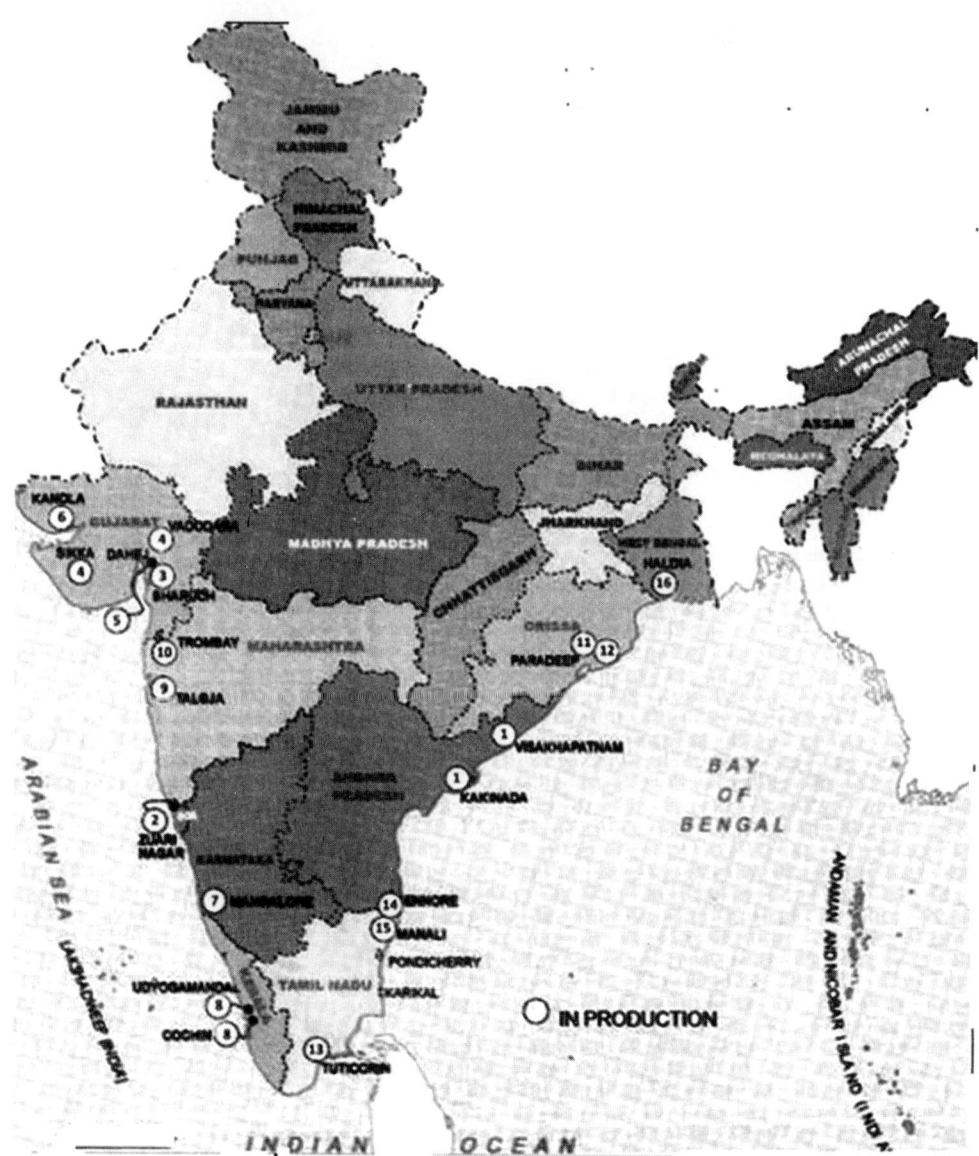

Fig. A.3: Location of complex fertilizer plants

Table A.3: Methodology for quick testing of fertilizer

Fertilizer	Method
Macro nutrient fertilizer	
Urea	Take 1 g urea fertilizer in a test tube. Heat the sample, complete melting ensures good quality/ Take 1 g urea fertilizer in test tube. Add 5 ml normal water. Mix it. Add 5–6 drops of 1% $AgNO_3$. Appearance of white coloured solution ensures presence of adulterant.
DAP	Pure DAP granules are not completely round shaped. If the DAP granules on heating doubles its size, it ensures good quality. To test the presence of nitrogen in DAP add lime with one gram of DAP. If there is bad odour /pungency of NH_3 that ensures presence of nitrogen.
SSP	Take 1 g SSP fertilizer in a test tube. Add 5 ml normal water. Filter it. Add one drop of NaOH and one drop of $AgNO_3$ in the filtrate. If there is yellow precipitate, it ensures presence of phosphate in the fertilizer.
MOP	In presence of fire/heat if it converts to yellow coloured substance it ensures presence of adulterant. Crystals of MOP are completely soluble in water with the red part floating in water.
Micro nutrient fertiliser	
Zinc sulphate	White crystalline powder of $ZnSO_4$ is not completely soluble in water and on dissolving in water does not impart cooling effect. Take 1 g $ZnSO_4$ fertilizer in a test tube. Add 5 ml normal water. Filter it. Add eight to ten drops of NaOH in the filtrate. If there is white jelly like formation and subsequently further addition of 8–10 drops of NaOH, the jelly dissolves which ensures right grade of $ZnSO_4$.

Glossary

Absorption: The movement of a pesticide from the surrounding environment into an organism through the surface of the organism.

Acid Equivalent (ae): For those pesticides that are acids, acid equivalent, abbreviated as ae, is the amount of active ingredientexpressed in terms of the parent acid.

Acid-Forming: A product that tends to make the soil more acid.

Active Ingredient (ai): Component of a pesticide formulation contributing to the direct or indirect biological activity against pests and diseases, or in regulating metabolism/growth.

Acute Toxicity: Ability of a substance to cause adverse effects within a short period following dosing or exposure.

Adjuvant: Formulant designed to enhance the activity or other properties of a pesticide mixture.

Adsorption: The accumulation of a pesticide on the surface of an organism. See also absorption

Aerosol: System of fine solid or liquid particles (<39 µm dia.) dispersed in a gas. Aerosol cans using an inert compressed propellant are a common means of dispensing insecticides for domestic use.

Agrochemicals: Another word for agricultural chemicals used in crop and food production. Agrochemicals include pesticides, feed additives, veterinary medicines and related compounds

Allelopathy: The adverse effect on the growth of plants or microorganisms caused by the action of chemicals produced by other living or decaying plants .

Ammoniation: A process wherein ammonia (anhydrous, aqua or a solution containing ammonia and other forms of nitrogen) is used to treat superphosphate to form ammoniated superphosphate, or to treat a mixture of fertilzer ingredients (including superphosphate) in the manufacture of a multiple-nutrient fertilizer.

Ammonium Nitrate (NH_4NO_3): A product containing approximately 33.5 percent nitrogen, one half of which is in the ammonium form and one half in the nitrate form. Ammonium nitrate is water soluble and is also used in fertilizer solutions.

Ammonium Sulfate ($(NH_4)_2SO_4$): A solid material manufactured by reacting ammonia with sulfuric acid, typically containing 20.5 percent-21 percent nitrogen.

Analytical Standard: Pesticide reference material of high and defined purity (generally >95%) used for preparation of calibration standards in pesticide analysis.

Anhydrous Ammonia (NH_3): A gas containing approximately 82% nitrogen. Under pressure, ammonia gas is changed to a liquid and is stored and transported in this form.

Anion: A monoatomic or polyatomic species having one or more elementary charges of the electron.

Antidote: Substance used as a medical treatment to counteract pesticide poisoning.

AOAC: Association of official analytical chemists.

Attractant: Chemical or substance intentionally used to attract organisms for monitoring or other purposes related to control.

Available (nutrient): Form of a nutrient that can be taken up by a crop immediately or within a short period, so acting as an effective source of that nutrient for the crop.

Basic Slag: A by-product in the manufacture of steel, containing lime, phosphate and small amounts of the plant food elements such as sulfur, manganese and iron. Basic slags may contain 10–17 percent phosphate (P_2O_5), 35–50 percent calcium oxide (CaO), and 2–10 percent magnesium oxide (MgO).

Batch: A quantity of material which is produced under uniform conditions.

Best Management Practices: In agriculture and fertilizer industry, best management practices (BMPs) are measures taken to prevent air and water pollution during the manufacture, transport, storage, and use of crop inputs such as fertilizer.

Bioaccumulation: The progressive increase in the amount of a substance in an organism or part of an organism because the organism takes up the substance at a faster rate than it is removed from the organism.

Bioactivation: Transformation of a pesticide within an organism into a more biochemically active metabolite.

Bioavailability: The extent to which a pesticide residue can be taken up into an organism from its food and environment and the rate at which this occurs.

Biofertilizers: Microorganisms that increase the amount of nutrients available to plants.

Biogas: Typically refers to a gas produced by the biological breakdown of organic matter in the absence of oxygen. Biogas originates from biogenic material and is a type of biofuel.

Biopesticides: Pesticides of biological origin including pheromones and other semiochemicals, microorganisms such as *Bacillus thuringiensis*, fungi, protozoa, viruses, viroids), plant extracts such as rotenone and pyrethrum, and other novel alternative products

Bonemeal: Raw bonemeal is cooked bones ground to a meal without any of the gelatine or glue removed.

Borax ($Na_2B_4O_7.10H_2O$): A salt used in fertilizer as a source of the plant nutrient element boron. Fertilizer borax contains about 11 percent boron.

Broadcast: Application of fertilizer or other material to the soil surface.

Calcareous Soil: Soil that is alkaline due to the presence of free calcium carbonate or magnesium carbonate or both.

Calcite: Limestone containing mostly calcium carbonate, $CaCO_3$. A more common name is simply ground agricultural limestone.

Calcium Ammonium Nitrate: A product formed by reacting calcium carbonate and ammonium nitrate, typically contains 25 percent nitrogen.

Carcinogen: Agent (chemical, physical, or biological) that is capable of increasing the incidence of malignant neoplasms or cancer in animals.

Cation Exchange Capacity: Capacity of the soil to hold cations by electrostatic forces. Cations are held at exchange sites mainly on clay particles and organic matter.

Cation: Monatomic or polyatomic species having one or more elementary charges of the proton.

Chlorosis: A condition caused by low chlorophyll content and characterized by yellowing of the leaves of affected plants. Often a symptom of nutrient deficiency.

Clay: Finely divided inorganic crystalline particles in soils, less than 0.002 mm in diameter.

Colloidal: Referring to a state of subdivision, implying that the molecules or polymolecular particles dispersed in a medium have at least in one direction a dimension roughly between 1 nm and 1 µm, or that in a system discontinuities are found at distances of that order compartment (e.g., of the environment), or (sub-) population.

Compost: Organic material produced by aerobic decomposition of biodegradable organic materials.

Compost: Relatively stable humus material that is produced through controlled biological decomposition of organic material in the presence of air.

Concentrated Superphosphate: Frequently referred to as triple superphosphate (TSP). Manufactured by reacting phosphoric acid with phosphate rock. This produces a product with a P_2O_5 equivalent to 44–48 percent, depending upon the ratio of the acids used. The material contains only a minor amount of gypsum.

Contaminant: Minor impurity in a substance.

Copper Sulfate ($CuSO_4.5H_2O$): Most common source of copper for fertilizer, 25 percent copper. Also used as an insecticide and fungicide. A common name is blue vitriol.

Copperas (Green vitriol, $FeSO_4.7H_2O$): Ferrous sulfate used as a source of iron, especially in alkaline soils.

Crop Available Nitrogen: The total nitrogen content of organic manure that is available for crop uptake in the growing season in which it is spread on land.

Cumulative Effect: Overall adverse change which occurs when repeated doses of a pesticide have biological consequences which are additive.

Degradation: The process by which a pesticide is broken down to simpler substances. The process is also referred to as breakdown and decomposition.

Desorption: The release of a substance from or through the surface of an organism. The opposite of adsorption or absorption.

Detoxification: The chemical processes which make a pesticide less toxic.

Diffusion: Spreading or scattering of a gaseous or liquid material.

Diluent: An inert substance used to dilute.

Dioxin: Colloquial (short) name of a toxic by-product (and sometimes contaminant) of chlorophenol-derived herbicides.

Dolomite: Made by grinding dolomitic limestone which contains both magnesium carbonate– $MgCO_3$, and calcium carbonate– $CaCO_3$.

Emulsifier: A surfactant used to facilitate dispersion of one liquid in another liquid with which it does not normally mix.

EPA: Environment protection agency

Erosion: Movement (transport) of the soil by running water or wind.

Eutrophication: Enrichment of ecosystems by nitrogen or phosphorus. In water it causes algae and higher forms of plant life to grow too fast. This disturbs the balance of organisms present in the water and the quality of the water concerned. On land, it can stimulate the growth of certain plants which then become dominant.

Exposure: The amount of a pesticide that reaches the target population, organism, tissue or cell, usually expressed in numerical terms of concentration, duration and frequency.

FAO: Food and agriculture organisation of the United Nations.

Farmyard Manure (FYM): Livestock excreta that is mixed with straw bedding material that can be stacked in a heap without slumping.

Fate: Pattern of distribution of an agent, its derivatives or metabolites in an organism, system.

Fertilizer: Any material or mixture used to supply one or more of the essential plant nutrient elements.

Fluid Fertilizer: Pumpable fertiliser in which nutrients are dissolved in water (solutions) or held partly as very finely divided particles in suspension.

Formulant: Any added material in a pesticide formulation other than the biologically active ingredients.

Good Agricultural Practice (GAP): The nationally authorised safe uses of pesticides under conditions necessary for effective and reliable pest control .

Good Laboratory Practice (GLP): The formalised process and conditions under which laboratory studies on pesticides are planned, performed, monitored, recorded, reported and audited.

Grade: The guaranteed analysis of a fertilizer containing one or more of the primary plant nutrient elements. Grades are stated in terms of the guaranteed percentages of total nitrogen (N), available phosphate (P_2O_5), and soluble potash (K_2O) in that order. For example, a 10-10-10 grade would contain 10 percent total nitrogen, 10 percent available phosphate, and 10 percent soluble potash.

Granular Fertilizer: Fertiliser in which particles are formed by rolling a mixture of liquid and dry components in a drum or pan. Typically, particles are in the 2–4 mm diameter range.

Greenhouse Effect: Process whereby greenhouse gases released into the atmosphere cause heat to be trapped in the atmosphere rather than escaping into space. The greenhouse gases form an insulating blanket around the planet. This blanket allows light and heat from the sun through, but prevents some of the heat, which radiates back from the earth from escaping.

Ground Water: The water present in the saturated subsurface zone of the soil profile, where all open spaces/pores in the sediment and rock are filled with water .

Guano: Decomposed dried excrement of birds and bats. The most commonly known guano comes from islands of the coast of Peru and is derived from the excrement of sea fowl. It is high in nitrogen and phosphate, and at one time was a major fertilizer in this country.

Guarantee: Amount of active ingredient contained in a product, expressed as either a percentage or a concentration.

Gypsum ($CaSO_4.2H_2O$): The common name for calcium sulfate, a mineral used in the fertilizer industry as a source of calcium and sulfur. Gypsum also is used widely in reclaiming alkali soils in the western United States. Another common name is landplaster. When pure it contains approximately 18.6 percent sulfur.

Haber-Bosch Process: An industrial process used in the manufacture of anhydrous ammonia.

Half-Life: The time taken for the concentration of a pesticide in a particular environment to decline by one half.

Hazard: The inherent properties of a pesticide which gives potential for adverse effects to man or the environment during its production, use or disposal, depending on the degree of exposure.

Heavy Metal: Cadmium, copper, lead, mercury, nickel or zinc. Elements that are potentially toxic to mammals above critical levels. Copper, nickel and zinc are required by plants in a very small amounts.

Hydrolysis: Reaction in which a chemical bond is cleaved and a new bond formed with the oxygen atom of a molecule of water.

Hygroscopic: A term applied to a material which tends to absorb moisture from the atmosphere. Many materials used for fertilizer are hygroscopic and may require special treatment to prevent caking.

Immobilization: The process of converting inorganic N to organic form (typically by microbes which incorporate the N into their own proteins), making the N unavailable to plants.

Impurity: A by-product of the manufacture or storage of a pesticide. Impurities require definition, evaluation and regulation, if they are toxicologically significant.

Inert Ingredient: An ingredient in a formulation which by itself does not add materially to the effectiveness of the formulation.

Integrated Pest Management (IPM): A pest management system that makes use of all suitable techniques and methods in as compatible a manner as possible to maintain the pest populations at levels below those causing economically unacceptable damage or loss.

IUPAC: International union of pure and applied chemistry.

Leaching: The process by which a pesticide moves downward through the soil profile in the aqueous phase.

Lime Requirement: Amount of standard limestone needed in tonnes/ha to increase soil pH from the measured value to a higher specified value (often 6.5 for arable crops). Can be determined by a laboratory test or inferred from soil pH.

Liming: Application of lime to a field as a soil amendment to raise the soil pH in the field.

Lot: The quantity of material which is assumed to be a single population for sampling purposes. See also batch.

Lysimeter: A device for measuring leaching losses from a column or block of soil.

Magnesium Carbonate ($MgCO_3$): A principal component of dolomitic limestone is calcite ($CaCO_3$) or high Mg calcite [$(Ca, Mg) CO_3$] (See also dolomite and liming materials).

Major Nutrient: Nitrogen, phosphorus and potassium that are needed in relatively large amounts by crops.

Manufactured Fertilizer: Any fertiliser that is manufactured by an industrial process. Includes conventional straight and NPK products (solid or fluid), organo-mineral fertilisers, rock phosphates, slags, ashed poultry manure, liming materials that contain nutrients.

Marl: A calcium-rich mud made mostly of clay and calcium carbonate, used as a soil amendment. Agricultural use of marl was more widespread before the rise of commercial fertilizers.

Maximum Residue Level (MRL): The maximum concentration of a pesticide residue (expressed as mg/kg) legally permitted in or on food commodities and animal feeds.

Metabolism: Sum total of all physical and chemical processes that take place within an organism.

Metabolite: The set of all the chemical reactions that goes on inside a living plant or animal is called its metabolism. When chemicals are broken down by metabolisms, any new chemicals produced inside the plant or animal are metabolites.

Methane: An odourless, highly explosive gas formed during manure's anaerobic decomposition.

Micronutrient: Boron, Copper, Iron, Manganese, Molybdenum, Zinc that are needed in very small amounts by crops.

Mineralisation: The conversion of an element from an organic form to an inorganic form.

Mineralisation: Microbial breakdown of organic matter in the soil, releasing nutrients in crop-available, inorganic forms.

Molybdenum: One of the essential micronutrients, especially for legumes which have nitrogen-fixing bacteria.

Monoammonium Phosphate: See ammonium phosphate.

Muriate of Potash (KCl): The principal source of potassium for fertilizer. Muriate of potash, the chemicl name of which is potassium chloride, usually sold on the basis of a material containing 95–99 percent KCl, with a K_2O equivalent of 60–62 percent.

Nebulisation: Formation of an aerosol of very small liquid particles (fog) or solid particles (smoke) from a pesticide formulation, generally for fumigation of an enclosed space such as a glass-house.

Neutralizing Value (NV): Percentage calcium oxide (CaO) equivalent in a material. 100 kg of a material with a neutralising value of 52% will have the same neutralising value as 52 kg of pure CaO. NV is determined by a laboratory test.

Nitrification: A process whereby bacteria form nitrates from ammonium nitrogen.

Nitrous Oxide (N_2O): A potent greenhouse gas that is emitted naturally from soils. The amount emitted is related to supply of mineral nitrogen in the soil, so increases with application of anures and fertilisers, incorporation of crop residues and growth of legumes and is greater in organic and peaty soils than in other soils.

Nonpoint Source Pollution: Pollution, usually water pollution, that cannot be traced to a single "point source" such as an effluent pipe or spill.

Normal Superphosphate: Manufactured by mixing together sulfuric acid and finely ground phosphate rock which produces a material containing principally monocalcium phosphate and gypsum. Small amounts of unreacted rock and phosphoric acid may also be present. Normal superphosphate has a P_2O_5 equivalent of 18–22 percent.

OC: Organochlorine pesticide. A generic term for pesticides containing chlorine but commonly used to refer to older persistent materials including aldrin, BHC, chlordane, DDT, dieldrin, heptachlor, lindane and toxaphene.

Organic Fertilizer: Strictly speaking, an organic material is one containing carbon. This includes urea and calcium cyanamide which are manufactured synthetically. The term generally applies to products derived from plant or animal materials, such as manure, sewage slude, castor pomace and process tankage.

Organic Manure: Any bulky organic nitrogen source of livestock, human or plant origin, including livestock manures.

Organic Soil: Soil containing 10–20% organic matter .

Parts per Billion (PPB): Ratio of amounts expressed as parts of pesticide per 1,000,000,000 parts of sample.

Parts per Million (PPM): Ratio of amounts expressed as parts of pesticide per 1,000,000 parts of sample.

Peaty Soil (peat): Soil containing more than 20% organic matter.

Permaculture: The development of agricultural ecosystems intended to be sustainable and self-sufficient.

Persistence: The extent to which a pesticide remains in a particular environment.

Persistent Organic Pollutant (POPs): POPs are chemicals which do not break down easily in the environment. This means that the amounts in the environment can increase over time.

Pest: An organism that attacks food and other materials essential to mankind or which affects human beings adversely.

Pesticide: Any substance, preparation or organism prepared or used for controlling or destroying a pest. 'Pesticide' is a broad term, covering a range of products that are used to control pests. The slug pellets, ant powder, weed killers, and rat and mouse baits used in everyday life, are all pesticides.

Pesticide Formulation: The combination of active substances and other ingredients that make up the end-user product.

Pesticide Residue: The traces of a pesticide which remains in or on a feed or food commodity, or soil, air or water following use of the pesticide.

pH: This term, an abbreviation for potential hydrogen, expresses a measurement of hydrogen ion activity or concentration in a solution. More simply, pH is a scale from 1 to 14, used to denote the relative intensity of acidity or alkalinity. A neutral solution (or soil) has a pH of 7.0. Values below 7.0 denote progressively more intense acid conditions, those above 7.0 similarly more intense alkaline conditions.

Phosphoric Acid (H_3PO_4): An inorganic acid used in the manufacture of concentrated superphosphates, ammonium phosphates and sometimes for direct application.

Photolysis: A chemical reaction caused by light in which the bonds between atoms in a chemical compound are broken, resulting in the breakdown of the compound.

Photosynthesis: The process by which carbon dioxide (from the air) and water (from the soil) are combined under the influence of light to form complex sugars in a plant

Placement: Application of fertiliser to a zone of the soil usually close to the seed or tuber.

Plant Extracts: There is a large spectrum of plant extracts, i.e. unprocessed extracts representing a 'cluster of substances' or highly refined containing one active substance.

Plant Growth Regulator (PGR): A naturally occurring or synthetic substance which influences but has no nutritive value.

Pre-Emergence: The period before a specific crop or pest has emerged.

Prilled Fertilizer: Fertiliser in which particles (prills) are formed by allowing molten material to fall as droplets in a tower.

Registration: The process whereby the responsible national government authority approves the sale and use of a pesticide, following the evaluation of scientific data demonstrating that the pesticide is effective for the purposes intended and poses no significant risks to human health, animals or the environment.

Residue: The small amounts of pesticides present in vegetable and animal products following the application of pesticides. They may not only include the pesticide that was applied but also degradation or reaction products and metabolites that may be of toxicological significance. The levels or amounts of residues present are expressed in milligrams of the chemical in a kilogram of crop/food/commodity (mg/kg), or parts per million.

Resistance: Sometimes when pesticides are used repeatedly to control specific pests or diseases, those pests and diseases can develop tolerance of a pesticide, generally through natural selection, which makes the pesticide less effective.

Risk: The probability of any specific hazard occurring from exposure to a pesticide under specific conditions.

Safener: A substance added to a pesticide formulation to eliminate or reduce phytotoxic effects of the pesticide to certain crops.

Salt Index: An index used to compare solubilities of chemical compounds. Most nitrogen and potash compounds have a high index, and phosphate compounds have a low index. When applied too close to seed or on foliage, the ones with high indexes can cause salt injury.

Secondary Nutrient: Magnesium, sulphur, calcium or sodium that are needed in moderate amounts by crops.

Slow-release Fertilizer: Fertilizers that will release nutrients gradually with time. Slow-release fertilizers can be inorganic or organic. Examples of inorganic slow-release fertilizers are sulfur-coated urea and nitroform.

Sodium Molybdate ($Na_2MoO_4, 2H_2O$): Common source of the micronutrient, molybdenum.

Soil Incorporation: The application of a pesticide to soil by mixing or through injection into the soil body.

Soil Organic Matter: The organic fraction of the soil, including both fresh and older material (humus) of biological origin.

Soil Organic Matter: Often referred to as humus. Composed of organic compounds ranging from undecomposed plant and animal tissues to fairly stable brown or black material with no trace of the anatomical structure of the material from which it was derived.

Soil Solution: Water residing in the soil.

Sorption: Removal of pesticide from solution by soil or sediment via mechanisms of adsorption and absorption.

Sticker: A substance which increases the adhesiveness of a formulation applied to a surface. It may be part of the formulation or added at the point of application in a tank mix.

Surface Band: Fertilizer applied in a relatively narrow band along the surface, where seed will be planted.

Surfactant: A formulant for reducing surface tension, thereby increasing the emulsifying, spreading, dispersability or wetting properties of liquids or solids.

Systemic Pesticide: A pesticide that can be translocated to sites other than where it was absorbed, in sufficient quantities to be biologically effective.

Target: Any organism, organ, tissue, cell or cell constituent that is subject to the action of a pesticide or its residue.

Threshold: The concentration of a pesticide in an organism or particular environment below which an adverse effect is not expected

Toxicology: Toxicology is the science of adverse effects of chemicals on living organisms (plants and animals).

Ultra Low Volume (ULV) Spray: Signifies that the total volume rate of spray application is very low (5 litres per hectare or less).

Urea $CO(NH_2)_2$: A solid synthetic organic material containing approximately 45 percent nitrogen. In the soil its nitrogen changes first to the ammonium form, then to the nitrate form.

Volatilisation: The evaporation of a pesticide into the atmosphere from a solid or liquid form/loss of nitrogen as ammonia from the soil to the atmosphere.

Watershed: The geographical boundaries which divide one water/river catchment area from another.

Water-soluble Phosphate: Phosphate, expressed as P_2O_5, that is measured by the statutory method for fertiliser analysis.

Wetting Agent: A surfactant for use in spray formulations to assist dispersion of a powder in the diluent or spreading of spray droplets on surfaces.

Xylem: The part of the plant's vascular system which transports water and dissolved nutrients from the roots to other parts of the plant.

Zero Waste: The goal of developing products and services, managing their use and deployment, and creating recycling systems and markets to eliminate the volume and toxicity of waste and materials, and to conserve and recover all resources.

Zinc Sulfate ($ZnSO_4.7H_2O$): White vitriol, a solid material used as a source of zinc for plants (36 percent zinc).

References

Brown RH and Kerry BR. Eds. *Principles and Practices of Nematode Control in Crops*, Academic Press, Marrikville, 1987.

Büchel KH. Ed. *Chemistry of Pesticides*, John Wiley & Sons, New York, 1983.

Corbett JR, Wright K and Baillie AC. *The Biochemical Mode of Action of Pesticides*, Academic Press, New York, 1984.

Fertilizer Association of India. *Handbook on Fertilizer Technology*. FAI House, 10, Shaheed Jit Singh Marg, New Delhi, 2010.

Gruzdyev GS. Ed. *The Chemical Protection of Plants*, Mir Publishers, Mascow, 1988.

Gy Matolesy, Nadasy M and Andorsk V. *Pesticide Chemistry*, Elsevier, New York, 1988.

He Z and Hailin Z. Eds. *Applied Manure and Nutrient Chemistry for Sustainable Agriculture and Environment*, Springer, Dordrecht, 2014

http://agricoop.nic.in/seed/Fertiliser241209.pdf

http://agritech.tnau.ac.in/org_farm/orgfarm_index.html

http://ncof.dacnet.nic.in/

http://www.fertilizer.org/

http://www.gov.uk/government/uploads/system/uploads/attachment_data/file/69469/rb209-fertiliser-manual-110412.pdf

International Fertilizer Development Center, Fertiliser manual, UN Industrial Development Organization, p.615, Springer Science & Business Media, 1998.

Jacobson M and Crosby DG. Eds. *Naturally Occurring Insecticides*, Marcel Dekker, New York, 1971.

Jeppson LR, Kaifer HH and Baker EW. In: *Mite Injurious to Economic Plants*, University of California Press, Berkeley, 1975.

Valkenburg WV. *Pesticide Formulations*, Marcel Dekker, New York, 1973.

Index

314